Sports Medicine: Principles and Practice

Sports Medicine: Principles and Practice

Editor: Ray Keller

Callisto Reference

www.callistoreference.com

Callisto Reference,
118-35 Queens Blvd., Suite 400,
Forest Hills, NY 11375, USA

Visit us on the World Wide Web at:
www.callistoreference.com

ISBN: 978-1-64116-138-1 (Hardback)

The publisher's policy is to use permanent paper from mills that operate a sustainable forestry policy. Furthermore, the publisher ensures that the text paper and cover boards used have met acceptable environmental accreditation standards.

Printed in China.

Cataloging-in-Publication Data

Sports medicine : principles and practice / edited by Ray Keller.
p. cm.
Includes bibliographical references and index.
ISBN 978-1-64116-138-1
1. Sports medicine. 2. Sports sciences. I. Keller, Ray.
RC1210 .S66 2019
617.102 7--dc23

Table of Contents

Preface

Every book is initially just a concept; it takes months of research and hard work to give it the final shape in which the readers receive it. In its early stages, this book also went through rigorous reviewing. The notable contributions made by experts from across the globe were first molded into patterned chapters and then arranged in a sensibly sequential manner to bring out the best results.

Sports medicine is a specialized branch of medicine that deals with the treatment and prevention of sports related injuries and emergencies. Various treatment interventions for injuries pertaining to muscles, ligaments, tendons and bones are under the medical domain of sports medicine. Injuries such as concussion, muscle cramps, sprains, tears and splints are common occurrences in sports. Practitioners also deal with the treatment of chronic illnesses that potentially affect performance like asthma and diabetes. They also recommend appropriate exercise and other physical activity regimes for the management and prevention of injuries. This book is a compilation of chapters that discuss the most vital concepts and emerging trends in the field of sports medicine. It aims to shed light on some of the unexplored aspects of this discipline and the recent researches in this field. Scientists and students actively engaged in the area of sports medicine will find this book helpful.

It has been my immense pleasure to be a part of this project and to contribute my years of learning in such a meaningful form. I would like to take this opportunity to thank all the people who have been associated with the completion of this book at any step.

Editor

1

Consensus on measurement properties and feasibility of performance tests for the exercise and sport sciences: a Delphi study

Sam Robertson[1,2*], Peter Kremer[1], Brad Aisbett[3], Jacqueline Tran[1] and Ester Cerin[3,4]

Abstract

Background: Performance tests are used for multiple purposes in exercise and sport science. Ensuring that a test displays an appropriate level of measurement properties for use within a population is important to ensure confidence in test findings.

The aim of this study was to obtain subject matter expert consensus on the measurement and feasibility properties that should be considered for performance tests used in the exercise and sport sciences and how these should be defined. This information was used to develop a checklist for broader dissemination.

Methods: A two-round Delphi study was undertaken including 33 exercise scientists, academics and sport scientists. Participants were asked to rate the importance of a range of measurement properties relevant to performance tests in exercise and sport science. Responses were obtained in binary and Likert-scale formats, with consensus defined as achieving 67% agreement on each question.

Results: Consensus was reached on definitions and terminology for all items. Ten level 1 items (those that achieved consensus on all four questions) and nine level 2 items (those achieving consensus on ≥2 questions) were included. Both levels were included in the final checklist.

Conclusions: The checklist developed from this study can be used to inform decision-making and test selection for practitioners and researchers in the exercise and sport sciences. This can facilitate knowledge sharing and performance comparisons across sub-disciplines, thereby improving existing field practice and research methodological quality.

Keywords: Performance tests, Sports testing, Reliability, Validity, Responsiveness, Assessment, Delphi

Key points

- Traditional measurement properties such as re-test reliability, rater reliability, content validity and discriminant validity were agreed to be important in all applications.
- Items not commonly considered in the literature as integral to performance tests were also agreed upon as important, including test feasibility, interpretability and duration.
- The checklist developed in this study can be used to inform performance test development or selection by exercise and sport scientists.

* Correspondence: sam.robertson@vu.edu.au
[1]Centre for Exercise and Sport Science, Deakin University, Geelong, Victoria, Australia
[2]Institute of Sport Exercise and Active Living (ISEAL), Victoria University, Footscray Park campus, PO Box 14428, Melbourne, Victoria 8001, Australia
Full list of author information is available at the end of the article

Background

In the exercise and sport sciences, a performance test can be defined as a measurement or series of measurements that help to determine the health status, physical fitness or sport-specific ability of an individual [1–4]. Performance tests serve a variety of purposes in exercise and sport scenarios, including assessing the effectiveness of researcher- or practitioner-implemented interventions [5–7] or monitoring participant progress within a prescribed exercise programme [3, 8]. These tests can also be used to gather objective evidence of a participant's strengths and weaknesses [9, 10] or provide diagnostic information relating to the health (e.g., injury) status of an individual [3, 11, 12]. In sport, performance tests are also used to inform the identification and selection of talented young participants, which may assist governing bodies when prioritising the time and financial contributions they invest into their athletes [13, 14].

The importance of physical performance tests displaying adequate measurement properties has received considerable attention in the exercise and sports science literature. Measurement properties such as reliability [1, 4, 15, 16], validity [1, 17] and responsiveness [1, 4, 18] have all been investigated with respect to their importance. Various industry and governing bodies have also published ethical guidelines for the undertaking of such testing [19, 20]. Despite this, no specific recommendations or guidelines exist to inform the selection or the design of a performance test based on its measurement properties and feasibility. This is an important consideration on many levels. For instance, multiple tests are often available to measure the same performance construct, each with their own relative strengths and limitations. For example, maximal oxygen uptake during exercise can be estimated using running [21, 22], walking [23], step [24] and cycling-based [24] tests. Such tests can also vary in both their content and purpose (i.e., to discriminate participants, identify talent or assess the effect of an intervention). The use of an unsuitable test may lead to a variety of adverse consequences. These could include a risk of incorrect conclusions being reached on an individual's physical status, increased assessment error, non-evidence-based practice and a lack of comparative data across exercise disciplines, sports or research studies. In the worst case scenario, it may also mean that clients, patients, research participants and athletes are put at risk during testing procedures.

Similar problems have recently been addressed in other disciplines, most notably medicine [25], health [26] and physical activity [27]. However, despite the success of these approaches for their target disciplines, the large number of redundant items in these studies with respect to exercise and sport science means that their direct application may not be appropriate. As an example, previous manuals developed in health, rate questionnaires on their cross-cultural validity and the ability to be translated into multiple languages [28], which may be less relevant for many of the exercise and sport sciences.

Previous research has utilised the Delphi technique to obtain the consensus needed by content experts in order to develop such a set of standardised guidelines [28–30]. The Delphi approach utilises groups of subject matter experts responding anonymously to a series of subsequent questionnaires, with repeated feedback used in order to reach consensus among the group [31, 32]. Recent work in other disciplines has successfully undertaken this task (e.g. quality of life research [28, 33], medicine [34] and nursing [29]) developing user-friendly and easily applicable checklists based on the resulting findings [33]. For example, publications from the COSMIN framework (a manual developed to help assess the measurement properties of health reporting questionnaires) have experienced considerable citations (over 500) in the 5 years since its 2010 inception [26, 28, 35, 36]. In order to improve physical performance testing quality and quality control, along with standardisation of test selection (thereby allowing comparison across sub-disciplines), a specific framework for use in exercise and sport sciences is needed.

The primary aim of this study was to obtain subject matter expert consensus on which measurement and feasibility properties should be considered for performance tests used in the exercise and sport sciences, as well as how these should be defined. A secondary aim was to develop a checklist which can be implemented to inform performance test development or selection.

Methods

Participants

Three types of exercise and sport scientists were recruited for participation in this Delphi study. These were defined as (i) clinical exercise scientists/exercise physiologists, (ii) sport scientists and (iii) academics. These groups were specifically targeted for inclusion in the study given their potential application of the findings in their work environment. Participants may have fit more than one category in some instances, however indicated their 'primary' affiliation at the start of the survey process. Data collection was undertaken via internet-based questionnaires, with the exact number of rounds dependent on the rate with which consensus on specific items was achieved.

Participants were recruited via methods shown previously to produce highest response rates in Delphi studies [37], including contacting personal industry contacts and cold contacting via publicly provided email addresses. Inclusion criteria for participants were set as follows. Clinical exercise scientists/exercise physiologists were required to (a) maintain current accreditation with their relevant accrediting body and (b) have ≥5 years' experience in the clinical exercise or exercise physiology industry. Sport scientists were required to be currently employed by a professional sporting club or institution. Those undertaking senior management roles were specifically targeted. For academics, a background of publications relating to measurement properties of testing in exercise or sport (≥3 articles) was required.

Although a variety of methods can be used when implementing Delphi studies [28], it is preferable for a minimum of 15 subject matter experts to be recruited [32, 38]. In accounting for potential non-response, a total of 136 individuals were contacted for participation in the Delphi procedure. Of these, 13 declined to participate, 90 did not respond and 33 (24% of total invited) agreed to participate. Following provision of written consent, panel members provided an information letter via email outlining specific details relating to the overall aims, study procedures and requirements of the study.

Delphi study—round 1

All rounds of the Delphi questionnaire were developed and administered to participants via a commercial survey provider (SurveyMonkey Inc, CA, USA). Prior to the first Delphi round, a steering committee was created [29], comprising all five authors. Information relating to physical performance test measurement properties and their definitions were primarily developed by the first author, with revisions made based on feedback from the steering committee. The questionnaire items were based upon content extracted from previous systematic reviews undertaken in exercise and sport science, as well as other disciplines. Once finalised, the initial taxonomy administered to participants grouped the 20 items into four distinct categories (Fig. 1). All participants were presented with this list (including reference support for each item) which also included a range of questions relating to each item.

Specifically, for each item included in the first round of the questionnaire, participants were asked (i) whether it should be considered when evaluating the quality of a performance test and (ii) whether they agreed with the terminology and definition used to describe the item. In interpreting the latter question, 'terminology' referred to the name of the item itself, whereas 'definition' comprised the explanation assigned to each item. Additionally, using a 5-point Likert scale, participants were also asked to (iii) rate the importance of each item for determining the quality of an exercise and sports performance test, with 1 indicating 'not at all important' and 5 considered 'extremely important'. The final question for each item also required a second 5-point Likert response, asking (iv) the participant's attitude to the item with 1 indicating 'I never consider this item' and 5 indicating 'I always consider this item'. The Likert scale responses were used to guard against information loss which can occur when experiencing response dichotomisation [39]. For all four questions, participants were permitted to provide explanation and/or justification for their response using a text box inserted into the questionnaire.

The questionnaire was left open for 15 weeks in order to facilitate the largest response rate possible. Following this, all participant responses were exported for further analysis. Based on the summation of scores received, all items were then ranked by the steering committee. Newly suggested items recommended for addition to the list were arranged in order of the frequency with which they were suggested. In order for an item to achieve consensus, a minimum of 67% agreement was required from the participants with respect to the four questions [28, 32]. For the two Likert-scale responses, this constituted a minimum of 67% of participants rating the item as 4 or 5 for both questions.

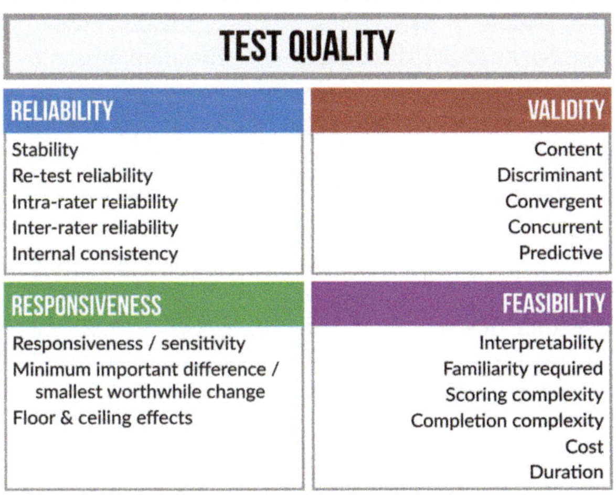

Fig. 1 Taxonomy including the initial measurement properties and feasibility as sent to participants as part of the first Delphi round

Delphi questionnaire—round 2

In the second Delphi round, participants received (i) a summary of results from the previous round, (ii) a transcript of written responses from other participants, and (iii) a list of proposed revisions as determined by the steering committee based on these responses. Each participant also received a link to the next round of the questionnaire. At this point, participants were asked to provide a binary 'yes' or 'no' response to each proposed revision, whilst also being able to consider the responses from other participants and results from the preceding round [32].

Results

Participants

Of the 33 individuals that provided consent for participation in the study, a total of 28 (response rate (RR) 21% of total approached, RR 85% of those who agreed and consented) provided responses to round 1. The 28 participants consisted of 14 academics, eight sport scientists and six clinical exercise scientists/exercise physiologists. The names of all panel members who completed at least one round are presented in the "Acknowledgements" section.

Round 1

Results relating to the four questions asked of each item are shown in Table 1. All 20 items proposed in the initial

Table 1 Results relating to round 1 of the Delphi study, including specific percentage of consensus reached for each of the four questions

Group	Item	Q1	Q2	Q3		Q4	
		Consider the item?	Definition and terminology	Importance to quality (mean)	% responses level 4 or 5	Attitude to item (mean)	% responses level 4 or 5
Reproducibility/reliability	Stability	71.4	68.2	3.62	65.4[a]	3.62	69.2
	Re-test reliability	92.9	96.0	4.5	85.7	4.43	85.7
	Intra-rater	100.0	92.9	4.5	92.9	4.46	89.3
	Inter-rater	100.0	92.9	4.46	89.3	4.5	89.3
	Internal consistency	67.9	100.0	3.39	50.0[a]	3.29	46.4[a]
Validity	Content validity	100.0	89.3	4.68	96.4	4.64	96.4
	Discriminant validity	100.0	92.9	4.21	82.1	4.14	75.0
	Convergent validity	78.6	91.3	3.14	28.6[a]	3.11	28.6[a]
	Concurrent validity	82.1	88.9	3.25	32.1[a]	3.25	35.7[a]
	Predictive validity	85.7	91.7	3.79	64.3[a]	3.71	60.7[a]
Responsiveness	Responsiveness	100.0	89.3	4.5	85.7	4.37	81.5
	Sensitivity	92.9	85.7	4.25	85.7	4.14	78.6
	Min. important diff.	92.9	88.9	4.04	71.4	3.96	67.9
	Floor and ceiling	89.3	96.2	3.54	53.6[a]	3.39	46.4[a]
Feasibility	Interpretability	100.0	89.3	4.21	82.1	4.18	82.1
	Familiarity required	78.6	95.7	3.79	71.4	3.75	71.4
	Scoring complexity	92.6	96.2	3.75	57.1[a]	3.86	60.7[a]
	Completion complexity	85.7	96.3	3.54	57.1[a]	3.64	60.7[a]
	Cost	89.3	88.9	3.61	64.3[a]	3.75	67.9
	Duration	92.9	100.0	3.75	67.9	3.93	75.0

Q1 refers to question one and so forth
[a]Consensus not reached on the question for the corresponding item

questionnaire achieved a minimum 67% consensus with respect to whether the item should be considered (range = 68 to 100%), whilst terminology and definitions reported similar levels of agreement (68 to 100%). Of the 20 items, 10 also achieved consensus with respect to the participants' rating of item importance and attitude (via the Likert-scale responses).

Three main actions were proposed by the steering committee based on round 1 results and participant feedback. First, a definition of 'test quality' was provided for round 2. Quality was defined as 'the standard of something as measured against other things of a similar kind; the degree of excellence of something' [40] and was included in round 2 of the questionnaire. Second, the uniform use of 'exercise and sport sciences' nomenclature was introduced into definitions and examples to help overcome instances of perceived ambiguity. Third, there were discrepancies in that some items achieved consensus for all questions whereas others did not; written participant feedback expressed that the relevance of certain measurement properties in a test may depend on the context of its use (i.e. laboratory vs. applied settings). Thus, it was determined that the development of level 1 and level 2 levels be used to distinguish between these items. Level 1 items were defined as those achieving group consensus (>67%) in all four questions, and therefore by inference were deemed essential for consideration when selecting or developing any exercise and sport science performance test. Level 2 items included those achieving partial consensus across the four questions. Specifically, this meant that the item was required to have achieved consensus in at least two of the four questions. For example, a level 2 item may have reached consensus on its definition and terminology, however, may not have reached consensus on the Likert-based importance and/or attitude questions. These items were deemed relevant for consideration in some cases; for example, depending on the test's intended use (i.e. laboratory based or in the field).

Despite achieving consensus on terminology and definitions, the steering committee nonetheless recommended a number of minor revisions for consideration based on written participant feedback. The majority of these related to changes to wording of definitions; however, two additional recommendations relating to items were also proposed. First, it was accepted that minor differences existed between the corresponding definitions for responsiveness and sensitivity to change. Specifically, sensitivity to change referred to 'the ability of test to detect change, regardless of noise, relevance or meaningfulness' and responsiveness 'the ability of a test to detect worthwhile and 'real' improvements over time'. However, in the interest of usability, the two items were consolidated as a single item for the checklist (see final definition in Table 2). Second, it was apparent that a number of terms existed in the literature were interchangeable in their use and meaning. In addition to the initially proposed 'minimum important difference', this also included 'smallest worthwhile change' and 'smallest worthwhile difference'. Consequently, it was recommended that these also be consolidated into a single item (minimum important difference/smallest worthwhile change).

Round 2

Of the 28 respondents participating in round 1, 20 (71%) also completed round 2 of the questionnaire. This consisted of eight academics, eight sport scientists and four clinical exercise scientists. This was slightly lower than the typically expected 75% retention rate [28] seen in similar studies. Results from the second round revealed that all three main recommendations by the steering committee achieved consensus, along with the minor revisions relating to terminology and definitions. Final definitions and terminology are shown in Table 2, along

Table 2 Final list of items ranked by level; corresponding definitions are also included

	Item	Definition
Level 1	Re-test reliability	The consistency of performers(s) results over repeated rounds of testing conducted over a period of typically days or weeks. This represents the change in a participant's results between repeated tests due to both systematic and random error, rather than true changes in performance [27, 36, 46]
	Intra-rater	The agreement (consistency) among two or more trials administered or scored by the same rater [4, 47]
	Inter-rater	The level of agreement (consistency) between assessments of the same performance when undertaken by two or more raters [4, 46, 47]
	Content validity	How well a specific test measures that which it intends to measure [4, 27]
	Discriminant validity	The extent to which results from a test relate to results on another test which measures a different construct (i.e., the ability to discriminate between dissimilar constructs) [42, 48, 49]
	Responsiveness/sensitivity to change	The ability of a test to detect worthwhile and 'real' improvements over time (e.g., between an initial bout of testing and subsequent rounds) [42, 50–54]
	MID/SWC	The smallest change or difference in a test result that is considered practically meaningful or important [55–58]
	Interpretability	The degree to which practical meaning can be assigned to a test result or change in result [25, 28]
	Familiarity required	The need to undertake a test familiarisation session with all participants prior to main testing in order to reduce or eliminate learning or reactivity effects [4]
	Duration	Expected and/or actual duration of the testing protocol [59, 60]
Level 2	Stability	The consistency of performer(s) results over repeated rounds of testing conducted over a period of months or years [40, 42, 61, 62]
	Internal consistency	The degree of inter-relatedness among test components that intend to measure the same construct/characteristic [28]
	Convergent validity	The extent to which results from tests that theoretically should be related to each other are, in fact, related to each other [42, 49]
	Concurrent validity	The extent to which the test relates to an alternate, previously validated measure of the same construct administered at the same time [42, 63]
	Predictive validity	The extent to which the test relates to a previously validated measure of a theoretically similar construct, administered at a future point in time [42, 63]
	Floor and ceiling effects	The ability of a test to distinguish between individuals at the lower and upper extremities of performance (i.e., ability to distinguish between high results (ceiling effect) and low results (floor effect)) [28, 64]
	Scoring complexity	The ease with which a test can be conducted and scored in a practical setting by the test administrator [65, 66]
	Completion complexity	The ease with which a test can be completed by a participant [65–67]
	Cost	The total amount of resources required for test administration including equipment, time, and administrator expertise/experience [25]

Reference support for each definition has also been provided
MID minimum important difference, *SWC* smallest worthwhile change

with relevant reference support. Figure 2 represents a taxonomy of the final list of items.

A checklist derived from the findings of the Delphi questionnaire (at the completion of round 2) has been included as Table 3. The checklist can be implemented by users to record information relating to the measurement properties and feasibility characteristics of a given test, using existing results in the literature. Results from users' testing on a sample population of interest can also be documented.

Discussion

This study primarily aimed to obtain subject matter expert consensus on which measurement and feasibility properties should be considered for performance tests used in the exercise and sport sciences, along with their terminology and definitions. Ten items, including re-test reliability, content validity and responsiveness were considered essential by respondents. A further ten, including stability, predictive validity and concurrent validity, though recognised as important, were considered more context-specific. A secondary aim was to develop a checklist of the agreed upon properties which can inform performance test development or selection.

It was notable that all of the 20 items originally proposed in the first round of the questionnaire were accepted at some level. This suggests that experienced practitioners and academics in the exercise and sport sciences have an appreciation for the importance of measurement quality, but also that there are many components that come together to make a 'high-quality measure'. The findings also demonstrate that the list was comprehensive, particularly as no additional items were suggested for inclusion by any of the participants. Specifically, commonly reported measurement properties such as re-test reliability, discriminant validity and responsiveness were all included as relevant items based on the final results, thereby confirming their importance for consideration when using a performance test. Based on these results, it would appear that these items be considered by researchers and practitioners alike in a variety of contexts. Measurement properties such as stability and concurrent validity, whilst included in the framework as level 2 items may not necessarily be relevant however under all circumstances. It is worth noting here that the likelihood of a given test displaying an appropriate level of each of these properties will depend largely on the user's ability to administer it appropriately. Despite these conclusive findings in the participant sample, an increased number of participants from each of the three types of subject matter experts may have allowed for the investigation of whether statistical differences in the responses of these three subgroups existed and more generalisable results overall.

Comparison of the findings of this study also revealed some similarities with work undertaken in other disciplines. Previous checklists developed from research undertaken in the COSMIN project (used in health-related patient-reported test outcomes) also included measurement properties such as reliability, content validity, criterion-related validity, responsiveness and interpretability [28, 41]. The current findings also build additionally on previous work undertaken in exercise and sport science that has espoused the importance of many of the measurement properties included here [1, 4, 15, 16]. Further, in addition to 'traditional' measurement properties, this study also considered often overlooked items relating to feasibility in performance testing, which may be particularly important for users working in field environments. Whilst not considered measurement properties per se, items such as test duration, cost and complexity of completion were all deemed important considerations based on results of the current study.

The development of level 1 and level 2 criteria in this study represents a novel addition to previous work from other disciplines. Specifically, these criteria provide the user with flexibility in application of the findings. This is particularly useful as the relative importance of any item may differ depending on the intended use of, or context for, the test [27]. For example, the costs of administering a test may be a critical factor if financial resources are limited, but this may not be a constraint in all settings. Similarly, convergent validity may not be assessable in scenarios whereby a similar measure for comparison is not available.

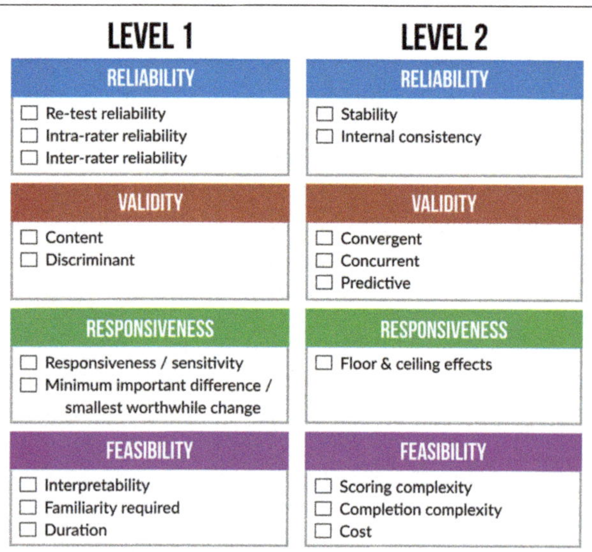

Fig. 2 Final taxonomy displaying the 19 level 1 and 2 items important for consideration in evaluating an exercise and sport science performance test

Table 3 User checklist based on the final results of the Delphi study

Performance test name:

Level 1 Item	Assessed?	Source	Results	Comments
1. Re-test reliability	☐			
2. Intra-rater reliability	☐			
3. Inter-rater reliability	☐			
4. Content validity	☐			
5. Discriminant validity	☐	*i.e., journal citation, book chapter reference*	*i.e., re-test reliability: r = 0.85*	*i.e., results higher/lower than similar alternatively available test*
6. Responsiveness /Sensitivity to change	☐			
7. MID / SWC	☐			
8. Interpretability	☐			
9. Familiarity required	☐			
10. Duration	☐			

Level 2 Item	Assessed?	Source	Results	Comments
11. Stability	☐			
12. Internal consistency	☐			
13. Convergent validity	☐			
14. Concurrent validity	☐			
15. Predictive validity	☐			
16. Floor & ceiling effects	☐			
17. Scoring complexity	☐			
18. Completion complexity	☐			
19. Cost	☐			

All items achieving consensus in the questionnaire are included under the respective 'level 1' or 'level 2' categories. The user can list previous findings relating the measurement properties and feasibility of a test and/or record their own results

The development of the checklist based on the findings from this study represents the main practical application of this work. The checklist consists of the 19 level 1 and level 2 criteria from the Delphi questionnaire, which can be used to assess an existing or newly developed performance test. Specifically, when selecting a test for implementation, the user can directly assess its quality based on existing results reported in the literature. These results can be recorded and easily compared against different test options or with newly developed alternative. The checklist also allows for the user to add their own testing results to compare directly with previous findings. This is important because although a test may display appropriate measurement properties and feasibility in one setting, this does not guarantee the same results when applied to a new scenario or population [25, 42]. It is hoped that this feature of the checklist prompts users to undertake their own measurement property and feasibility assessments when using a performance test.

Some limitations of the study should also be stated. The Delphi approach has been criticised due to its potential for researcher bias, its potential issues in achieving appropriate expert selection and has also been considered a restrictive communication method [43]. Further, the authors also acknowledge that the use of a face-to-face method (whilst difficult to facilitate) may have elicited different results to those seen here. Also, participants involved in the Delphi questionnaire were all of a single nationality and an even distribution from each of the three sub-groups was also noted. This may have meant that consensus was easier to achieve, given participants may have had similar conditions in their work environments and also experienced similar socio-cultural norms. There is a potential that engaging an international sample or a different sampling procedure altogether may have elicited different results to those observed here. Further, it is worth noting that the sample was recruited based on their expertise in sport and exercise rather than in measurement. As such, results may have differed somewhat to one that included statisticians or measurement experts.

In addition to addressing some of these limitations, future work in this area may also focus on the development of a user manual to be used as a supplement to the checklist. This manual could include specific practical examples of each item in order to increase the interpretability and increase the practical utility of the checklist for a wider user population. This may also allow for wider dissemination of the checklist to non-academic audiences. Further work may also look to evaluate the properties of the checklist itself. For instance, an evaluation of the uptake of the checklist after a period of time post-implementation may allow for identification of areas in need of further development. The measurement properties of the checklist itself are also still to be determined. For instance, the inter-rater reliability of user implementation of the checklist to rate particular tests may represent an appropriate starting point [36]. Follow-up studies may also look to determine the most appropriate statistical methods available in order to evaluate each item included in the checklist. This would serve to define the actual quantitative quality criteria relating to each item. For instance, in the case of a specific validity item, a minimum level of a particular statistical measure (i.e. correlation statistic) may be determined in order to provide a more specific representation of test quality. This approach, already undertaken in other disciplines [44, 45], could be a valuable addition to exercise and sport science research and practice.

Conclusions

The aim of the current study was to obtain subject matter expert consensus on which measurement and feasibility properties should be considered for exercise and sport science performance tests. Respondents agreed with the terminology and definitions for all 20 items proposed. Traditional measurement properties such as re-test reliability, content validity and responsiveness were considered essential (level 1) by respondents. Items such as stability, predictive validity and concurrent validity were considered to be more context-specific (level 2) in their application. Establishing a two-level hierarchy for measurement properties is a step-forward in the consensus literature, building on previous research in medicine and health. The checklist developed from the results should serve as a prompt for researchers and practitioners to overtly consider measurement properties in their exercise and sports science practice. Evaluating the implementation, use and measurement properties of the checklist itself is an obvious next step to further assist rigorous and transferable exercise and sports science research and practice.

Abbreviations

COSMIN: Consensus-based standards for the selection of health measurement instruments; RR: Response rate

Acknowledgements

This study was supported by a Deakin University Faculty of Health Research Development Grant. Ester Cerin is supported by an ARC Future Fellowship (FT#140100085). The authors would like to acknowledge the contributions of the 28 participants involved in at least one round of the Delphi questionnaire. These have been listed below in alphabetical order (affiliations in brackets). Mr John Baker (Australian Institute of Sport), Dr Jon Bartlett (Western Bulldogs/Victoria University), Professor Stephen Bird (Royal Melbourne Institute of Technology), Dr Lyndell Bruce (Royal Melbourne Institute of Technology), Dr Darren Burgess (Port Adelaide Football Club), Professor Jill Cook (Monash University), Dr Stuart Cormack (Australian Catholic University), Mr Matt Cutler (Golf Australia), Dr Dan Dwyer (Deakin University), Professor Damian Farrow (Australian Institute of Sport/Victoria University), Dr Guy Gregory Haff (Edith Cowan University), Dr Shona Halson (Australian Institute of Sport), Mr Chris Hume (Australian Sports Commission), Mr Brad James (Golf Australia), Associate Professor David Jenkins (University of Queensland), Mr David Joyce (Greater Western Sydney AFL Club), Mr Vince Kelly (University of Queensland), Associate Professor Justin Keogh (Bond University), Associate Professor Anthony Leicht (James Cook University), Dr Kevin Netto (Curtin University), Associate Professor Denny Meyer (Swinburne University), Dr Ian McKeown (Port Adelaide Football Club), Dr Derek Panchuk (Australian Institute of Sport), Professor Warren Payne (Victoria University), Professor Remco Polman (Victoria University), Professor David Pyne (Australian Institute of Sport), Dr Tony Sparrow (Victoria University), Associate Professor Michael Spittle (Victoria University) and Associate Professor Warren Young (Federation University).

Authors' contributions

SR, PK, BA and EC contributed to the study concept and design. SR and JT contributed to the acquisition of data. SR, PK, BA, JT and EC contributed to the analysis and interpretation of the data. SR, PK, BA, JT and EC contributed to the drafting of the manuscript. SR contributed to the statistical analysis. All authors read and approved the final manuscript.

Competing interests

Sam Robertson, Peter Kremer, Brad Aisbett, Jacquie Train and Ester Cerin declare that they have no conflict of interest.

Author details

[1]Centre for Exercise and Sport Science, Deakin University, Geelong, Victoria, Australia. [2]Institute of Sport Exercise and Active Living (ISEAL), Victoria University, Footscray Park campus, PO Box 14428, Melbourne, Victoria 8001, Australia. [3]Centre for Physical Activity and Nutrition Research, Deakin University, Burwood, Victoria, Australia. [4]School of Public Health, The University of Hong Kong, Hong Kong, China.

References

1. Currell K, Jeukendrup AE. Validity, reliability and sensitivity of measures of sporting performance. Sports Med. 2008;38:297–316.
2. Bartels B, de Groot JF, Terwee C. The six-minute walk test in chronic pediatric conditions: a systematic review of measurement properties. Phys Ther. 2013;93:529–41.
3. Tanner R, Gore C. Physiological tests for elite athletes. Lower Mitcham: Human Kinetics; 2001.
4. Robertson S, Burnett A, Cochrane J. Tests examining skill outcomes in sport: a systematic review of measurement properties and feasibility. Sports Med. 2014;44:501–18.
5. Duncan MJ, Taylor S, Lyons M. The effect of caffeine ingestion on field hockey skill performance following physical fatigue. Res Sports Med. 2012; 20:25–36.
6. Currell K, Conway S, Jeukendrup AE. Carbohydrate ingestion improves performance of a new reliable test of soccer performance. Int J Sport Nutr Exerc Metab. 2009;19:34–46.
7. Russell M, Benton D, Kingsley M. The effects of fatigue on soccer skills performed during a soccer match simulation. Int J Sports Physiol Perform. 2011;6:221–33.
8. Gabbett TJ, Georgieff B. The development of a standardized skill assessment for junior volleyball players. Int J Sports Physiol Perform. 2006;1:95–107.
9. Pyne DB, Gardner AS, Sheehan K, et al. Fitness testing and career progression in AFL football. J Sci Med Sport. 2005;8:321–32.
10. Robertson SJ, Burnett AF, Newton RU. Development and validation of the Approach-Iron Skill Test for use in golf. Eur J Sport Sci. 2013;13:615–21.

11. Robertson S, Gupta S, Kremer P, et al. Development and measurement properties of a putting skill test for high-level golf. Eur J Sport Sci. 2015;15: 125–33.
12. Robertson S, Burnett AF, Gupta R. Two tests of approach-iron golf skill and their ability to predict tournament performance. J Sport Sci. 2014;32:1341–9.
13. Ali A. Measuring soccer skill performance: a review. Scand J Med Sci Sports. 2011;21:170–83.
14. Lidor R, CôTé JE, Hackfort D. ISSP position stand: to test or not to test? The use of physical skill tests in talent detection and in early phases of sport development. Int J Sport Exerc Psychol. 2009;7:131–46.
15. Hopkins WG. Measures of reliability in sports medicine and science. Sports Med. 2000;30:1–15.
16. Atkinson G, Nevill AM. Statistical methods for assessing measurement error (reliability) in variables relevant to sports medicine. Sports Med. 1998;26: 217–38.
17. Hopkins W, Marshall S, Batterham A, Hanin J. Progressive statistics for studies in sports medicine and exercise science. Med Sci Sport Exer. 2009;41:3.
18. Haskell WL. What to look for in assessing responsiveness to exercise in a health context. Med Sci Sport Exer. 2001;33:S454–8.
19. ESSA in 2014. Exercise and Sports Science Australia. Code of Professional Conduct and Ethical Practice. Queensland; 2014. https://www.essa.org.au/wp-content/uploads/2014/06/Code-of-Professional-Conduct-and-Ethical-Practice_FINAL2014.pdf. Accessed 27 Jan 2016.
20. ASCA in 2012. Australian Strength & Conditioning Association. Professional standards and guidelines. 2012. https://www.strengthandconditioning.org/professional-coaches-scheme. Accessed 27 Jan 2016.
21. Ramsbottom R, Brewer J, Williams C. A progressive shuttle run test to estimate maximal oxygen uptake. Brit J Sport Med. 1988;22:141–4.
22. Leger LA, Lambert J. A maximal multistage 20-m shuttle run test to predict VO2 max. Eur J Appl Physiol O. 1982;49:1–12.
23. Cahalin LP, Mathier MA, Semigran MJ, et al. The six-minute walk test predicts peak oxygen uptake and survival in patients with advanced heart failure. Chest. 1996;110:325–32.
24. Fitchett MA. Predictability of VO2 max from submaximal cycle ergometer and bench stepping tests. Brit J Sport Med. 1985;19:85–8.
25. Lohr KN. Assessing health status and quality-of-life instruments: attributes and review criteria. Qual Life Res. 2002;11:193–205.
26. Mokkink LB, Terwee CB, Knol DL, et al. Protocol of the COSMIN study: COnsensus-based Standards for the selection of health Measurement INstruments. BMC Med Res Methodol. 2006;6:2.
27. Terwee CB, Mokkink LB, van Poppel MN, et al. Qualitative attributes and measurement properties of physical activity questionnaires: a checklist. Sports Med. 2010;40:525–37.
28. Mokkink LB, Terwee CB, Patrick DL, et al. The COSMIN checklist for assessing the methodological quality of studies on measurement properties of health status measurement instruments: an international Delphi study. Qual Life Res. 2010;19:539–49.
29. Hasson F, Keeney S, McKenna H. Research guidelines for the Delphi survey technique. J Adv Nurs. 2000;32:1008–15.
30. Miró J, Huguet A, Nieto R. Predictive factors of chronic pediatric pain and disability: a Delphi poll. J Pain. 2007;8:774–92.
31. Jones J, Hunter D. Consensus methods for medical and health services research. Brit Med J. 1995;311:376.
32. Vergouw D, Heymans MW, de Vet HC, et al. Prediction of persistent shoulder pain in general practice: Comparing clinical consensus from a Delphi procedure with a statistical scoring system. BMC Fam Pract. 2011;12:63.
33. Lohr KN, Aaronson NK, Alonso J, et al. Evaluating quality-of-life and health status instruments: development of scientific review criteria. Clin Ther. 1996; 18:979–92.
34. Meijer R, Ihnenfeldt D, Vermeulen M, et al. The use of a modified Delphi procedure for the determination of 26 prognostic factors in the sub-acute stage of stroke. Int J Rehabil Res. 2003;26:265–70.
35. Mokkink LB, Terwee CB, Knol DL, et al. COSMIN checklist for evaluating the methodological quality of studies on measurement properties: a clarification of its content. BMC Med Res Methodol. 2010;10:22.
36. Mokkink LB, Terwee CB, Gibbons E, et al. Inter-rater agreement and reliability of the COSMIN (COnsensus-based Standards for the selection of health status Measurement Instruments) checklist. BMC Med Res Methodol. 2010;10:82.
37. Cook C, Heath F, Thompson RL. A meta-analysis of response rates in web-or internet-based surveys. Educ Pyschol Meas. 2000;60:821–36.
38. Delbecq AL, Van de Ven AH, Gustafson DH. Group techniques for program planning: a guide to nominal group and Delphi processes. Glenview: Scott, Foresman; 1975.
39. MacCallum RC, Zhang S, Preacher KJ, et al. On the practice of dichotomization of quantitative variables. Psychol Methods. 2002;7:19.
40. Fowler HW, Fowler FG, Crystal D. The Concise Oxford Dictionary: The Classic First Edition. Oxford: Oxford University Press; 2011.
41. Mokkink LB, Terwee CB, Patrick DL, et al. The COSMIN study reached international consensus on taxonomy, terminology, and definitions of measurement properties for health-related patient-reported outcomes. J Clin Epidemiol. 2010;63:737–45.
42. Streiner DL, Norman GR, Cairney J. Health measurement scales: a practical guide to their development and use. Oxford: Oxford University Press; 2014.
43. Vernon W. The Delphi technique: a review. Int J Ther Rehabil. 2009;16:69–76.
44. Terwee CB, Bot SD, de Boer MR, et al. Quality criteria were proposed for measurement properties of health status questionnaires. J Clin Epidemiol. 2007;60:34–42.
45. Mokkink LB, Terwee CB, Stratford PW, et al. Evaluation of the methodological quality of systematic reviews of health status measurement instruments. Qual Life Res. 2009;18:313–33.
46. Bartlett JW, Frost C. Reliability, repeatability and reproducibility: analysis of measurement errors in continuous variables. Ultrasound Obst Gyn. 2008;31: 466–75.
47. Baumgartner TA, Jackson AS. Measurement for evaluation in physical education and exercise science. 5th ed. Michigan: Brown & Benchmark; 1998.
48. Russell M, Benton D, Kingsley M. Reliability and construct validity of soccer skills test that measure passing, shooting, and dribbling. J Sports Sci. 2010; 28:1399–408.
49. Munro BH. Statistical methods for health care research. 5th ed. Philadelphia: Lippincott, Williams & Wilkins; 1999.
50. Beaton DE, Bombardier C, Katz JN, et al. A taxonomy for responsiveness. J Clin Epidemiol. 2001;54:1204–17.
51. Guyatt G, Walter S, Norman G. Measuring change over time: assessing the usefulness of evaluative instruments. J Chronic Dis. 1987;40:171–8.
52. Corzillius M, Fortin P, Stucki G. Responsiveness and sensitivity to change of SLE disease activity measures. Lupus. 1999;8:655–9.
53. Liang MH. Evaluating measurement responsiveness. J Rheumatol. 1995;22:1191–2.
54. Fritz JM. Sensitivity to change: a letter to the editor. Phys Ther. 1999;79:420–2.
55. Herbert R. Practical evidence-based physiotherapy. Philadelphia: Butterworth Henemann, Elsevier Health Sciences; 2005.
56. Ferreira ML, Herbert RD, Ferreira PH, et al. A critical review of methods used to determine the smallest worthwhile effect of interventions for low back pain. J Clin Epidemiol. 2012;65:253–61.
57. Copay AG, Subach BR, Glassman SD, et al. Understanding the minimum clinically important difference: a review of concepts and methods. Spine. 2007;7:541–6.
58. Donoghue D, Stokes EK. How much change is true change? The minimum detectable change of the Berg Balance Scale in elderly people. J Rehabil Med. 2009;41:343–6.
59. Streiner DL. A checklist for evaluating the usefulness of rating scales. Can J Psychiatry. 1993;38:140–8.
60. Bartlett J, Smith L, Davis K, et al. Development of a valid volleyball skills test battery. J Phys Educ Rec Dance. 1991;62:19–21.
61. Terwee CB, Mokkink LB, Knol DL, et al. Rating the methodological quality in systematic reviews of studies on measurement properties: a scoring system for the COSMIN checklist. Qual Life Res. 2012;21:651–7.
62. Schmidt FL, Le H, Ilies R. Beyond alpha: an empirical examination of the effects of different sources of measurement error on reliability estimates for measures of individual-differences constructs. Psychol Methods. 2003;8:206.
63. Packham T, Macdermid JC, Henry J, et al. A systematic review of psychometric evaluations of outcome assessments for complex regional pain syndrome. Disabil Rehabil. 2012;34:1059–69.
64. Wang L, Zhang Z, McArdle JJ, et al. Investigating ceiling effects in longitudinal data analysis. Multivariate Behav Res. 2009;43:476–96.
65. Stevens B, Gibbins S. Clinical utility and clinical significance in the assessment and management of pain in vulnerable infants. Clin Perinatol. 2002;29:459–68.
66. Stinson JN, Kavanagh T, Yamada J, et al. Systematic review of the psychometric properties, interpretability of self-report pain measures for use in clinical trials in children and adolescents. Pain. 2006;125:143–57.

2

Exercise Training but not Curcumin Supplementation Decreases Immune Cell Infiltration in the Pancreatic Islets of a Genetically Susceptible Model of Type 1 Diabetes

Leandro Kansuke Oharomari[1*], Camila de Moraes[2] and Anderson Marliere Navarro[1]

Abstract

Background: The main mechanism involved in the pathogenesis of autoimmunity is an uncontrolled inflammatory response against self-antigens. Therefore, anti-inflammatory factors, such as the intake of bioactive compounds and a physically active lifestyle, may decrease or cease the development of autoimmune diseases. Type 1 diabetes (T1D) is an autoimmune disease characterized by pancreatic β cell destruction. The non-obese diabetic (NOD) mouse is a model of spontaneous T1D and is the model most similar to human disease.

Methods: To determine the effects of exercise training and curcumin supplementation on T1D progression, 48 NOD mice, 5 weeks old, were randomly divided into four groups: control, curcumin supplementation, trained, and trained plus curcumin. Every 2 weeks, blood glucose was measured using a glucometer. At the end of 20 weeks, a histopathological procedure was used to assess immune cells infiltration into pancreatic β cells (insulitis).

Results: Moderate intensity exercise training has the potential to protect pancreatic β cells against an immune response in vivo. However, curcumin supplementation failed to attenuate insulitis in NOD mice.

Conclusions: These data provide evidence that exercise training can mitigate T1D development in genetically susceptible mice.

Keywords: Autoimmunity, Type 1 diabetes, Insulitis, Exercise training, Bioactive compound, Curcumin

Key Points

- Exercise training decreased immune cells infiltration in vivo in a spontaneous mouse model of type 1 diabetes.
- Curcumin supplementation did not attenuate insulitis alone or improve exercise training effects.
- The effect of exercise training is present regardless of IL-6 and TNF-alpha alteration.

* Correspondence: lkansuke@hotmail.com
[1]Department of Food and Nutrition, Pharmaceutical Sciences College, Araraquara, São Paulo, Brazil
Full list of author information is available at the end of the article

Background

Intense inflammatory response is a main feature of autoimmune diseases. Type 1 diabetes (T1D), for instance, occurs due to a chronic inflammatory response with enough severity to destroy most of the pancreatic β cells [1]. The incidence of some autoimmune diseases, including T1D, has been increasing worldwide over the past decades [2–5], and environmental factors are the most accepted explanation for this phenomenon. For example, vitamin D status [6] and the hygiene hypothesis [7] are being investigated. Currently, physical inactivity and processed food intake during childhood appear to be linked to the development of chronic [8–10] and inflammatory disease [11] in early stages of life. Furthermore, the Overload Hypothesis suggests an association between a modern lifestyle and beta cell overload, which could make these cells more vulnerable to an autoimmune response [12].

Intervention using functional foods with anti-inflammatory properties could decrease or halt the autoimmune response, leading to a delay or even prevention of autoimmunity. Dietary patterns characterized by high bioactive compounds, such as a Mediterranean diet, promote an "anti-inflammatory environment" in humans [13]. Among several compounds, curcumin, a polyphenol found in the rhizome of *Curcuma longa*, is one of the most studied bioactive compounds due to its anti-inflammatory properties [14–16]. Additionally, studies have shown that physical exercise also promotes anti-inflammatory responses through several mechanisms, such as increasing antioxidant activity [17], releasing myokines and hormones [18], modulating immune cell metabolism [19], and decreasing inflammation signaling [20].

Currently, the non-obese diabetic (NOD) mouse, a model of spontaneous T1D, is the model that is most similar to human T1D [21]. Over the last 30 years, it has been used in research to improve the science of autoimmunity [22]. As in humans, T1D occurs in NOD mice due to immune cell infiltration into pancreatic islets (insulitis) and subsequent destruction of β cells. Additionally, it has been demonstrated by ample literature that TNF-α, a pro-inflammatory cytokine, has an important role in the pathogenesis of T1D in NOD mice [23–27].

Some studies have tested bioactive compounds in NOD mice. Supplementation with cocoa flavonoids or green tea catechin reduced diabetes incidence in this animal model [28, 29]. However, no studies have tested the potential of exercise training to prevent T1D in NOD mice. Therefore, this study aimed to investigate the effects of exercise training and curcumin supplementation on T1D progression in NOD mice.

Methods

Animals

Forty-eight female NOD mice, 5 weeks old, were randomly divided into four groups ($n = 12$): control (C), curcumin supplementation (CUR), trained (T), and trained + curcumin supplementation (TC). The experimental protocol lasted 20 weeks. Animals were housed collectively (four animals per cage) and kept in conventional conditions (22–24 °C and 12-h light-dark cycle) with unlimited access to water and food, which was a pelletized AIN-93G diet [30]. Food intake was monitored three times a week. Body weight was measured weekly. Blood glucose was measured every 14 days using a drop of tail blood and a glucometer (FreeStyle Lite–Abbott). Mice were considered diabetic when their blood glucose level was higher than 250 mg/dL. Diabetic animals that lost more than 25% of their body weight were killed before 20 weeks. All procedures were reviewed and approved by the Ethics Committee on Animal Use in Research (CETEA-FMRP, protocol no. 190/2014) in compliance with the Ethical Principles in Animal Research adopted by the National Council for the Control of Animal Experimentation (CONCEA) and following the guidelines for the care and use of laboratory animals [31].

Sample Size

Sample size was calculated based on the primary outcome in this study, which was immune cell infiltration into pancreatic islets (insulitis). As insulitis is a nominal qualitative variable, the sample size was determined using the following equation:

$$\frac{(\text{p1.q1} + \text{p2.q2}).(Z\alpha/2 + Z\beta)^2}{(\text{p1-p2})^2}$$

Considering that each section of pancreas has approximately 10 islets and that in control groups, approximately 60% have some level of insulitis even in the absence of T1D [32], sample size was established to reach statistical significance when the applied interventions reduced the number of islets with some level of insulitis at least by half (30%).

Curcumin Supplementation

The AIN-93 diet was prepared twice a week, protected from light, and kept frozen. The food offered to the CUR and TC groups had curcumin added (500 mg/kg). Curcumin was purchased from Sigma-Aldrich (St. Louis, MO, USA). Considering the daily food intake of the mice, the curcumin dose reached approximately 65 mg/kg per day.

Exercise Training Protocol

All mice from the T and TC groups performed a maximal incremental running test at the beginning of the experimental protocol. This test began at 10 m/min and increased by 1.7 m/min every 2 min until exhaustion (determined when the animal touched the bottom of the bay five times within 1 min). The speed at which exhaustion occurred was considered 100%. Adjustment of exercise load was done every 4 weeks by repeating the same incremental test. According to the animals' performance in the incremental test, they were divided into three running groups (best, middle, and lower) to guarantee that exercise intensity was maintained and to respect the differences in mouse performance.

Exercise training was carried out for 20 weeks, 5 days a week. All exercise sessions were performed in the morning. The exercise session consisted of a 5-minute warm-up followed by 60 min of running at training intensity and a 2-min cool down. Training intensity varied during week sessions. On Monday, Wednesday, and Friday, the mice ran at 60% of their maximal speed reached in the incremental test; on

Tuesday and Thursday, mice had recovery sessions running at 30% of the maximal speed.

Cytokine and Insulin Concentration

Following overnight fasting, the animals were euthanized by decapitation 48 h after the last exercise session, without previous anesthetic. The serum obtained was used to determine glucose concentration by the colorimetric method (Labtest, Lago Santa, Brazil), and frozen samples (−70 °C) were used to measure insulin, TNF-α, and IL-6 using Luminex xMAP® technology with a Milliplex® kit (Millipore Corporation) analyzed on MAGPIX®; the standard curve of all analytes had $R^2 = 1$.

A homeostatic model assessment of insulin resistance (HOMA-IR) was calculated to estimate insulin resistance as previously described [33].

Insulitis

Pancreas was fixed in formalin (10%), embedded in paraffin, and stained with hematoxylin-eosin. Images were taken on an optical microscope (Olympus BX61VS). Three sections of each pancreas were analyzed. Islets were counted as previously described [34] and labeled as: No Insulitis (absence of immune cells), Pre-Insulitis (few immune cells around the islet), and Insulitis (>25% of cells infiltrated and destruction of islet architecture). Counts were performed manually by two independent researchers (blinded). Insulitis extension was calculated as previously described [35]:

$$\frac{(N^{\circ}\text{No Insulitis}) + (N^{\circ}\text{ Pre Insulitis} \times 2) + (N^{\circ}\text{Insulitis} \times 3)}{N^{\circ}\text{Total Islets}}$$

Statistics

Data are presented as the means ± standard deviation. Analysis of variance (one-way ANOVA) followed by a Tukey post hoc test was performed, except for HOMA-IR and IL-6, which did not have a normal distribution and were analyzed using a Kruskal-Wallis test. Weekly blood glucose was analyzed using a repeated measure ANOVA. A log-rank test was used to compare diabetes incidence. A Chi-square test was used to compare insulitis distribution. The level of significance adopted was $p < 0.05$.

Results

Although the daily food intake was approximately 10% greater in the trained group than in the control group, body weight gain was approximately 41% lower in the trained mice after 20 weeks. Only four animals developed T1D, two each in groups C and CUR. Insulin levels tended to be lower in CUR and T, but the difference only reached a statistical level of significance in the TC group. HOMA-IR was not modified by curcumin or exercise training (Table 1). Blood glucose was similar among groups during the 20 weeks, as seen in Fig. 1.

Despite the low incidence of T1D, insulitis was seen in all groups but in different levels. The trained and trained + curcumin groups had 50% less immune cell infiltration in pancreatic islets than the sedentary groups (Fig. 2a). In addition, insulitis extension was also reduced with exercise training (Fig. 2b). Regarding cytokine levels, IL-6 and TNF-α were not modified by curcumin or exercise training (Fig. 3).

Discussion

To the best of our knowledge, this study is the first to show that exercise training has the potential to protect pancreatic β cells against an immune response in vivo. However, curcumin supplementation failed to attenuate insulitis in NOD mice.

Curcumin is a polyphenolic compound that exhibits low bioavailability [36]. The route of administration and the dose of curcumin used in this study were established based on previous studies that aimed to simulate a rich polyphenol diet [36–39]. Although chronic oral curcumin (500 ppm in diet) reached detectable concentrations in plasma (0.035 μg/ml) and in brain tissue (0.469 μg/ml) in a dose-dependent study [37], our study indicates that this concentration was not enough to prevent an immune response against pancreatic β cells. However, intraperitoneal curcumin supplementation (25 mg/kg body weight) inhibited leucocyte infiltration in accelerated murine models of T1D [40]. These data suggest that the concentration of curcumin required to modulate immune function could not be reached using dietary strategies.

The low incidence of T1D observed was expected because animals were fed a gluten-free diet and were not

Table 1 Food intake, weight gain, T1D incidence, insulin level, and HOMA-IR after the 20-week experimental protocol

Group	Food intake (g/day)	Weight gain (g)	T1D incidence (%)	Insulin (μU/mL)	HOMA-IR
Control	3.05 ± 0.23	12.40 ± 5.02	16.66	28.07 ± 25.53	4.97 ± 4.79
Curcumin	3.13 ± 0.20	9.30 ± 3.30	16.66	15.06 ± 13.15	2.32 ± 1.95
Trained	3.39 ± 0.26[a]	6.73 ± 1.68[a]	0.00	9.60 ± 15.88	1.80 ± 2.95
Trained + curcumin	3.31 ± 0.21	7.25 ± 1.48[a]	0.00	8.27 ± 6.08[a]	1.71 ± 1.17
P value	0.0006	0.0006	0.5078	0.0400	0.1172

Data are the mean ± standard deviation
[a]Different from control

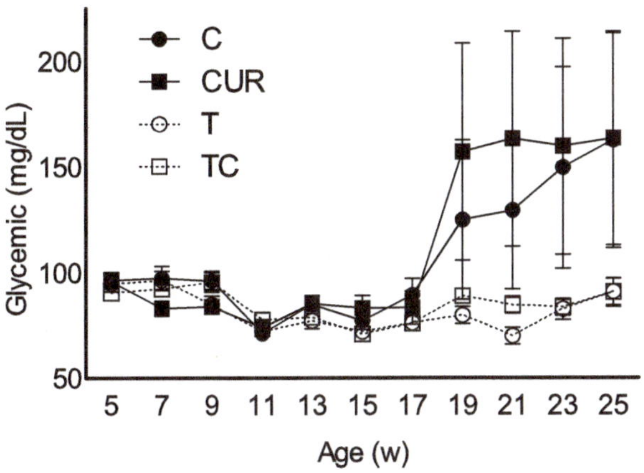

Fig. 1 Blood glucose during the 20-week experimental protocol from control (*C*), curcumin (*CUR*), trained (*T*), and trained + curcumin (*TC*). NOD mice were 5 weeks old at the beginning. Data are mean ± standard deviation

in a germ-free environment [41, 42]. However, NOD mice present ~60% immune cell infiltration in islets even in the absence of T1D [32], which is consistent with our findings. Exercise training lowered this rate to 30%.

The effect of exercise training in diminishing body weight gain is well documented and was observed in the present study, showing the importance of physical exercise for caloric balance. Lower body weight gain could be one mechanism that explains the reduction of insulitis in the T and TC groups. Since obesity induces chronic inflammation [43] and the Overload Hypothesis proposes that environment factors, such as obesity, increase T1D risk [12], this line of thought is strengthened.

Another possible mechanism to explain the effects of exercise training is through dendritic cells modulation. It is well known that dendritic cells modulate both innate and adaptive immune responses, and the role of these cells on the development of T1D was recently demonstrated [44]. Several studies have shown that exercise training decreases the number of dendritic cells or diminishes their response [45–48]. Thus, exercise could mitigate autoimmunity by shaping dendritic cell activation.

Regarding cytokine signaling, IL-6 has been recognized as one of the myokines produced during exercise training [49]. In 2010, exercise training was documented as an anti-inflammatory approach, which is able to prevent type 2 diabetes, cardiovascular diseases, cancer, and dementia [50]. Although no significant differences were seen in cytokine levels, the CUR, T, and TC groups exhibited an IL-6 concentration more than twofold higher than the C group ($p = 0.07$). In an ex vivo study, the pancreas of trained animals had fewer apoptosis biomarkers than sedentary animals. When an IL-6 blocker was added to the trained animals' pancreas, the apoptosis biomarkers rose to sedentary levels. The authors concluded that the benefit of exercise training on pancreatic β cell survival is through the IL-6 pathway [51]. However, the results of the present study cannot reinforce the role of IL-6 in preventing insulitis because the CUR group had the same insulitis markers as the C group, which suggests that the effect of exercise training is due to other mechanisms.

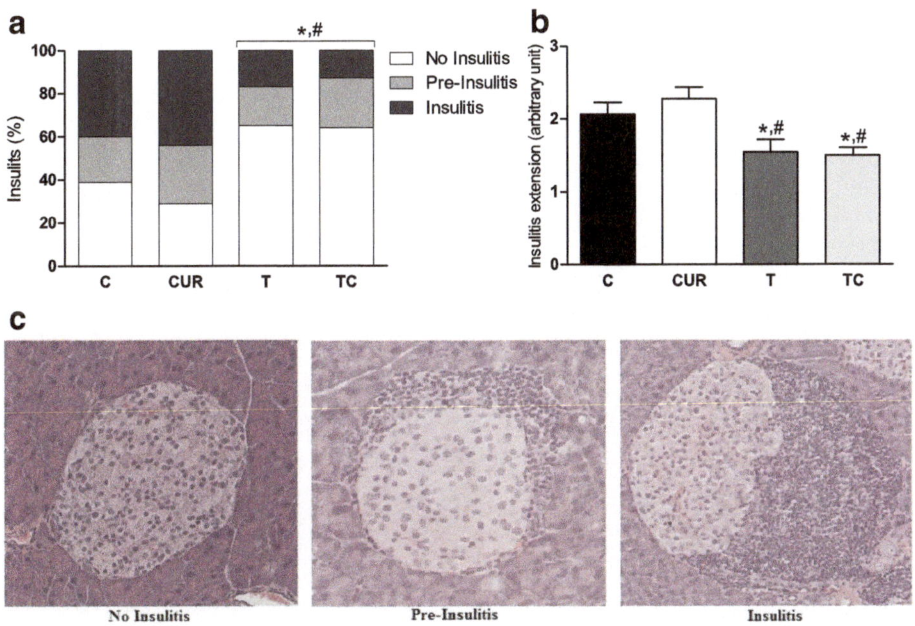

Fig. 2 Quantitative/representative analysis of insulitis. Insulitis distribution (**a**), insulitis extension (**b**), and representative image used to label insulitis level (**c**). Control (*C*), curcumin (*CUR*), trained (*T*), and trained + curcumin (*TC*).*Different from control; #different from curcumin

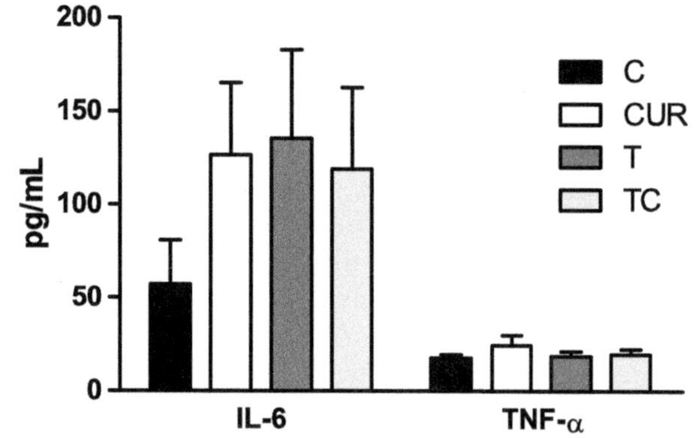

Fig. 3 Cytokine levels after the 20-week experimental protocol from control (*C*), curcumin (*CUR*), trained (*T*), trained plus curcumin (*TC*) NOD mice

Conclusions

In conclusion, moderate intensity exercise training has the potential to protect pancreatic β cells against an immune response in NOD mice. The limitation of the present study is a lack of mechanisms that establish a causal effect, as well as the lack of an evaluation of other inflammatory markers, and both pancreatic and blood oxidative stress, epinephrine levels, and the characterization of infiltrating immune cells. Those measurements are an important area of future research. Therefore, additional and prospective studies are needed to uncover the mechanisms that explain the link between exercise training and autoimmunity.

Abbreviations

AIN: American Institute of Nutrition; ANOVA: Analysis of variance; C: Control; CONCEA: Conselho Nacional de Controle de Exeperimentação Animal; CUR: Curcumin; FMRP: Faculdade de Medicina de Ribeirão Preto; HOMA-IR: Homeostatic model assessment of insulin resistance; IL: Interleukin; NOD: Non-obese diabetic; T: Trained; T1D: Type 1 diabetes; TC: Trained + curcumin; TNF: Tumor necrosis factor

Funding

No financial support was received for the conduct of this study or preparation of this manuscript.

Authors' Contributions

LKO conceived, designed the study, performed the experiments, analyzed the data, and wrote the paper. CDM and AMN conceived and designed the study, contributed to discussions, and edited the manuscript. All authors reviewed the manuscript. All authors read and approved the final manuscript.

Competing Interests

Author L.K.O., Author C.D.M., and Author A.M.N declare no conflict of interest.

Author details

[1]Department of Food and Nutrition, Pharmaceutical Sciences College, Araraquara, São Paulo, Brazil. [2]School of Physical Education and Sport of Ribeirão Preto, University of São Paulo, Ribeirão Preto, São Paulo, Brazil.

References

1. Wållberg M, Cooke A. Immune mechanisms in type 1 diabetes. Trends Immunol. 2013;34:583–91.
2. Cooper GS, Stroehla BC. The epidemiology of autoimmune diseases. Autoimmun Rev. 2003;2:119–25.
3. The autoimmune diseases coordinating committee (ADCC). Progress in Autoimmune Diseases Research Progress. Bethesda: National Institutes of Health; 2005. p. 1–129.
4. Forlenza GP, Rewers M. The epidemic of type 1 diabetes: what is it telling us? Curr Opin Endocrinol Diabetes Obes [Internet]. 2011;18:248–51. Available from: http://www.ncbi.nlm.nih.gov/pubmed/21844707.
5. Egro FM. Why is type 1 diabetes increasing? J Mol Endocrinol. 2013;51:R1–13.
6. Antico A, Tampoia M, Tozzoli R, Bizzaro N. Can supplementation with vitamin D reduce the risk or modify the course of autoimmune diseases? A systematic review of the literature. Autoimmun Rev. 2012;12:127–36.
7. Bach JF, Chatenoud L. The hygiene hypothesis: an explanation for the increased frequency of insulin-dependet diabetes. Cold Spring Harb Perspect Med. 2012;2:1–10.
8. Ludwig DS. Relation between consumption of sugar sweetened drinks and childhood obesity: a prospective observational analysis. Lancet. 2001;357:505–8.
9. Ayer J, Charakida M, Deanfield JE, Celermajer DS, Ng M, Fleming T, et al. Lifetime risk: childhood obesity and cardiovascular risk. Eur Heart J. 2015;36:1371–6.
10. Downing KL, Hnatiuk J, Hesketh KD. Prevalence of sedentary behavior in children under 2 years: a systematic review. Prev Med (Baltim). 2015;78:105–14.
11. Noutsios GT, Floros J. Childhood asthma: causes, risks, and protective factors; a role of innate immunity. Swiss Med Wkly. 2014;144:w14036.
12. Dahlquist G. Can we slow the rising incidence of childhood-onset autoimmune diabetes? The overload hypothesis. Diabetologia. 2006;49:20–4.
13. Bonaccio M, Pounis G, Cerletti C, Donati MB, Iacoviello L, de Gaetano G. Mediterranean diet, dietary polyphenols and low-grade inflammation: results from the moli-sani study. Br J Clin Pharmacol. 2016;83:107–13.
14. Sahebkar A. Are curcuminoids effective C-reactive protein-lowering agents in clinical practice? Evidence from a meta-analysis. Phyther Res. 2014;28:633–42.
15. Shehzad A, Rehman G, Lee YS. Curcumin in inflammatory diseases. BioFactors. 2013;39:69–77.
16. Srivastava RM, Singh S, Dubey SK, Misra K, Khar A. Immunomodulatory and therapeutic activity of curcumin. Int Immunopharmacol. 2011;11:331–41.
17. Ji LL, Zhang Y. Antioxidant and anti-inflammatory effects of exercise: role of redox signaling. Free Radic Res. 2013;48:1–9.
18. Nielsen S, Pedersen BK. Skeletal muscle as an immunogenic organ. Curr Opin Pharmacol. 2008;8:346–51.
19. Wasinski F, Gregnani MF, Ornellas FH, Bacurau AVN, Câmara NO, Araujo RC, et al. Lymphocyte glucose and glutamine metabolism as targets of the anti-inflammatory and immunomodulatory effects of exercise. Mediators Inflamm. 2014;2014:1–10.
20. Ringeis R, Eder K, Mooren FC, Kruger K. Metabolic signals and innate immune activation in obesity and exercise. Exerc Immunol Rev. 2015;21:58–68.
21. Driver JP, Serreze DV, Chen Y-G. Mouse models for the study of autoimmune type 1 diabetes: a NOD to similarities and differences to human disease. Semin Immunopathol. 2011;33:67–87.
22. Pearson JA, Wong FS, Wen L. The importance of the non obese diabetic (NOD) mouse model in autoimmune diabetes. J Autoimmun. 2016;66:76–88.
23. Ventura-Oliveira D, Vilella CA, Zanin ME, Castro GM, Moreira Filho DC, Zollner RL. Kinetics of TNF-alpha and IFN-gamma mRNA expression in islets and spleen of NOD mice. Brazilian J Med Biol Res. 2002;35:1347–55.
24. Wang JL, Qian X, Chinookoswong N, John L, Chow G, Theill LE, et al. Polyethylene glycolated recombinant TNF receptor I improves insulitis and reduces incidence of spontaneous and cyclophosphamide-accelerated diabetes in nonobese diabetic mice. Endocrinology. 2002;143:3490–7.
25. Kägi D, Ho A, Odermatt B, Zakarian A, Ohashi PS, Mak TW. TNF receptor 1-dependent beta cell toxicity as an effector pathway in autoimmune diabetes. J Immunol. 1999;162:4598–605.
26. Pakala SV, Chivetta M, Kelly CB, Katz JD. In autoimmune diabetes the transition from benign to pernicious insulitis requires an islet cell response to tumor necrosis factor alpha. J Exp Med. 1999;189:1053–62.
27. Chee J, Angstetra E, Mariana L, Graham KL, Carrington EM, Bluethmann H, et al. TNF receptor 1 deficiency increases regulatory T cell function in nonobese diabetic mice. J Immunol. 2011;187:1702–12.

28. Fu Z, Yuskavage J, Liu D. Dietary flavonol epicatechin prevents the onset of type 1 diabetes in nonobese diabetic mice. J Agric Food Chem. 2013;61:4303–9.
29. Fu Z, Zhen W, Yuskavage J, Liu D. Epigallocatechin gallate delays the onset of type 1 diabetes in spontaneous non-obese diabetic mice. Br J Nutr. 2011; 105:1218–25.
30. Reeves PG, Nielsen FH, Fahey GC. AIN-93 purified diets for laboratory rodents: final report of the american institute of nutrition ad hoc writing committee on the reformulation of the AIN-76A rodent diet. J Nutr. 1993; 123:1939–51.
31. National Research Council (US) Committee for the Update of the Guide for the Care and Use of Laboratory Animals. Guide for the Care and Use of Laboratory Animals. 8th edition. Washington (DC): National Academies Press (US); 2011. Available from: https://www.ncbi.nlm.nih.gov/books/NBK54050/. doi:10.17226/12910.
32. Reddy S, Chai RCC, Rodrigues JA, Hsu TH, Robinson E. Presence of residual beta cells and co-existing islet autoimmunity in the NOD mouse during longstanding diabetes: a combined histochemical and immunohistochemical study. J Mol Histol. 2008;39:25–36.
33. Matthews DR, Hosker JP, Rudenski AS, Naylor BA, Treacher DF, Turner RC. Homeostasis model assessment: insulin resistance and β-cell function from fasting plasma glucose and insulin concentrations in man. Diabetologia. 1985;28:412–9.
34. Zhang C, Todorov I, Lin C-L, Atkinson M, Kandeel F, Forman S, et al. Elimination of insulitis and augmentation of islet beta cell regeneration via induction of chimerism in overtly diabetic NOD mice. Proc Natl Acad Sci USA. 2007;104:2337–42.
35. Signore A, Annovazzi A, Giacalone P, Beales PE, Valorani MG, Vestri AR, et al. Reduced cumulative incidence of diabetes but not insulitis following administration of chimeric human IL-15-murine IgG2b in NOD mice. Diabetes Metab Res Rev. 2003;19:464–8.
36. Anand P, Kunnumakkara AB, Newman RA, Aggarwal BB, Anand P, Kunnumakkara AB, et al. Bioavailability of curcumin: problems and promises. Mol Pharm. 2007;4:807–18.
37. Begum AN, Jones MR, Lim GP, Morihara T, Kim P, Heath DD, et al. Curcumin structure-function, bioavailability, and efficacy in models of neuroinflammation and Alzheimer's disease. J Pharmacol Exp Ther. 2008; 326:196–208.
38. Prasad S, Gupta SC, Tyagi AK, Aggarwal BB. Curcumin, a component of golden spice: from bedside to bench and back. Biotechnol Adv. 2014;32:1053–64.
39. Zhang D-W, Fu M, Gao S-H, Liu J-L. Curcumin and diabetes: a systematic review. Evid Based Complement Alternat Med. 2013;2013:1–6.
40. Castro CN, Barcala Tabarrozzi AE, Winnewisser J, Gimeno ML, Antunica Noguerol M, Liberman AC, et al. Curcumin ameliorates autoimmune diabetes. Evidence in accelerated murine models of type 1 diabetes. Clin Exp Immunol. 2014;177:149–60.
41. Marietta EV, Gomez AM, Yeoman C, Tilahun AY, Clark CR, Luckey DH, et al. Low incidence of spontaneous type 1 diabetes in non-obese diabetic mice raised on gluten-free diets is associated with changes in the intestinal microbiome. PLoS One. 2013;8:1–9.
42. Hoorfar J, Buschard K, Dagnaes-Hansen F. Prophylactic nutritional modification of the incidence of diabetes in autoimmune non-obese diabetic (NOD) mice. Br J Nutr. 1993;69:597–607.
43. Odegaard JI, Chawla A. Pleiotropic actions of insulin resistance and inflammation in metabolic homeostasis. Science. 2013;339:172–7.
44. Pane JA, Fleming FE, Graham KL, Thomas HE, Kay TWH, Coulson BS. Rotavirus acceleration of type 1 diabetes in non-obese diabetic mice depends on type I interferon signalling. Sci Rep. 2016;6:1–12.
45. Morgado JM, Rama L, Silva I, Inácio De Jesus M, Henriques A, Laranjeira P, et al. Cytokine production by monocytes, neutrophils, and dendritic cells is hampered by long-term intensive training in elite swimmers. Eur J Appl Physiol. 2012;112:471–82.
46. Nickel T, Emslander I, Sisic Z, David R, Schmaderer C, Marx N, et al. Modulation of dendritic cells and toll-like receptors by marathon running. Eur J Appl Physiol. 2012;112:1699–708.
47. Deckx N, Wens I, Nuyts AH, Hens N, De Winter BY, Koppen G, et al. 12 weeks of combined endurance and resistance training reduces innate markers of inflammation in a randomized controlled clinical trial in patients with multiple sclerosis. Mediators Inflamm. 2016;2016:1–13. Hindawi Publishing Corporation.
48. MacKenzie B, Andrade-Sousa AS, Oliveira-Junior MC, Assumpção-Neto E, Alves-Rangel MB, Silva Renno A, et al. Dendritic cells are involved in the effects of exercise in a model of asthma. Med Sci Sport Exerc. 2016;48:1459–67.
49. Pedersen BK, Toft AD. Effects of exercise on lymphocytes and cytokines. Br J Sports Med. 2000;34:246–51.
50. Pedersen BK, Brandt C. The role of exercise-induced myokines in muscle homeostasis and the defense against chronic diseases. J Biomed Biotechnol. 2010;2010:1–6.
51. Paula FMM, Leite NC, Vanzela EC, Kurauti MA, Freitas-Dias R, Carneiro EM, et al. Exercise increases pancreatic β-cell viability in a model of type 1 diabetes through IL-6 signaling. FASEB J. 2015;29:1805–16.

3

Neck Muscle EMG-Force Relationship and Its Reliability During Isometric Contractions

Riccardo Lo Martire[1,2,3*], Kristofer Gladh[1,2], Anton Westman[1,2,4] and Björn O. Äng[1,5]

Abstract

Background: Susceptible to injury, the neck is subject to scientific investigations, frequently aiming to elucidate possible injury mechanisms via surface electromyography (EMG) by indirectly estimating cervical loads. Accurate estimation requires that the EMG-force relationship is known and that its measurement error is quantified. Hence, this study examined the relationship between EMG and isometric force amplitude of the anterior neck (AN), the upper posterior neck (UPN), and the lower posterior neck (LPN) and then assessed the relationships' test-retest reliability across force-percentiles within and between days.

Methods: EMG and force data were sampled from 18 participants conducting randomly ordered muscle contractions at 5–90% of maximal voluntary force during three trials over 2 days. EMG-force relationships were modeled with general linear mixed-effects regression. Overall fitted lines' between-trial discrepancies were evaluated. Finally, the reliability of participants' fitted regression lines was quantified by an intraclass correlation coefficient (ICC) and the standard error of measurement (SEM).

Results: A rectilinear model had the best fit for AN while positively oriented quadratic models had the best fit for UPN and LPN, with mean adjusted conditional coefficients of determination and root mean square errors of 0.97–0.98 and 4–5%, respectively. Overall EMG-force relationships displayed a maximum 6% between-trial discrepancy and over 20% of maximal force, and mean ICC was above 0.79 within day and 0.27–0.61 between days across areas. Corresponding SEM was below 12% both within and between days across areas, excluding UPN between days, for which SEM was higher.

Conclusions: EMG-force relationships were elucidated for three neck areas, and provided models allow inferences to be drawn from EMG to force on a group level. Reliability of EMG-force relationship models was higher within than between days, but typically acceptable for all but the lowest contraction intensities, and enables adjustment for measurement imprecision in future studies.

Keywords: Biomechanics, Cervical spine, Electromyography, Moment, Muscle activity, Semispinalis capitis, Splenius capitis, Sternocleidomastoideus, Torque

Key Points

- Of the studied relationships, a linear relationship was best suited for the anterior neck while exponential relationships were best suited for the upper and lower posterior neck.
- Overall EMG-force relationships were similar between trials which suggests that they are stable over time.
- Provided models can be used to draw inferences from EMG to force on a group level.

Background

The human neck allows head movements and load-bearing while protecting vital neural structures and stabilizing the visual and vestibular systems [1]. Its flexibility [2], combined with the heavy head weight relative to the neck muscles' force capacity [3, 4], however, makes the area susceptible to pain and injury. Neck pain is the fourth leading cause of disability globally [5], with an average one-year prevalence of 37% in the general population [6].

* Correspondence: riccardo.lo.martire@ki.se
[1]Division of Physiotherapy, Department of Neurobiology, Care Sciences, and Society, Karolinska Institutet, Alfred Nobels allé 23 100, Huddinge 141 83, Sweden
[2]Department of Physiology and Pharmacology, Karolinska Institutet, Stockholm, Sweden
Full list of author information is available at the end of the article

During athletics, where rapidly changing conditions result in high demands on the spine, the neck is also prevalently injured, sometimes gravely [7–11]. Consequently, the area is subject to scientific investigations, not least within the sport sciences [12–14].

From a functional perspective, the neck can be viewed as a three-part stabilizing system in which support is provided by passive spinal structures, while stability is regulated according to demands via the neck muscles in a feedback-driven neural control scheme [1]. To coordinate swift variations in spinal posture and loads, a highly optimized system which stabilizes the spine in both static and dynamic situations is required [1]. Two neural control strategies have been identified for maintaining cervical spine stability in an upright neutral posture: reciprocal muscle activation, which is direction-specific to postural perturbations, and co-contraction of agonistic and antagonistic muscles [15]. In the sagittal plane, these strategies presumably function primarily via four main neck force-generating muscles, which include the sternocleidomastoids, the semispinalis capitis, and the splenius capitis [2]. These muscles are all near their maximum force-generating capacity in a neutral spine posture [2], wherein perturbations are commonly countered under quasi-isometric conditions [15], and are frequently targeted in studies of the neck [12–14]. It is therefore relevant to investigate them in a neutral spine posture during isometric contractions.

Surface electromyography (EMG) is a technique frequently used to examine forces and activation patterns during direct and indirect perturbations to the head [12–14]. EMG allows indirect estimation of internal loads via Newton's laws of motion when the EMG-force relationship is characterized, which is essential to injury mechanism elucidation, as direct measurements of internal loads are both infeasible and ethically undesirable. It is generally accepted that the EMG-force relationship is positive; however, reported relationship shapes vary and need to be established separately for individual muscles due to the many factors that influence EMG measurements [16, 17]. To our knowledge, five studies have, to various extents, examined the EMG-force relationship of the neck during isometric contractions in a neutral spine posture [18–22]. Reported results have incongruities, but suggest a rectilinear relationship for measurements over sternocleidomastoids and semispinalis capitis, and a curvilinear relationship over splenius capitis. However, because none of these studies provided models, information from the EMG-force relationship cannot be extrapolated. In addition, methodological limitations such as small sample sizes, insufficient statistical analyses, contraction intensities below 50% of maximal force, or ramp contractions, which incorporate incremental speed of contraction intensity as a confounding variable, impede the results' dependability. Hence, further investigation of the neck muscle EMG-force relationship is necessary to facilitate interpretation of studies based on EMG measurements and to provide a basis for accurate biomechanical models. To adjust for imprecision in force estimation, it is also essential to assess the EMG-force relationship's reliability. This study therefore examined the neck muscle EMG-force relationship and quantified this relationship's test-retest reliability.

Methods

Research Design and Subjects

In three trials distributed over two days within a two-week period, neck muscle EMG-force relationships were examined across seven submaximal contraction intensities during sustained isometric constant-force contractions for neck flexion and neck extension. Following approval by the Regional Committee for Medical Research Ethics, a convenience sample of eighteen participants was recruited through personal communication. Inclusion criteria were being healthy and aged 18–65 years; exclusion criteria were neck or shoulder pain within the last three months and known patch allergy. Nine males and nine females with a mean (SD; min-max) age of 29 (7; 20–48) years, height of 1.70 (0.08; 1.53–1.81) m, and weight of 66 (10; 45–84) kg enrolled for participation and signed a written informed consent. Eleven participants reported that they had trained for muscle strength or cardiovascular fitness more than three times per week over the past 12 months. All participants were requested to refrain from alcohol and physical training of the neck and shoulders for 72 h preceding measurements.

Protocol

EMG activity was monitored bilaterally in three areas (Fig. 1): the anterior neck (AN) – centered on the belly of the sternocleidomastoid muscle, approximately one third of the length above the sternal attachment [21], the upper posterior neck (UPN) – centered over the most superficial splenius capitis muscle area, between the sternocleidomastoid and upper trapezius muscles [19–21], and the lower posterior neck (LPN) – over the lower semispinalis capitis, 20 mm lateral to the median line in level with the C7 spinous process [20]. Reference electrodes were placed over sternum and spinous processes. In accordance with current recommendations [23], electrode placement areas were meticulously shaved, abraded, and disinfected with alcohol. Disposable, self-adhesive, pregelled Ag/AgCl electrodes with a conductive diameter of 10 mm (Blue Sensor N-00-S, Medicotest A/S, Ølstykke, Denmark) were attached pairwise with an inter-electrode distance of 20 mm, and secured with surgical tape. Skin potential offset was allowed to stabilize for 20 min preceding measurements, after which electrode-

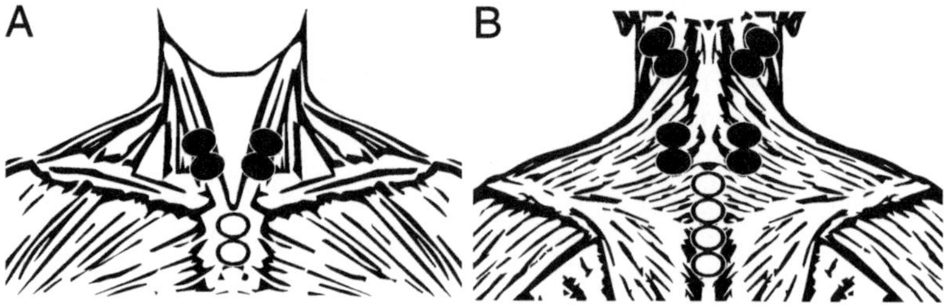

Fig. 1 Electrode placement for the anterior (**a**) and the posterior (**b**) neck. *Filled* and *unfilled circles* mark detection and reference electrodes, respectively

skin impedance was consistently below 5 kΩ. To obtain temporally synchronized data, differentially amplified EMG (bandwidth 8–500 Hz, input impedance = 10 GΩ, CMRR = 110 dB at 50 Hz, input noise <1.6 μV_{RMS}, gain = 305) and force signals (TB5 tension load cell, Lahti Precision Ltd, Lahti, Finland; maximal load = 500 kg, error <0.02%, sensitivity <0.1%) were digitized by a 14-bit A/D converter with a sampling frequency of 1000 Hz and stored in an integrated system (Biomonitor ME6000, Mega Electronics Ltd, Kuopio, Finland).

Subjects were seated in a standardized position on a fixed, height-adjustable stool, with a rigid square block stabilizing the torso in a neutral spine posture, and the extremities placed to prevent them from aiding during trials (Fig. 2a). A rigid strap connected to a fixed force transducer was placed over the supraorbital ridge and reference values were acquired through three maximal voluntary contractions for each contraction direction, during which subjects pushed their head against the strap. Subjects were carefully instructed as to the correct technique. To obtain accurate reference values, maximal contractions were rehearsed before trials, verbal encouragement and visual feedback of the force output was provided during trials, and the highest 1-s average of the highest contraction was selected. Reference values were used to calculate submaximal target contraction intensities equivalent to 5, 10, 20, 30, 50, 70, and 90% of maximal force.

Following a 30-min rest, participants met target contraction intensities aided by live visual feedback of produced force. When subjects did not reach target intensities, they were permitted an additional trial. Software malfunction resulted in two cases failing to meet this criterion: one being 18% instead of 20%, and one 26% instead of 30%; both included in the analyses below. Total time for the submaximal protocol was 40 min, followed by a one-hour break with electrodes retained, after which the submaximal contraction procedure was repeated. The same 40-min sampling procedure was repeated again 5–14 days after the first day, with identical preparatory steps. To avoid systematic bias due to muscular fatigue, contraction direction and intensities were conducted in random order, sustained for approximately five seconds, and separated by 2-min rest periods. Data sampling took place in a university motion laboratory, and was carried out by a trained physiotherapist with prior experience of the protocol.

Data Management and Statistics

Data management was conducted in MATLAB (v8.1, The MathWorks Inc., Natick, MA, USA). Unprocessed signals were visually inspected in time and frequency domains. EMG and force signals were then respectively band-passed at 20–400 Hz and low-passed at 25 Hz, with a fourth-order zero phase Butterworth filter. Next,

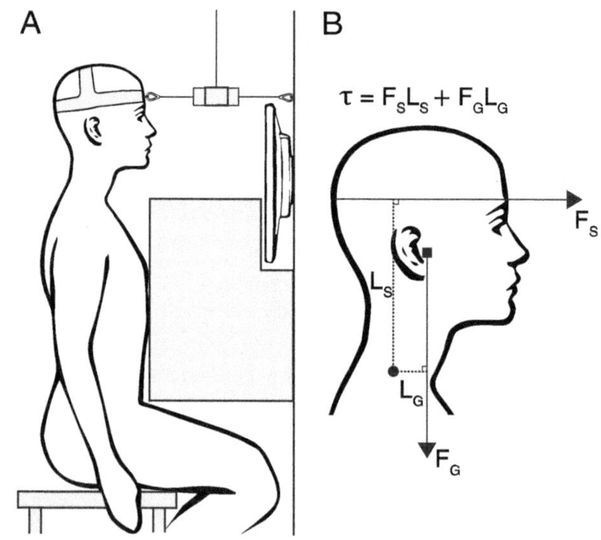

Fig. 2 Schematic diagrams of the data sampling setup and torque calculation. **a** shows body positioning during neck extensions with a square block stabilizing the spine in a neutral posture, arms hanging slack beside the torso, and legs placed to prevent them from aiding during trials. A wall-attached force transducer, supported by a sling from the roof, is fixed to a strap that is level with the supraorbital ridge. Visual feedback is provided by a monitor on the wall. During neck flexions, subjects are reversed 180°, facing an additional monitor (not shown in figure). **b** shows the neck extension torque (τ) formula along with a visual description of its variables: the resistance force of the strap (F_S), the force on the center of mass of the head and neck (*filled square*) due to gravitational acceleration (F_G), and their respective lever arms (l_S and l_G) originating from the axis of rotation between the C7–T1 spinous process (*filled circle*)

EMG signals were full-wave rectified, and both EMG and force signals were smoothed by a centered 1-s moving average with a 1-ms lag. The signal-to-noise ratio was calculated as the ratio of desired EMG signal power to the noise signal power obtained during rest to provide a measure of EMG signal quality. Automated functions were employed to extract submaximal values from the smoothed data by selecting the most stable second of force data within ±5% of the target intensity, followed by extraction of the coinciding EMG amplitude. All selected values were visually controlled to confirm their adequacy. Torques were calculated for neck flexion and extension from force data, and for gravity on the mass of the head and neck [20], using a constant of 7.9% of body weight [3]. Gravitational torque was then subtracted from neck flexion and added to neck extension. The torque calculation details are provided in Fig. 2b. Because target contraction intensities did not account for gravity, data below 20% of maximal target force in some cases ($n = 16$ for 5%, $n = 6$ for 10%, and $n = 1$ for 20% of target intensity) corresponded to neck flexion torques below zero. These values were discarded in the following analyses, since it was uncertain whether they were related to the examined exertion or to gravity alone. Submaximal force and EMG values were normalized as the percentage of maximal force (% MVC), and maximal voluntary excitation (% MVE), respectively. Finally, to decrease random bias related to measurement error [24], EMG data averaged between both muscle sides and trials were used for EMG-force relationship analyses, whereas EMG data averaged between muscle sides were used for the reliability analysis.

Statistical analyses were conducted in R (v3.1.3, R Core Team 2015, R Foundation for Statistical Computing, Vienna, Austria). EMG-force relationships were visually inspected and modeled with general linear mixed-effects regression via a top-down strategy [25]: following selection of fixed effects, random effects were iterated one by one, and last, fixed effects were reduced until the most parsimonious model was identified. Maximum likelihood estimation was used to fit models in which the number of fixed effects differed, while restricted maximum likelihood estimation was used to fit models in which random effects differed. Akaike's information criterion and Schwarz's Bayesian information criterion aided in the model selection [26], and the Pratt-adjusted coefficient of determination [27, 28] and the root mean square error [29] were used as measures of the models' fit to the data. Statistical assumptions were assessed visually [25]. The influence of antagonistic muscle activity was tested for all sampling areas.

Test-retest reliability of individual subjects' modeled EMG-force relationships were examined within and between days across sampling areas. The final EMG-force relationship models were refitted for each of the three trials, and the participant-specific regression lines were extracted from the refitted models and compared between trials per percentile across the contraction intensity range. Changes in the mean were presented graphically. An intraclass correlation coefficient (ICC) based on a single measurement two-way random effects model of absolute agreement was utilized to examine test-retest correlation [30, 31], and the standard error of measurement (SEM; i.e., the within-subject standard deviation between trials) [31] was used to investigate within-subject variation. Alpha was set at 0.05 for all analyses.

Results

Non-Normalized Force and EMG Data

Noticeable intersex differences were observed for maximal force with average female/male force ratios of 0.5 for neck flexion and 0.6 for neck extension. In absolute numbers, mean (SD) measured torques of 16 (5) Nm vs. 34 (13) Nm for flexion and 34 (4) Nm vs. 60 (14) Nm for extension were registered for females and males, respectively.

Signal-to-noise ratio calculations revealed that LPN had a markedly lower signal amplitude than other sampling areas. The mean (SD; min-max) reference contractions' signal-to-noise ratios were 48 (6; 38–61) dB for AN, 44 (5; 32–54) dB for UPN, and 31 (3; 22–36) dB for LPN.

EMG-Force Relationship

Visual inspection of individual subjects' EMG-force curves suggested multiple patterns within the same sampling area, with observations noticeably more homogenous for UPN and LPN than for AN. Two-thirds of all cases appeared rectilinear for AN. In contrast, for UPN and LPN, approximately one third of the curves had a distinct positively oriented quadratic shape, one third suggested a piecewise linear pattern with a breakpoint at roughly 25% MVC, and one third could fit both profiles.

Figure 3 displays the fitted models juxtaposed on the sampled data, while Table 1 provides details for the final models. First-order models had the best fit for AN, whereas second-order models had the best fit for UPN and LPN. Goodness-of-fit indices were consistent, in that incorporating the intercept and slope as random effects (i.e., allowing by-subject variation of the intercept and slope) substantially improved models across all sampling areas (Table 1); no other random effects improved final models. Point estimates of the adjusted conditional coefficient of determination and root mean square error both demonstrated excellent model fit for all sampling areas, with 97–98% of the variance accounted for by the

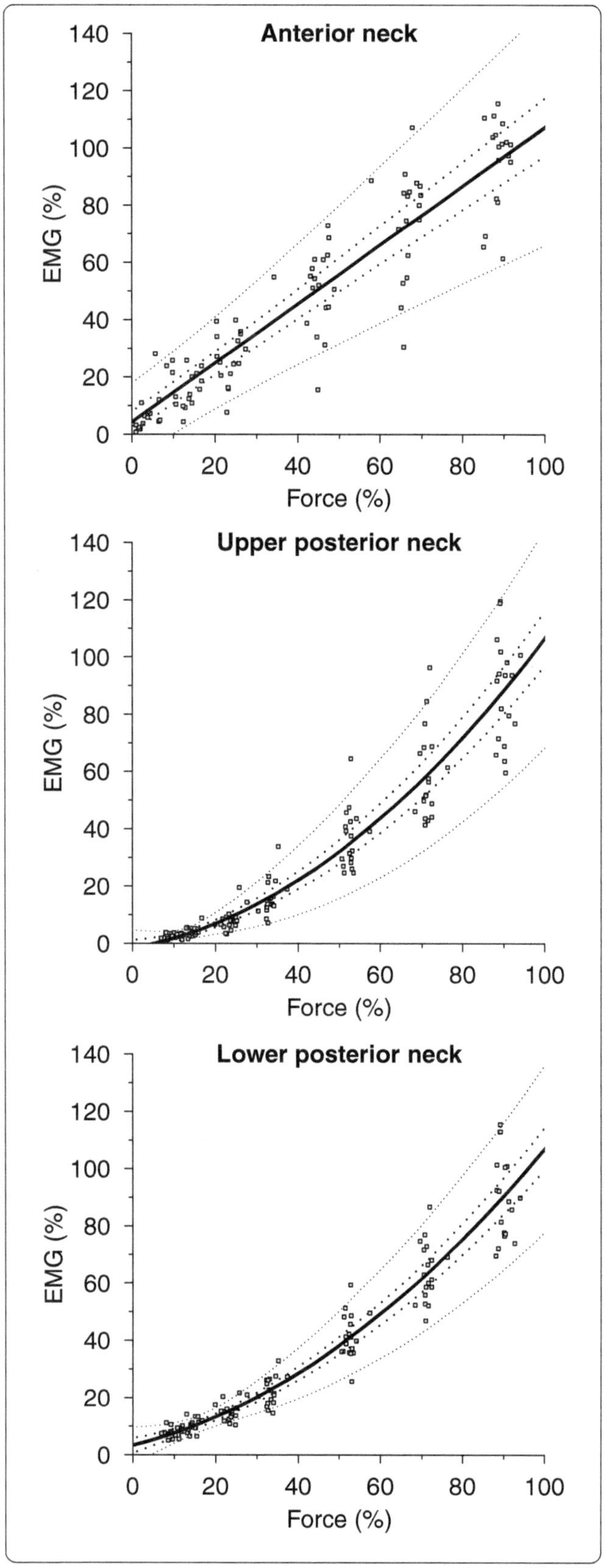

Fig. 3 Final EMG-force relationship models. *Solid lines* denote the fitted regression line on the sampled data points (*gray squares*). Inner and outer dotted lines mark the 95% confidence interval of the fitted lines computed via the delta method, and the 95% prediction interval generated via parametric bootstrap with 10,000 replicates, respectively

models, and absolute errors of 4–5% MVE. Mean antagonistic EMG activity during neck flexion was 20–42% and 17–133% for UPN and LPN, respectively, relative to AN EMG activity, whereas that of AN during neck extension was 4–30% and 5–10% relative to UPN and LPN activity, respectively. With the exception of the UPN activity during neck flexion, which had a U-shaped pattern, relative antagonistic activity decreased with contraction intensity. Antagonistic muscle activity did not remain in any of the final models, as no significant effect was observed with its inclusion.

EMG-Force Relationship Reliability

To provide a measure of the between-trial changes in the mean, Fig. 4 shows the fitted line for each of the three trials. In absolute numbers, mean force differences were below 6% for all sampling areas, with UPN having the largest between-trial discrepancies (within-day: AN ≤ 1%, UPN ≤ 3%, LPN ≤ 4%; between-day: AN ≤ 3%, UPN ≤ 6%, LPN ≤ 6%). Figure 5 shows test-retest reliability estimates of individual participants' fitted EMG-force relationship regression lines within and between days through 0–100% of MVC. Both ICC and SEM estimates tended to be unstable from 0–20% MVC. From 20–100% MVC, mean ICC for within-day was 0.79 or higher (AN ≥ 0.89, UPN ≥ 0.83, LPN ≥ 0.79), whereas it for between-day was 0.27–0.61 (AN ≥ 0.61, UPN ≥ 0.27, LPN ≥ 0.38), with the lower 95% confidence boundary frequently below zero. Over the same force range, the mean SEM was below 12% of the corresponding EMG magnitude for all sampling areas (within-day: AN ≤ 6%, UPN ≤ 9%, LPN ≤ 6%; between days: AN ≤ 12%, LPN ≤ 10%), with the exception of the UPN between days, for which this applied above 42% MVC.

Discussion

This study examined neck muscles' EMG-force relationships and assessed the modeled relationships' test-retest reliability. The main findings were that relationships were rectilinear for the anterior neck (AN) and the upper shoulders (US), and curvilinear for the upper (UPN) and lower posterior neck (LPN). Group-level relationships were similar between trials, and relationship reliability for individual participants was acceptable over most contraction intensities, albeit less reliable between than within days.

Consistent with previous findings [18, 21], AN displayed a near one-to-one rectilinear relationship between EMG

Table 1 Final EMG-force relationship models

	Anterior neck		Upper posterior neck		Lower posterior neck	
	Est	95% CI	Est	95% CI	Est	95% CI
FE						
b_0	4.2×10^0	0.6×10^0, 7.8×10^0	-1.7×10^0	-4.3×10^0, 1.1×10^0	3.3×10^0	0.9×10^0, 5.7×10^0
b_1	1.0×10^0	0.9×10^0, 1.1×10^0	2.7×10^{-1}	0.1×10^{-1}, 4.2×10^{-1}	3.6×10^{-1}	2.3×10^{-1}, 4.9×10^{-1}
b_1^2	–	–	8.2×10^{-3}	6.9×10^{-3}, 9.5×10^{-3}	6.8×10^{-3}	5.7×10^{-3}, 7.8×10^{-3}
RE						
σ_{b0}	7.4×10^0	4.6×10^0, 10.4×10^0	2.8×10^0	$0.8e^0$, $4.5e^0$	3.3×10^0	1.6×10^0, 5.1×10^0
σ_{b1}	2.0×10^{-1}	1.3×10^{-1}, 2.8×10^{-1}	2.3×10^{-1}	1.4×10^{-1}, 3.1×10^{-1}	1.8×10^{-1}	1.2×10^{-1}, 2.4×10^{-1}
σ_ε	4.3×10^0	3.6×10^0, 5.1×10^0	4.6×10^0	4.1×10^0, 5.4×10^0	3.7×10^0	3.2×10^0, 4.3×10^0
R^2M_{adj}	0.84	0.80, 0.85	0.89	0.87, 0.90	0.92	0.91, 0.93
R^2C_{adj}	0.98	0.97, 0.98	0.97	0.95, 0.97	0.98	0.97, 0.98

b_0, intercept. b_1, first-order term (slope). b_1^2, second-order term (curvature). σ_{b0}, standard deviation of the intercept. σ_{b1}, standard deviation of the slope. σ_ε, standard deviation of the within-subject residual. R^2M_{adj}, adjusted marginal coefficient of determination. R^2C_{adj}, adjusted conditional coefficient of determination
Est point estimate, *95% CI* 95% confidence interval, *FE* fixed effects, *RE* random effects

and force, and the model provided a good data fit which accounted for 98% of the total variance. This model can therefore aid interpretation of EMG studies when inferences are to be linked to force on a group level and have an accuracy within a 4% mean error margin. In contrast, both UPN and LPN displayed curvilinear relationships and force values were considerably higher than EMG values over most contraction intensities. Assuming a one-to-one relationship for these muscles would therefore lead to underestimated force values if inferences were to be drawn from EMG data. The final models for UPN and LPN had an excellent fit to the data, with 97–98% of the total variance accounted for, and an accuracy level within an average 4–5% error margin. Our UPN results are in agreement with the findings of three prior investigations [19, 20, 22], whereas a fourth study reported a rectilinear relationship [21]. The standardized weights used to derive the latter study's results, however, corresponded to a limited range of low intensities in our study, for which, in isolation, the relationship could also be interpreted as rectilinear. In sum, our results for UPN are supported by findings in the literature and therefore likely reflect the actual EMG-force relationship for the electrode placement area. For LPN, one previous study reported a curvilinear relationship [20], whereas three prior studies reported rectilinear relationships [18, 19, 21], contrariwise to our results. This incongruity is probably a result of the limited contraction range investigated in two of these studies [19, 21]. Indeed, upon visual inspection of the LPN EMG-force relationship curves in the 0–50% range (Fig. 3), it is apparent that a linear curve could be fitted to the data and likely provide an accurate predictive measure, but the measures could not be extrapolated beyond that range, whereas our curve provides predictive values over nearly the whole force range. In the third study [18], the few subjects (five) combined with the limited number of investigated contraction intensities (three) is unlikely to have provided the proper resolution to elucidate the curvilinearity of the relationship. In the study in agreement with our results, contractions were measured over 3–75% range for 10 females. The larger contraction range examined likely provides the explanation for the agreement. In sum, our results agree with those presented in the literature, with the difference that our measurements over nearly the full contraction range combined with our sample size of 18 allowed us to elucidate the EMG-force relationship over a larger interval and to a more specific degree. Visual inspection of LPN data suggested that piecewise linear models may have a better fit for some individuals. However, a greatly increased complexity rendered the implementation of such models impractical.

Overall EMG-force relationships displayed a maximum 6% between-trial discrepancy, with the rectilinear model being more similar between trials than curvilinear models across most of the contraction range (Fig. 4). No clear systematic biases accounting for these discrepancies were observed, and we therefore assume that they are the result of random variation which needs to be considered when inferences are to be drawn from EMG to force on group-level test-retest investigations of similar sample sizes. No analogous data exists for EMG-force relationship reliability on an individual level, and guidelines for relevant point estimate evaluation have therefore not yet been established. However, universal guidelines have previously defined ICC estimates of 0.00–0.39, 0.40–0.59, 0.60–0.74, and 0.75–1.00 as poor, fair, good, and excellent, respectively [32], and SEM estimates for acceptable reliability range from 7.5–20% of the measured variable, with 15% being the most common

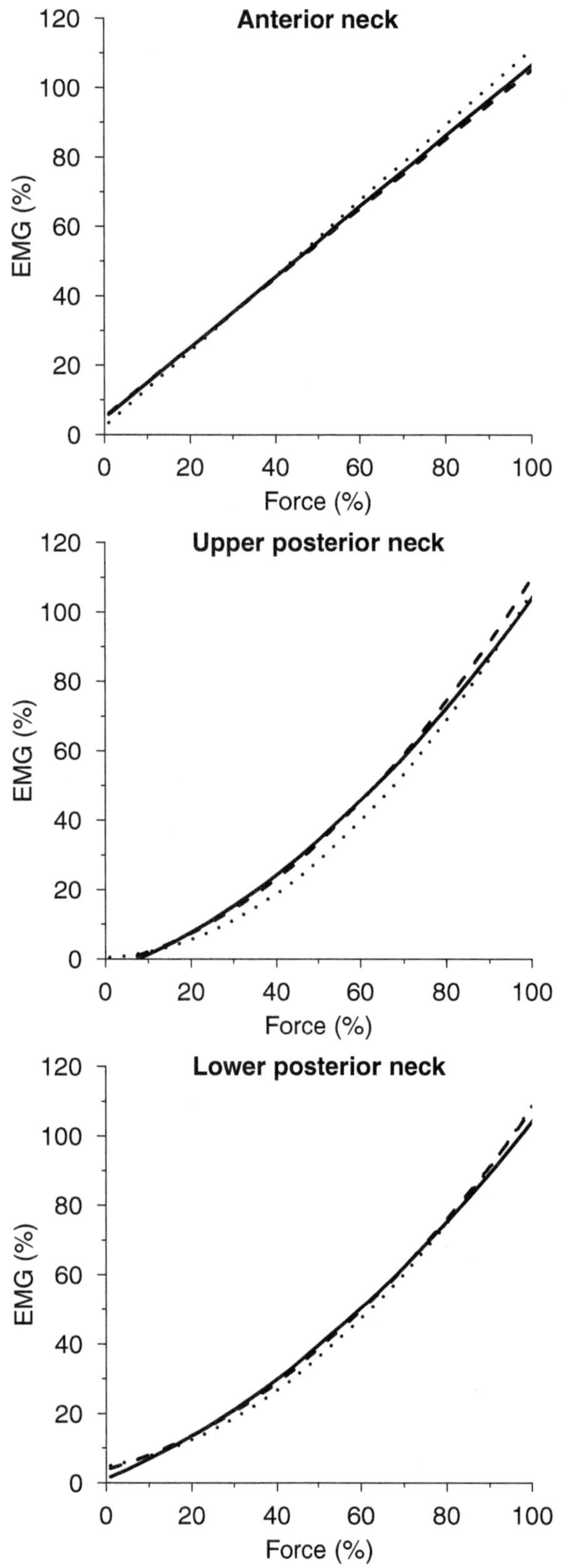

Fig. 4 By-trial fitted regression lines. *Solid, dashed,* and *dotted lines* denote by-trial fitted regression lines for the first day's morning session, the first day's afternoon session, and the second day's morning session, respectively

cutoff [33]. Interpreting ICC and SEM point estimates in light of these guidelines, within-day and between-day reliability for individual AN EMG-force relationships was excellent over 9 and 12% MVC, respectively. For UPN and LPN, within-day reliability was excellent over 20% MVC, whereas between-day reliability was fair over 58 and 33% MVC, respectively. Hence, reliability was unacceptably low at low contraction intensities, and consistently higher within rather than between days, which supports that individual EMG-force relationships are stable over most contraction intensities within the same day, but can vary considerably for between-day measurements. Universal standards should be interpreted with caution, as they may have considerable limitations when generalized. ICC estimates are context-specific, as magnitude of ICC is inversely related to sample homogeneity [30, 31]. In this study, the mean between-subject coefficient of variation following 20% MVC ranged from 17–27% across sampling areas and was 10–18% lower from first- to second-day trials. The lower second-day sample variance therefore provides a partial explanation for the large reduction in ICC estimates between days that was not consistently reflected in the SEM estimates. In contrast to ICC, which suggested that relationship agreement was unacceptably low between trials over certain force intensities, SEM showed that absolute differences remained within an acceptable level. A less conservative interpretation based on absolute between-trial differences alone therefore suggests acceptable reliability for UPN between days over 58% MVC and for LPN past 10% MVC both within and between days. AN and LPN can therefore likely be reliably measured both within and between days for all but the lowest contraction intensities, whereas UPN is limited to within-day measurements over 20% MVC and between-day measurements over 28% MVC.

This study has some limitations. The measurements obtained should be construed as location-specific rather than muscle-specific due to the various factors influencing EMG measurements [17]. One major factor was EMG activity contributions due to co-contraction of adjacent muscles [17], which was of particular concern for the UPN measurements, owing to its proximity to the antagonist AN. In contrast, force measurements were limited in that only the net force effect was obtained, while antagonistic activity added to internal loads; however, including antagonistic activity as a covariate in regression models did not improve them, thus indicating their influence to be inconsistent. The complexity of the neck muscle anatomy [34] rendered

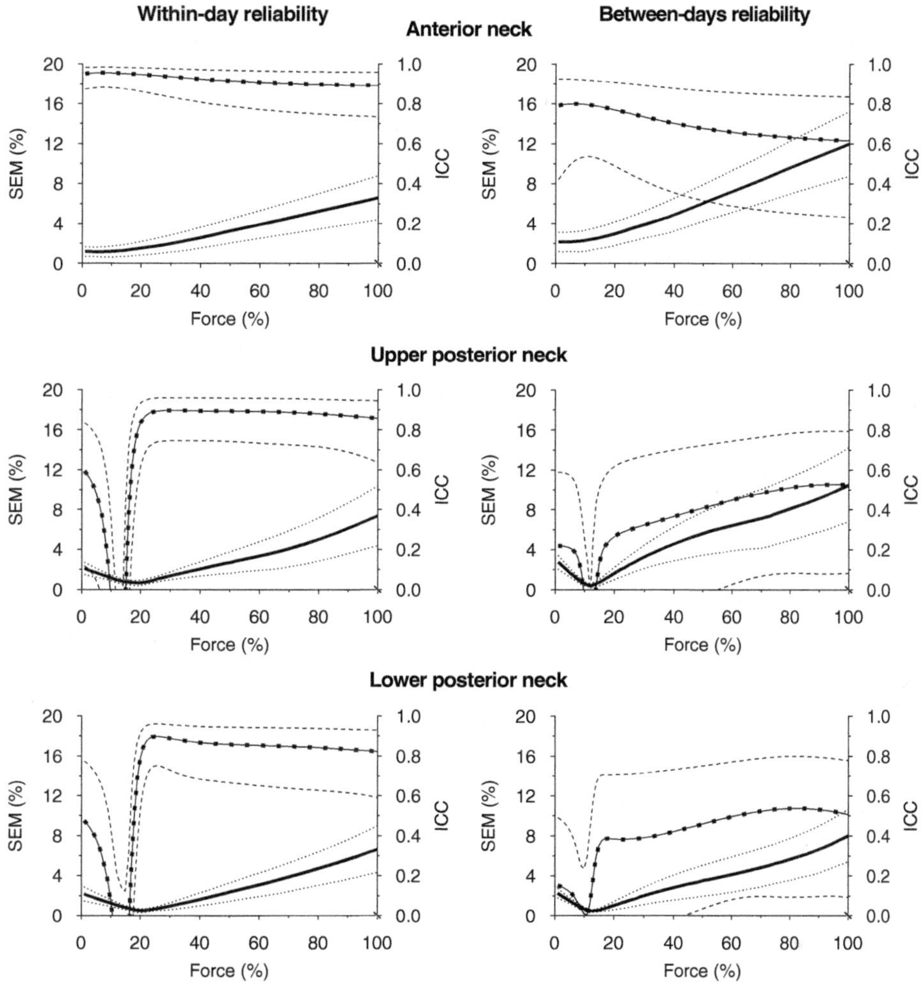

Fig. 5 Test-retest reliability of the EMG-force relationship over the full force range. *Solid lines* denote point estimates of the standard error of measurement (SEM), and *dotted lines* its 95% confidence interval (CI). *Lines with squares marks* point estimates of the intraclass correlation coefficient (ICC), and *dashed lines* its 95% CI

precise electrode placement challenging, and likely decreased signal quality in some measurements. LPN signal amplitude was lower relative to other sampling areas and is attributable to the tendinous structures below the electrodes. The high signal stability and good regression model fit, however, support that valuable information can be extracted from this location, and it is questionable whether upwards relocation of electrodes would improve signal quality, as prior research has also reported low signal amplitudes on posterior muscles at the C4-level [35].

The EMG-force relationship models provided permit inferences to be drawn from isometric neck muscle EMG measurements to force on a group level, and enable cervical loads to be estimated during activities in EMG-driven biomechanical models. In total, three force estimation models were derived: one for neck flexion and two for neck extension. Of the two latter models, the higher accuracy of the LPN model makes it the better choice for estimating neck extension forces. In addition, the between-trial differences in mean EMG-force relationships suggest that the models are stable over time. They do not, however, allow prediction of individual values, with maximum prediction errors ranging between approximately 30–60% force across sampling areas. Further, individual-level relationships showed insufficient reliability over the lower parts of the contraction range, which prevents meaningful analyses from being made for individuals over those intensities. Figure 3 allows force to be estimated visually, while the regression coefficients provided in Table 1 enable precise force calculation. In contrast to many laboratory studies, factors such as temperature, sound level, time of measurement, surrounding crowd, and exact electrode placement were allowed to deviate between trials to render results more representative of field measurements. Combined with the recruitment criteria, the sample's demography, and neck strength being similar to normative values [4], our results may be generalized to relatively fit and healthy adults between 20–50 years.

Conclusions

Of the studied models, a rectilinear model was best suited for the anterior neck while curvilinear models were best suited for the upper and lower posterior neck. All models had small between-trial variation in the mean and we therefore conclude they can be reliably used to estimate force from EMG on a group level. Models did not have sufficient accuracy for force prediction from single EMG values. However, EMG-force relationships for individual participants typically had acceptable reliability over most of the contraction range both within and between days, suggesting that individual-level relationships remain stable over time. Provided models enable inferences to be drawn from EMG to force on a group level, and reliability estimates facilitate adjustment for measurement imprecision.

Abbreviations

AN: Anterior neck; EMG: Electromyography; LPN: Lower posterior neck; UPN: Upper posterior neck

Acknowledgements

We thank Lea Constan for excellent feedback on the manuscript, Dr. Peter Lindholm for equipment contribution, Dr. Karl Garme for fruitful mathematical discussions, and the participants for contributing their time.

Funding

This study received funding from Gösta Fraenckel's Foundation for Medical Research (2013fobi38138).

Authors' Contributions

RLM was involved in the design, data collection, analysis, and article writing. KG participated in the design, data collection, and article reviewing. AW contributed to the design and article reviewing. BA was involved in the conception, design, and article reviewing. All authors read and approved the final manuscript.

Competing Interests

Riccardo Lo Martire, Kristofer Gladh, Anton Westman, and Björn O. Äng declare that they have no conflict of interest.

Author details

[1]Division of Physiotherapy, Department of Neurobiology, Care Sciences, and Society, Karolinska Institutet, Alfred Nobels allé 23 100, Huddinge 141 83, Sweden. [2]Department of Physiology and Pharmacology, Karolinska Institutet, Stockholm, Sweden. [3]Department of Aeronautical and Vehicle Engineering, KTH Royal Institute of Technology, Stockholm, Sweden. [4]Department of Anesthesia and Intensive Care, Karolinska University Hospital, Huddinge, Sweden. [5]School of Education, Health and Social Studies, Dalarna University, Falun, Sweden.

References

1. Panjabi MM. The stabilizing system of the spine. Part I. Function, dysfunction, adaptation, and enhancement. J Spinal Disord. 1992;5(4):383–9.
2. Vasavada AN, Li S, Delp SL. Influence of muscle morphometry and moment arms on the moment-generating capacity of human neck muscles. Spine (Phila Pa 1976). 1998;23(4):412–22.
3. Dempster WT, Gaughran GR. Properties of body segments based on size and weight. Am J Anat. 1967;120(1):33–54.
4. Jordan A, Mehlsen J, Bulow PM, Ostergaard K, Danneskiold-Samsoe B. Maximal isometric strength of the cervical musculature in 100 healthy volunteers. Spine (Phila Pa 1976). 1999;24(13):1343–8.
5. Vos T, Flaxman AD, Naghavi M, Lozano R, Michaud C, Ezzati M, et al. Years lived with disability (YLDs) for 1160 sequelae of 289 diseases and injuries 1990-2010: a systematic analysis for the Global Burden of Disease Study 2010. Lancet. 2012;380(9859):2163–96.
6. Fejer R, Kyvik KO, Hartvigsen J. The prevalence of neck pain in the world population: a systematic critical review of the literature. Eur Spine J. 2006; 15(6):834–48.
7. Sharma VK, Rango J, Connaughton AJ, Lombardo DJ, Sabesan VJ. The current state of head and neck injuries in extreme sports. Orthop J Sports Med. 2015;3(1):2325967114564358.
8. Freitag A, Kirkwood G, Scharer S, Ofori-Asenso R, Pollock AM. Systematic review of rugby injuries in children and adolescents under 21 years. Br J Sports Med. 2015;49(8):511–9.
9. Sikic M, Mikocka-Walus AA, Gabbe BJ, McDermott FT, Cameron PA. Bicycling injuries and mortality in Victoria, 2001-2006. Med J Aust. 2009;190(7):353–6.
10. Lystad RP, Pollard H, Graham PL. Epidemiology of injuries in competition taekwondo: a meta-analysis of observational studies. J Sci Med Sport. 2009; 12(6):614–21.
11. McIntosh AS, McCrory P. Preventing head and neck injury. Br J Sports Med. 2005;39(6):314–8.
12. Lo Martire R, Gladh K, Westman A, Lindholm P, Nilsson J, Ang BO. Neck muscle activity in skydivers during parachute opening shock. Scand J Med Sci Sports. 2016;26(3):307–16.
13. Bauer JA, Thomas TS, Cauraugh JH, Kaminski TW, Hass CJ. Impact forces and neck muscle activity in heading by collegiate female soccer players. J Sports Sci. 2001;19(3):171–9.
14. Eckner JT, Oh YK, Joshi MS, Richardson JK, Ashton-Miller JA. Effect of neck muscle strength and anticipatory cervical muscle activation on the kinematic response of the head to impulsive loads. Am J Sports Med. 2014; 42(3):566–76.
15. Danna-Dos-Santos A, Degani AM, Latash ML. Anticipatory control of head posture. Clin Neurophysiol. 2007;118(8):1802–14.
16. De Luca CJ. The use of surface electromyography in biomechanics. J Appl Biomech. 1997;13:135–63.
17. Farina D, Merletti R, Enoka RM. The extraction of neural strategies from the surface EMG. J Appl Physiol. 2004;96(4):1486–95.
18. Netto KJ, Burnett AF, Green JP, Rodrigues JP. Validation of an EMG-driven, graphically based isometric musculoskeletal model of the cervical spine. J Biomech Eng. 2008;130(3):031014.
19. Queisser F, Bluthner R, Brauer D, Seidel H. The relationship between the electromyogram-amplitude and isometric extension torques of neck muscles at different positions of the cervical spine. Eur J Appl Physiol Occup Physiol. 1994;68(1):92–101.
20. Schuldt K, Harms-Ringdahl K. E.m.g./moment relationships in neck muscles during isometric cervical spine extension. Clin Biomech. 1988;3(2):58–65.
21. Keshner EA, Campbell D, Katz RT, Peterson BW. Neck muscle activation patterns in humans during isometric head stabilization. Exp Brain Res. 1989;75(2):335–44.
22. Mayoux-Benhamou MA, Revel M. Influence of head position on dorsal neck muscle efficiency. Electromyogr Clin Neurophysiol. 1993;33(3):161–6.
23. Hermens HJ, Freriks B, Disselhorst-Klug C, Rau G. Development of recommendations for SEMG sensors and sensor placement procedures. J Electromyogr Kinesiol. 2000;10(5):361–74.
24. White E, Armstrong BK, Saracci R. Reducing measurement error and its effects. Principles of exposure measurement in epidemiology: collecting, evaluating, and improving measures of disease risk factors. 2nd ed. New York, USA: Oxford University Press; 2008. p. 1–30.
25. Bates D, Machler M, Bolker BM, Walker SC. Fitting linear mixed-effects models using lme4. J Stat Softw. 2015;67(1):1–51.

26. Grueber CE, Nakagawa S, Laws RJ, Jamieson IG. Multimodel inference in ecology and evolution: challenges and solutions. J Evol Biol. 2011;24(4):699–711.
27. Nakagawa S, Schielzeth H. A general and simple method for obtaining R2 from generalized linear mixed-effects models. Methods Ecol Evol. 2013;4(2):133–42.
28. Yin P, Fan X. Estimating R^2 shrinkage in multiple regression: a comparison of different analytical methods. J Exp Educ. 2001;69(2):203–24.
29. Chai T, Draxler RR. Root mean square error (RMSE) or mean absolute error (MAE)?—Arguments against avoiding RMSE in the literature. Geosci Model Dev. 2014;7:1247–50.
30. Weir JP. Quantifying test-retest reliability using the intraclass correlation coefficient and the SEM. J Strength Cond Res. 2005;19(1):231–40.
31. Hopkins WG. Measures of reliability in sports medicine and science. Sports Med. 2000;30(1):1–15.
32. Cicchetti DV. Guidelines, criteria, and rules of thumb for evaluating normed and standardized assessment instruments in psychology. Psychol Assessment. 1994;6(4):284–90.
33. Shechtman O. The coefficient of variation as an index of measurement reliability. In: Doi SAR, Williams GM, editors. Methods of clinical epidemiology. Berlin, Germany: Springer; 2013. p. 39–52.
34. Kamibayashi LK, Richmond FJ. Morphometry of human neck muscles. Spine (Phila Pa 1976). 1998;23(12):1314–23.
35. Moroney SP, Schultz AB, Miller JA. Analysis and measurement of neck loads. J Orthop Res. 1988;6(5):713–20.

4

Polygenic study of endurance-associated genetic markers *ACE I/D*, *ACTN3 Arg(R)577Ter(X)*, *CKMM A/G NcoI* and *eNOS Glu(G)298Asp(T)* in male Gorkha soldiers

Seema Malhotra[1], Kiran Preet[1], Arvind Tomar[2], Shweta Rawat[1], Sayar Singh[1], Inderjeet Singh[1], L. Robert Varte[1], Tirthankar Chatterjee[1], M. S. Pal[1] and Soma Sarkar[1*]

Abstract

Background: Gorkhas, a sub-mountainous population of the Himalayan region, are known for strength and bravery. In the present study when "Gorkha" is used without brackets, we are mentioning Gorkhas of Tibeto-Burman origin. Physical capability, strength and endurance are important components of fitness associated with genetic traits. The aim of this study was to examine the endurance potential of male Gorkha soldiers, based on endurance-related genetic markers *ACE I/D*, *ACTN3 Arg (R)577Ter(X)*, *CKMM A/G NcoI* and *eNOS Glu(G)298Asp(T)*.

Methods: Genotypic and allelic frequencies were determined in 374 male Gorkha soldiers (Tibeto-Burman). These frequencies were compared with frequencies obtained from Gorkha (Indo-Aryan), high-altitude natives (Tibeto-Burman) and Indian lowlanders (Indo-Aryan). "Total genotype score" (TGS) was calculated from accumulated combination of polymorphisms with maximum value "100" for theoretically "optimal" polygenic score. Probability of occurrence of "optimal" endurance profile was also determined.

Results: *ACE II* genotypic frequency was highest in Tamangs followed by Gurungs, Rais, Limbus and Magars. No statistical difference in genotypic and allelic frequency of *ACTN3 Arg(R)577Ter(X)* was noted within the groups. Rais showed the highest *CKMM A* allele frequency (0.908) compared to other Gorkha (Tibeto-Burman) groups. Limbus and Tamangs showed the highest *eNOS G* allele frequency (0.938 and 0.915, respectively) compared to that of other groups. Probability of male Gorkha soldiers possessing a theoretically optimal polygenic endurance profile for four candidate polymorphisms was ~3.35% (1 in 30). Four percent of the population of male Gorkha soldiers (15 in 374) exhibited an optimal TGS 100, and 16% exhibited TGS 87 for endurance compared to male Indian soldiers belonging to the lowland (Indo-Aryan) and Gorkha (Indo-Aryan) populations suggesting an overall more "favourable" polygenic profile in the male Gorkha soldier (Tibeto-Burman) population.

Conclusions: This study presents evidence of higher frequency of endurance-associated genes in the Gorkhas implying thereby that such genetically endowed individuals from the population may be selected and trained for achieving excellence in endurance-related elite sports activities.

Keywords: Polygenic, Endurance, Gorkha, Indian, *ACE*, *ACTN3*, *CKMM*, *eNOS*

* Correspondence: soma_sarkar2000@yahoo.com
[1]Defence Institute of Physiology and Allied Sciences (DIPAS), Ministry of Defence. Government of India, Lucknow Road, Delhi 110054, India
Full list of author information is available at the end of the article

Key points

- This study was conducted on male Gorkha soldiers of the Tibeto-Burman linguistic phyla wherein genetic studies are limited. The study reports for the first time the genotypic and allelic frequencies of four endurance-associated genetic markers in the male Gorkha soldiers.
- The study shows that nearly 4% of the male Gorkha soldiers exhibit an "optimal" total genotypic score (100) for endurance based on four polymorphisms, indicating the genetic potential of this population for achieving excellence in endurance-related elite sports activities.

Background

Gorkhas (also spelled as *Gurkhas*[1]) are a sub-mountainous population of the Himalayan region (Nepal) and make excellent soldiers. During the Anglo-Nepalese war of 1814–1816, the British were greatly impressed by the bravery of the Nepalese soldiers and started recruiting Nepalese to the Gurkha regiments of the British Indian Army [1]. The soldiers in the British army were mainly recruited from the "true Gorkha martial tribes" of *Gurung, Magar, Rai, Limbu, Thakur, Chhetri* and *Sunawar* [2]; the Indian Army continues to recruit from the same brigade of Gorkhas. *Gurungs, Magars, Rais, Limbus, Tamangs* and *Sherpas* are associated with Tibeto-Burmese cultural traditions and physical features conventionally labelled as Mongoloid while *Thakur* (*Brahmin*) and *Chhetri* castes are associated with Aryan cultural traditions and have physical features conventionally labelled as Caucasoid [3]. Gurkha Service opened an opportunity for the soldiers to settle in different parts of the British Empire including India, and their descendants are present in Assam, Sikkim, Darjeeling and Dehradun [3].

The Gorkha soldiers are best known for their physical strength, fighting tenacity, bravery and fearlessness in battle [1, 4]. Physical capability, strength and power are important components of fitness. Himalayan Sherpas are well known for their physical strength and endurance in the high-altitude terrain. Himalayan Sherpa elite climbers demonstrated high functional reserve with maximal oxygen uptake (VO_{2max}) of 66.7 ± 3.7 ml min^{-1} kg^{-1}, maximal cardiac frequency of 199 ± 7 beats min^{-1} and ventilatory anaerobic threshold of 62 ± 4% of VO_{2max} [5]. Higher frequency of *I* allele of *ACE* (angiotensin-converting enzyme gene, location: 17q23.3) have been reported in Sherpas [6]. *ACE I* allele is associated with endurance-related events [7, 8] and exercise performance in atmospheric hypoxia [9]. Predominance of *ACE II* genotype and *I* allele was demonstrated in male Gorkha soldiers [10]. Many other polymorphisms are associated with endurance-related performance [11]. *Arg(R)577Ter(X)* polymorphism of *ACTN3* (alpha actinin 3 gene, location: 11q 13.1) (functional *R* allele and non-functional *X* allele) is associated with generation of rapid forceful contractions [12] and muscle performance [13] with frequency of *XX*-null genotype (loss of alpha actinin 3) being higher in endurance athletes [14, 15]. In an earlier study, *XX* genotype of *ACTN3 Arg(R)577Ter(X)* polymorphism was observed to be present in 23% of Gorkhas [10]. The *A/G NcoI* polymorphism of *CKMM* (muscle-specific creatine kinase gene, location: 19q13.32) is associated with energy-buffering in the skeletal muscle fibres along with tolerance to skeletal muscle damage [16]. *A* allele and *AA* genotype were significantly higher in endurance athletes and were associated with high values of VO_{2max} [17]. Physical fitness test scores in military recruits were also associated with *A* allele [18]. *eNOS Glu(G)298Arg(T)* (endothelial nitric oxide gene, location: 7q36) polymorphism is linked with endurance performance and endurance elite status [19, 20]. *eNOS* encodes the rate-limiting enzyme for nitric oxide (NO) products [21]. Higher frequency of wild *G* allele of *eNOS Glu298Arg (G894T)* polymorphism was reported in high-altitude natives from Ladakh suggesting advantageous consequences in high-altitude environment [22, 23].

High functional reserve, physical strength and endurance in the hostile high altitudes coupled with higher frequency distribution of some of the endurance-related performance enhancing genetic markers in the mountain population indicates possibility of the mountain population being genetically endowed for endurance- related activities. This natural endowment would set the stage for investigation of prospects of the mountain people for distinctive performance in endurance-related elite sports activities. In the present study, we chose to investigate in male Gorkha soldiers, (i) the genotypic and allelic frequency distribution of four genetic variants associated with endurance performance: *ACE I/D (rs4646994), ACTN3 Arg(R)577Ter(X) (rs1815739 C/T), CKMM A/G NcoI (rs8111989 T/C)* and *eNOS Glu298Asp (rs1799983 G/T)*; (ii) determine the probability for the occurrence of an "optimal" polygenic endurance profile using the four polymorphisms in the population and assess whether individuals were likely to exist who harboured "preferable" genotypes for endurance; and (iii) generate a "total genotype score" (TGS) [11] for finding a likely distribution of genetic endurance potential of the male Gorkha soldiers and compare with virtual data of other populations of male Indian soldiers.

Methods

Study population and samples

(a) Three hundred ninety-four healthy male Gorkha individuals serving in the Gorkha regiment of Indian

Army, mean age 29 ± 8 years, participated in the study. The clan ties were determined based on self-report, and ethnic backgrounds were ascertained through ethno-linguistic questionnaire. Classification of linguistic phyla and clusters was as per van Driem [24]. For ascertaining that the individuals were unmixed, both parents had to belong to the same group. Based on the ethno-linguistic questionnaire, the male Gorkha soldier participants belonged to five ethnic groups of Tibeto-Burman linguistic phyla: *Gurungs* (28 participants were from Nepal and 47 were from India), *Magars* (25 participants were from Nepal and 101 were from India), *Rais* (37 participants were from Nepal and 37 were from India), *Tamangs* (36 participants were from Nepal and 18 were from India) and *Limbus* (25 participants were from Nepal and 40 were from India) (Table 1).

(b) Repository DNA samples from (i) Gorkhas belonging to the Indo-Aryan linguistic phylum, (ii) Indian lowlanders belonging to the Indo-Aryan linguistic phylum and (iii) high-altitude natives of Ladakh (elevation ~3500 m) belonging to Tibeto-Burman linguistic phylum were used for generating genotypic and allelic frequencies for comparison with male Gorkha soldiers (Tibeto-Burman). The repository DNA samples were from healthy male soldiers of Indian Army.

Physiological measurements

Body weight, height, and body mass index (BMI), heart rate, systolic and diastolic blood pressures were measured prior to blood draw. Height was measured with an anthropometer (GPM, Switzerland). Body weight and body mass index was measured by Body Composition Analyser (Tanita, Korea). Resting heart rate, resting systolic (SBP) and diastolic (DBP) blood pressures were measured with digital blood pressure monitor (M2 Model, Omron Health Care Company Limited, Japan). Hypertension was defined as BP ≥140/90 mmHg. Out of 394 individuals who initially participated (Table 1), 20 individuals were found to be hypertensive and were excluded from all further studies. The rest of the participants ($n = 374$) were normotensive and not on any medications. Of the normotensive participants, 122 volunteers consented for maximal oxygen uptake (VO_{2max}). VO_{2max} was assessed on a bicycle ergometer (Ergoline Gmbh, Lindenstr, Germany) using published protocol [25]. Briefly, the initial workload was 50 W, the increment was 25 $W \cdot min^{-1}$, and the target cadence was 60–70 rpm. Subjects kept the pedal rotational speed between 60–65 rpm throughout the test. After warm up for 2 min at 50 W, increments of 25 W were made every minute till exhaustion. The test was completed within 10–12 min including the warm up with maximum load of 200–225 W at 60 rpm. During the test, oxygen consumption (VO_2), carbon dioxide production (VCO_2) and heart rate (HR) were continuously recorded using a portable breath by breath gas analysis system ($K4b^2$, Cosmed Srl, Italy). Criteria for reaching VO_{2max} were assessed as reaching a plateau despite the increase in work rate or a respiratory exchange ratio value >1.1 or heart rate (HR) reaching >90% of age-predicted maximum HR. All subjects showed at least one of the above-mentioned criteria.

Table 1 Details of participants based on ethno-linguistic grouping ($n = 394$)

Group	Region of origin	Linguistic phylum and linguistic cluster[a]	*n*, males
Gurung	Nepal	TB, Tamangic	28
Gurung	India		47
Magar	Nepal	TB, Magaric	25
Magar	India		101
Rai	Nepal	TB, Kirantic	37
Rai	India		37
Tamang	Nepal	TB, Tamangic	36
Tamang	India		18
Limbu	Nepal	TB, Kirantic	25
Limbu	India		40

Note: Of the 394 participants, 20 individuals were hypertensive and excluded from subsequent studies. The participants were two *Gurungs* (one from Nepal and one from India), three *Magars* (two from Nepal and one from India), nine *Rais* (six from Nepal and three from India), one *Tamang* (from Nepal) and five *Limbus* (three from Nepal and one from India)
TB Tibeto-Burman
[a]Classification according to van Driem [24]

Genotyping

Venous blood samples (2–3 ml) were obtained at rest in EDTA anticoagulant vacutainers (Beckton Dickinson, CA, USA) and stored at −20 °C till further processing. Genomic DNA samples had $A_{260}/_{280}$ ratio of 1.8–1.9 and were adjusted to 20 ng/μl. ~100 to 150 ng of genomic DNA was used for polymerase chain reaction (PCR) amplification in a total volume of 25 μl. Gene variants studied for endurance status are shown in Table 2. Primer sequences and detection of polymorphism in *ACTN3 Arg(R)577Ter(X) (rs1815739), ACE Ins/Del (rs4646994)* and *eNOS Glu298Asp (rs1799983)* were performed as per published protocol [10, 23], and detection of polymorphism in *CKMM A/G (rs1803285)* was performed as per Rivera and co-workers [16]. PCR reaction was run on Gene Amp PCR system 9700 (Applied Biosystem). Samples found to have *ACE DD*and *ID* genotypes were reconfirmed by a second, independent PCR amplification having an insertion-specific sequence [26]. Genotypic profiling for *ACTN3 R577X, CKMM A/G NcoI* and *eNOS Glu298Asp* was performed on repository

Table 2 Gene variants studied for endurance status

Gene	Location	Polymorphism	Endurance-related marker	Minor allele frequency (MAF) (1000 Genomes)	Ancestral allele
ACE	17q23.3	*Alu I/D (rs1799752)*	*I*	NA	NA
ACTN3	11q13.1	*Arg(R)577Ter (X) (rs1815739 C/T)*	*577Ter (X)*	*T* = 0.4008	C
CKMM	19q13.32	*A/G NcoI (rs8111989 T/C)*	*A*	*C* = 0.3403	T
eNOS	7q36	*Glu 298Asp (rs1799983 G/T)*	*Glu298(G)*	*T* = 0.1763	G

DNA samples of Gorkhas (Indo-Aryan), Indian lowlanders (Indo-Aryan) and high-altitude natives of Ladakh (Tibeto-Burman). The experiments were conducted in accordance with the quality control measures at the Department of Molecular Biology, Defence Institute of Physiology and Allied Sciences, Delhi, which is an accredited laboratory (ISO 9001:2008).

Statistical analysis

Allele frequencies and genotype frequencies were calculated by allele counting and analysed by Pearson chi-square (χ^2) and Fisher's exact test, respectively. Deviations from the Hardy-Weinberg equilibrium (HWE) were tested for the polymorphisms by comparing observed and expected genotype frequencies with an exact goodness of fit test. For comparison of genotype frequencies within Gorkha sub groups, statistical significance was accepted at $p < 0.0025$ after adjustment with Bonferroni's correction (alpha = 0.05/20). For inter population comparisons, statistical significance was accepted at $p < 0.05$.

Comparison of maximal oxygen uptake (VO_{2max}) between the groups and association of VO_{2max} with genotypes and TGS was performed by one-way analysis of variance (ANOVA) using the software SPSS (Statistical Package for Social Sciences, version 17.0 for Windows; SPSS Inc., Chicago, IL, USA).

Probability of "optimal" polygenic profile for endurance in the Gorkha soldiers (Tibeto-Burman)

Probability of any given individual possessing the "optimal" genotype from one up to all four polymorphisms, ranked on official gene symbols placed in an alphabetical order, was calculated by using the typical frequency distribution of the genotypes. Based on the typical frequencies of the "optimal" genotypes in male Gorkha soldiers (Tibeto-Burman) and Indian lowlander soldiers (Indo-Aryan), a scale was generated indicating the probability of possessing the "optimal" genetic profile which was then applied to the population. The genetic potential for endurance phenotype of the population was computed by using the algorithm proposed by Williams and Folland [11], and a total genotype score (TGS) was produced. TGS is a bioinformatic approach using predictive algorithm "genotype score" for finding the probability of individuals carrying the preferable genotype for each polymorphism linked to a phenotype [27]. TGS modelling approach uses a simple algorithm resulting from the best accumulated combination of candidate gene polymorphisms. We chose this approach to provide a quantitative way of combining genotype data to predict a complex phenotype. Each genotype within each polymorphism was scored and a combined influence of polymorphisms was computed. A genotype score (GS) of 2 was assigned to the "optimal" homozygous genotype for endurance. A genotypic score of 0 was assigned to "less favourable" homozygous genotype for endurance while the heterozygous genotype received a score of 1. The genotype scores of each single genotype ($GS_{ACE} + GS_{ACTN3} + GS_{CKMM} + GS_{eNOS}$) were added up and a TGS was produced as follows:

$$TGS = (100/2n) \times (GS_{ACE} + GS_{ACTN3} + GS_{CKMM} + GS_{eNOS})$$

where n is the number of polymorphisms studied. As suggested by Williams and Folland [11], a TGS of 100 represents the "perfect" polygenic profile of endurance (all GS are 2) and a TGS of 0 represents the "not perfect" profile of endurance. Frequency distribution of the "optimal" endurance genotype in the Gorkha soldiers (Tibeto-Burman) obtained in the present study was compared with the frequency distribution of the optimal endurance genotype in other populations viz., Gorkhas (Indo-Aryan), high-altitude natives (HAN) from Ladakh (Tibeto-Burman), Indian lowlanders (Indo-Aryan), Indian Gujaratis from Houston (Indo-Aryan), HAN Chinese Beijing (Sino-Tibetan), Japanese from Tokyo and Caucasian (European ancestry) taken from published literature and databases.

To examine the distribution of TGS in the Gorkhas (Tibeto-Burman), we created a dataset of 100,000 virtual Gorkha (Tibeto-Burman) individuals from genotypic frequencies of the four polymorphisms obtained in the present study with randomly generated genotypes computed by online software GEMINI [28]. Similarly, a hypothetical data of 100,000 virtual individuals in each population of Gorkhas (Indo-Aryan), Indian lowlanders

(Indo-Aryan) and high-altitude natives (Tibeto-Burman) was computed with randomly generated genotypes based on the population-specific genotype frequencies. Distribution of TGS within these virtual populations was examined, and mean and kurtosis statistics were calculated using SPSS, v 17.0 for Windows. The TGS of simulated Gorkha (Tibeto-Burman) population was then compared to the average genotype score of the three hypothetical population datasets.

Results

Physiological characteristics

Of the 394 individuals, 151 were from Nepal and 243 were from India. The participants belonged to *Gurung, Magar, Rai, Tamang* and *Limbu* groups of Tibeto-Burman linguistic phyla (Table 1). Twenty individuals (3.26%) were found to be hypertensive [systolic blood pressure (SBP), 152.65 ± 10.08 mmHg; diastolic blood pressure (DBP), 98.25 ± 6.67 mmHg] and were excluded. Within the remaining population, systolic blood pressure and heart rate were observed to be statistically similar (Table 3). Body mass index and diastolic blood pressure (DBP) were significantly different within the population with Rais and Limbus showing the highest DBP (Table 3). Statistically significant difference in VO_{2max} was noted between the groups (Table 4). VO_{2max} was highest in Tamangs (55.80 ± 8.27) followed by Limbus (55.34 ± 6.26) (Table 4, Additional file 1: Table S1).

Genotypic and allelic frequency distribution of the studied polymorphisms

Overall genotypic frequency of the studied polymorphism in the male Gorkha soldiers is shown in Table 5. Distribution of homozygous *II* genotype was highest in Tamangs followed by Rais, Gurungs, Limbus and Magars; although, the difference was not statistically significant within the subgroups after Bonferroni correction ($p < 0.0025$). Genotypic frequency of *ACTN3 Arg(R)577Ter(X)* was statistically similar across the Gorkha subpopulation. Both *ACE Ins/Del* and *ACTN3 Arg(R)577Ter(X)* polymorphisms were in Hardy-Weinberg Equilibrium (HWE). Statistical difference was noted in allele frequency distribution of *ACTN3 Arg(R)577Ter(X)* between Gorkhas (Tibeto-Burman), Gorkhas (Indo-Aryan) and high-altitude natives ($p < 0.05$) (Table 6).

Higher frequency of *A* (major) allele of *CKMM A/G* and *G* (major) allele of *eNOS Glu298Arg*polymorphism was observed in the population (Table 5). Frequency of homozygous *AA* genotype of *CKMM A/G* was higher than homozygous mutant *GG* genotype in the population. Rais showed the highest *CKMM A* allele frequency compared to other Gorkha (Tibeto-Burman) groups. Frequency of homozygous *GG* genotype of *eNOS Glu298Arg* was also higher than homozygous mutant *TT* genotype. Limbus and Tamangs showed the highest *eNOS G* allele frequency compared to other groups. Homozygous mutant *TT* genotype of *eNOS Glu298Arg* was not observed in Tamang and Limbu groups (Table 5). Both the polymorphisms were in HWE. Of the 81 possible combinatorial genotypic profiles, 34 profiles were not observed. The predominant genotype combination was *ACE ID/ACTN3 RX/CKMM AA/eNOS GG* which was present in approximately 11.5% of the population (Additional file 2: Table S2). The optimal endurance-associated homozygous genotypic combination of *ACE II/ACTN3 XX/CKMM AA/eNOS GG* was present in nearly 4% of the male Gorkha soldier population (Additional file 2: Table S2). Although VO_{2max} values showed statistical difference within the subgroups, it did not show any statistically significant association with the genotypic profiles either individually or in combination (Additional file 3: Table S3 and Additional file 4: Table S4).

Probability of optimal polygenic profile for endurance performance in the Gorkha (Tibeto-Burman) population

Typical genotypic frequencies were used for calculating the probability of possessing optimal genetic profile for endurance in the male Gorkha soldiers (Tibeto-Burman) as compared to lowlander Indian population (Table 7). The typical genotypic frequencies of the four polymorphisms ranged

Table 3 Physiological characteristics of the male Gorkha soldiers (TB) ($n = 374$)

Characteristics	Overall ($n = 374$)	Gurung ($n = 73$)	Magar ($n = 123$)	Rai ($n = 60$)	Tamang ($n = 53$)	Limbu ($n = 65$)	*p*
Body weight (Kg)	64.51 ± 7.53	65.64 ± 6.8	63.43 ± 6.64	65.89 ± 7.95	63.19 ± 7.69	65.10 ± 9	0.057
Height (cm)	165.43 ± 5.01	165.65 ± 5.84	165.49 ± 4.91	164.24 ± 05.32	166.02 ± 4.29	165.73 ± 4.38	0.390
BMI (Kg/m^2)	23.49 ± 2.99	23.94 ± 3.59	23.00 ± 3.15	24.34 ± 2.28	22.9 ± 2.52	23.64 ± 2.69	*0.000*
SBP (mmHg)	121.10 ± 12.09	125.21 ± 11.75	121.91 ± 11.57	121.03 ± 13.02	117.80 ± 11.03	119.92 ± 12.27	*0.018*
DBP (mmHg)	73.79 ± 9.99	71.57 ± 11.5	71.16 ± 10.24	77.23 ± 10	72.30 ± 8.36	76.23 ± 8.02	*0.002*
HR (rate/min)	69.35 ± 12.37	69.75 ± 12.88	68.20 ± 11.5	71.10 ± 15.34	66.75 ± 11.11	70.85 ± 9.43	0.894

Values are mean ± SD, significant value <0.05. The significant *p* values are italicized
The values are from participants who were normotensive
BMI body mass index, *SBP* systolic blood pressure, *DBP* diastolic blood pressure, *HR* heart rate, *TB* Tibeto-Burman

Table 4 Comparison of VO_{2max} between Gorkha groups

	Group ID	Group	VO_{2max} (ml kg^{-1} min^{-1})	Group comparison	Level of significance (*p*)
Overall	–	–	50.82 ± 7.92		
	1	Gurung (31)	46.56 ± 8.18	1 vs 2	ns
	2	Magar (32)	47.97 ± 6.08	1 vs 3	*0.013*
	3	Rai (23)	52.86 ± 6.19	1 vs 4	*0.000*
	4	Tamang (18)	55.80 ± 8.27	1 vs 5	*0.000*
	5	Limbu (18)	55.34 ± 6.26	2 vs 3	ns
				2 vs 4	ns
				2 vs 5	*0.005*
				3 vs 4	ns
				3 vs 5	ns
				4 vs 5	ns

VO_{2max} values are mean ± SD. Level of significance calculated by one-way ANOVA with Tukey's post-hoc test. VO_{2max} values are from normotensive participants. Number in parenthesis indicates the number of participants in each group
p value <0.05 significant. The significant *p* values are italicized
ns not significant

from 25% for *II* genotype of *ACE* to 65% of *GG* genotype of *eNOS* in lowlanders and 43% for *II* genotype of *ACE* to 80% of *GG* genotype of *eNOS* in male Gorkha soldiers (Table 7). Probability of any given lowlander soldier possessing the "favourable" genotype for endurance at one locus (*II* genotype of *ACE*) was ~25% which was reduced to ~6.5% when the second polymorphism (*XX* genotype of *ACTN3*) was added. The probability of any lowlander possessing the optimal polygenic profile for endurance at all four loci further reduced to 1.88% with an approximate odds ratio of 1:78 (i.e., one in 78 individuals) (Table 7). In the male Gorkha soldiers (Tibeto-Burman), probability of possessing the favourable genotype for endurance for one polymorphism (*II* genotype of *ACE*) was ~43% which was reduced to ~6.5% when the second polymorphism (*XX* genotype of *ACTN3*) was added. The probability of any male Gorkha soldier possessing the optimal polygenic profile for endurance at all four loci was ~3.35% with an approximate odds ratio of 1:30 (i.e., one in 30 individuals) (Table 7). The typical endurance-associated optimal genotypic frequency in the male Gorkha soldiers (Tibeto-Burman) ranged from 15% for *XX* genotype of *ACTN3* to 80% of *GG* genotype of *eNOS* (Table 8). Frequency distribution of the optimal endurance genotype in the male Gorkha soldiers and other Asian and Caucasian populations is shown in Table 8.

The mean ± SD of total genotype score (TGS) was 69.05 ± 15.08 and kurtosis statistics 0.106 ± 0.252, and distribution was shifted towards the right in the male Gorkha soldiers (Fig. 1). About 4% of the male Gorkha soldiers (15 individuals out of 374) exhibited an optimal TGS (100) for endurance with another 16% of the population (60 individuals out of 374) showing a TGS of ~87 (Fig. 1, Additional file 5: Table S5). The lowest limit of genetic potential for endurance in male Gorkha soldiers was TGS ~25 with only 4 individuals having this score. On scrutiny, it was seen that two of these four individuals possessed *ACE DD*/*ACTN3 RR* genotypic combination, another possessed *ACE ID*/*ACTN3 RR* and the fourth one possessed *ACE DD*/*ACTN3RX* (Additional file 6: Table S6), genotypic combinations which are suggested to be favourably associated with muscle strength/power phenotypes [29]. Comparison of TGS (maximum 100 and minimum 25) with physiological characteristics (SBP, DBP and HR) and VO_{2max} did not show any statistical difference (Additional file 7: Table S7).

Frequency distribution of TGS calculated from the virtual samples is depicted in Fig. 2. In the simulated population of Gorkhas (Tibeto-Burman), mean ± SD TGS was 69.01 ± 15.40 and kurtosis statistics (–) 0.094 ± 0.015 (SE); 4% (4046 individuals out of 100,000) showed TGS 100 while 17.6% (17,591 individuals out of 100,000) had TGS 87 (Fig. 2) corroborating the observation obtained from the representative 374 participants of the present study (4% with TGS 100 and 16% with TGS of 87 (Fig. 1, Additional file 5: Table S5). In the simulated population of high-altitude natives, predicted mean ± SD TGS was 70.06 ± 15.66 and kurtosis statistics (–) 0.168 ± 0.015 (SE) with 5.2% (5174 individuals out of 100,000) having optimal TGS 100 and another 19.5% (19,487 individuals out of 100000) having TGS 87 (Fig. 2). In simulated Gorkha (Indo-Aryan) population, mean ± SD TGS was 67.44 ± 16.10 and kurtosis statistics (–) 0.176 ± 0.015 (SE); TGS 100 was observed in 3.8% (3761 out of 100,000 individuals), and TGS 87 was observed in 16.2% (16,199 individuals out of 100,000) (Fig. 2). In the simulated population of Indian lowlanders, the predicted mean ± SD TGS was 62.46 ± 16.66 and kurtosis statistics (–) 0.217 ± 0.015 (SE); TGS 100 was observed in 2.1% (2061 out of 100,000 individuals) and TGS 87 was in 10.5% (10530 individuals out of 100000) (Fig. 2). Number of Gorkha soldiers with

Table 5 Frequency distribution of the polymorphisms in the male Gorkha soldiers (Tibeto-Burman)

SNP	Variants		Overall Frequency	(1) Gurung	(2) Magar	(3) Rai	(4) Tamang	(5) Limbu	Comparison of groups Level of significance (p)	Genotypic[a] frequency	Allele[b] frequency
rs1799752	*ACE I/D*	Genotype									
		II	0.427	0.465	0.349	0.466	0.509	0.430	1 vs 2	0.14	0.04
		ID	0.467	0.438	0.471	0.466	0.452	0.507	1 vs 3	0.81	0.37
		DD	0.104	0.095	0.178	0.066	0.037	0.061	1 vs 4	0.45	0.38
		Allele							1 vs 5	0.62	0.99
		I	0.671	0.684	0.585	0.700	0.735	0.684	2 vs 3	0.08	0.03
		D	0.338	0.315	0.414	0.300	0.264	0.315	4 vs 2	0.02	0.007
									2 vs 5	0.07	0.05
		HWE p	0.381	0.893	0.751	0.389	0.230	0.156	3 vs 4	0.75	0.55
									3 vs 5	0.90	0.79
									4 vs 5	0.63	0.38
rs1815739 C/T	*ACTN3 Arg(R)577Ter(X)*	Genotype									
		RR	0.366	0.397	0.308	0.366	0.396	0.413	1 vs 2	0.33	0.13
		RX	0.478	0.465	0.487	0.466	0.471	0.492	1 vs 3	0.87	0.61
		XX	0.155	0.139	0.203	0.166	0.132	0.092	1 vs 4	0.99	0.97
		Allele							1 vs 5	0.71	0.58
		R	0.605	0.630	0.552	0.600	0.632	0.661	2 vs 3	0.69	0.39
		X	0.394	0.369	0.447	0.400	0.367	0.338	4 vs 2	0.38	0.16
									2 vs 5	0.10	0.04
		HWE p	0.970	0.99	0.882	0.829	0.917	0.423	3 vs 4	0.86	0.62
									3 vs 5	0.45	0.31
									4 vs 5	0.79	0.63
rs8111989 T/C	*CKMM A/G NcoI*	Genotype									
		AA	0.655	0.630	0.634	0.833	0.603	0.600	1 vs 2	0.89	0.86
		AG	0.296	0.287	0.300	0.150	0.377	0.369	1 vs 3	0.02	0.003
		GG	0.048	0.082	0.065	0.016	0.018	0.030	1 vs 4	0.22	0.72
		Allele							1 vs 5	0.31	0.83
		A	0.803	0.773	0.784	0.908	0.792	0.784	2 vs 3	0.02	0.003
		G	0.196	0.226	0.215	0.091	0.207	0.215	4 vs 2	0.32	0.86
									2 vs 5	0.44	0.99
		HWE p	0.244	0.280	0.221	0.442	0.283	0.456	3 vs 4	0.02	0.01
									3 vs 5	0.01	0.007
									4 vs 5	0.91	0.88
rs1799983 G/T	*eNOS Glu298Asp*	Genotype									
		GG	0.799	0.808	0.756	0.766	0.830	0.876	1 vs 2	0.59	0.30
		GT	0.184	0.178	0.211	0.216	0.169	0.123	1 vs 3	0.84	0.37
		TT	0.016	0.013	0.032	0.016	0.000	0.000	1 vs 4	0.68	0.63
		Allele							1 vs 5	0.41	0.21
		G	0.892	0.897	0.862	0.775	0.915	0.938	2 vs 3	0.82	0.98
		T	0.108	0.103	0.138	0.125	0.085	0.062	4 vs 2	0.31	0.16
									2 vs 5	0.09	0.02
		HWE p	0.387	0.770	0.211	0.941	0.499	0.597	3 vs 4	0.51	0.21
									3 vs 5	0.20	0.04
									4 vs 5	0.47	0.48

Significance is assumed when $p \leq 0.0025$ after Bonferroni's correction (alpha = 0.05/20, for four polymorphisms × five ethnic groups)
HWE Hardy -Weinberg Equilibrium
[a]Pearson values from chi-square test for genotypic frequency [http://www.physics.csbsju.edu/stats/contingency_NROW_NCOLUMN_form.html]
[b]p values from Fisher's exact test for allelic frequency [http://www.quantitativeskills.com/sisa/statistics/fisher.htm]

Table 6 Comparison of genotypic and allelic frequencies of studied polymorphisms in male soldiers belonging to Gorkha (TB), Gorkha (IA), HAN (TB) and Indian lowlander (IA)

			Gorkha (TB)	Gorkha (IA)	HAN (TB)	Indian lowlander (IA)	Gorkha (TB) vs Gorkha (IA)	Gorkha (TB) vs HAN (TB)	Gorkha (TB) vs Indian lowlander (IA) (TB)	Gorkha (IA) vs HAN lowlander (IA)	Gorkha (IA) vs Indian lowlander (IA)	HAN (TB) vs Indian
SNP	Variants		Frequency						Level of significance (*p*)*			
rs1799752	*ACE I/D*	Genotype										
		II	0.427	0.459[a]	0.408[a]	0.254[a]						
		ID	0.467	0.417[a]	0.551[a]	0.504[a]	0.525	0.291	*0.000*	0.130	*0.000*	*0.003*
		DD	0.104	0.122[a]	0.040[a]	0.240[a]						
		Allele										
		I	0.671	0.673[a]	0.683[a]	0.506[a]	0.676	0.664	*0.000*	0.849	*1.0E-6*	*0.001*
		D	0.338	0.326[a]	0.316[a]	0.493[a]						
rs1815739 C/T	*ACTN3 Arg(R)577Ter(X)*	Genotype										
		RR	0.366	0.287[a]	0.189	0.180[a]	0.094	*0.010*	*0.000*	0.116	0.160	0.197
		RX	0.478	0.490[a]	0.648	0.555[a]						
		XX	0.155	0.222[a]	0.162	0.263[a]						
		Allele										
		R	0.605	0.520[a]	0.513	0.458[a]	*0.03*	*0.037*	*1.0E-6*	0.89	0.149	0.240
		X	0.394	0.479[a]	0.486	0.541[a]						
rs8111989 T/C	*CKMM A/G NcoI*	Genotype										
		AA	0.655	0.475	0.594	0.455	*0.004*	0.608	*0.000*	0.289	0.245	0.065
		AG	0.296	0.445	0.351	0.388						
		GG	0.048	0.079	0.054	0.155						
		Allele										
		A	0.803	0.698	0.770	0.650	*0.001*	0.357	*1.0E-5*	0.133	0.317	*0.017*
		G	0.196	0.301	0.230	0.350						
rs1799983 G/T	*eNOS Glu298Asp*	Genotype										
		GG	0.799	0.653	0.682	0.648	*0.000*	0.223	*0.000*	0.674	0.094	0.861
		GT	0.184	0.287	0.292	0.333						
		TT	0.016	0.588	0.024	0.018						
		Allele										
		G	0.891	0.797	0.829	0.814	*4.9E-5*	0.09	*0.0002*	0.51	0.554	0.754
		T	0.108	0.202	0.170	0.185						

TB Tibeto-Burman, *IA* Indo-Aryan, *HAN* high-altitude native from Ladakh
*Significance for genotypic and allelic frequency is assumed when $p < 0.05$. The significant p values are italicized
[a]Data from [10]

Table 7 Probability of possessing "optimal" genetic profile by number of polymorphism in the male Gorkha (TB) and Indian lowlander (IA) soldiers

Polymorphisms influencing endurance performance	New gene included at each stage	Gorkha (Tibeto-Burman)			Indian lowlander		
		Typical frequency (%) of "optimal" genotype	Probability of possessing 'perfect' profile		Typical frequency (%) of "optimal" genotype	Probability of possessing "perfect" profile	
			% chance	Approximate odds ratio		% chance	Approximate odds ratio
1.	*ACE*	43	43.00	1:2	25[a]	25.00	1:4
2.	*ACTN3*	15	6.45	1:15	26[a]	6.50	1.15
3.	*CKMM*	65	4.19	1:23	45	2.99	1:35
4.	*eNOS*	80	3.35	1:30	65	1.88	1:78

Data obtained from a data set of 100,000 hypothetical male Gorkha (TB) and Indian lowlander (IA), each with a randomly generated genetic profile for all four polymorphisms based on the typical frequency of each genotype
TB Tibeto-Burman, *IA* Indo-Aryan
[a]Genotypic frequencies taken from [10]

Table 8 Frequency distribution of "optimal" endurance genotype in male Gorkha soldiers and other male Indian soldiers

Gene	Symbol	Polymorphism	Genotype (2 "optimal" endurance genotype)	Frequency (%)							
				Gorkha (TB)	Gorkha (IA)	HAN (TB)	Indian lowlander (IA)	Gujrati Houston (GIH, IA)	Han Chinese Beijing (CHB, ST)	JPT	Caucasian (CEU)
Angiotensin converting enzyme (Peptidyl dipeptidase A)	*ACE*	*287 bp I/D (rs1799752)*	0 = *DD*, 1 = *ID*, 2 = *II*	10, 47, 43	12, 42, 46[a]	04, 55, 41[a]	24, 51, 25[a]	–	12, 45, 43[d]	12,47,41[f]	30,51,19[g]
Alpha actinin 3	*ACTN3*	*Arg(R)577Ter(X) (rs1815739)*	0 = *RR*, 1 = *RX*, 2 = *XX*	37, 48, 15	25, 52, 23[a]	19, 65, 16	18, 56, 26[a]	14, 59, 27[c]	43, 39, 17[c]	21, 61, 17[c]	20, 58, 22 [c]
Creatine kinase, muscle	*CKMM*	*A/G NcoI (rs8111989)*	0 = *GG*, 1 = *AG*, 2 = *AA*	05, 30, 65	08, 45, 47	05, 35, 60	16, 39, 46	22, 39, 38[c]	04, 34, 61[c]	05, 27, 68[c]	05, 43, 51 [c]
Endothelial nitric oxide synthase	*eNOS*	*Glu 298Asp (rs1799983)*	0 = *TT*, 1 = *GT*, 2 = *GG*	02, 18, 80	06, 29, 65	02, 26, 72[b]	02, 33, 65	–	0, 22, 78[e]	14, 86, 0[c]	08, 51, 40 [c]

TB Tibeto-Burman, *IA* Indo-Aryan, *HAN* high-altitude natives from Ladakh, *ST* Sino-Tibetan, *CHB* Han Chinese, Beijing, *CEU* Utah residents with northern and western European ancestry, *GIH* Gujrati Indians in Houston, Texas, *JPT* Japanese in Tokyo, Japan

[a, b, d, f, g]Values from references [10, 23, 73–75]

[c]Data from HapMapPhase 3

[e]Data from the International HapMap Project

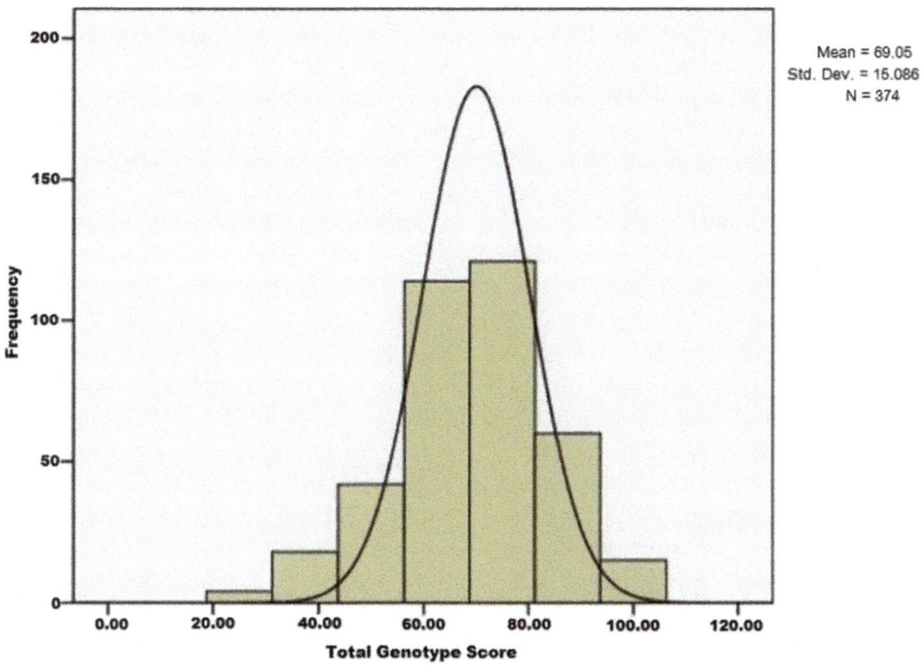

Fig. 1 Frequency distribution of total genotypes score (TGS) in male Gorkha soldiers ($n = 374$)

TGS 100 was significantly higher than the Indian lowlander soldiers with TGS 100 ($p < 0.0001$) (2×2 contingency table; www.graphpad.com/quickcalcs/contingency2/).

Discussion

The Gorkha population is largely an understudied population and genetic information on the population is scanty. This study reports for the first time the genotypic and allelic frequency distribution of endurance-related four polymorphic markers in the male Gorkha soldiers of Tibeto-Burman linguistic cluster and the polygenic endurance potential of the population. Ethnic heterogeneity with respect to *ACE I/D* polymorphism was noted with a trend of higher frequency of *ACE II* genotype and *I* allele in Tamangs. It may be mentioned here that the Gorkhas included in this study were main ethnics (tribes): Gurungs, Magars, Rais, Tamangs and Limbus. They look similar but are very different ethnics and could be having their own distinct genetic makeup. Thus, the frequency differences within the subgroups

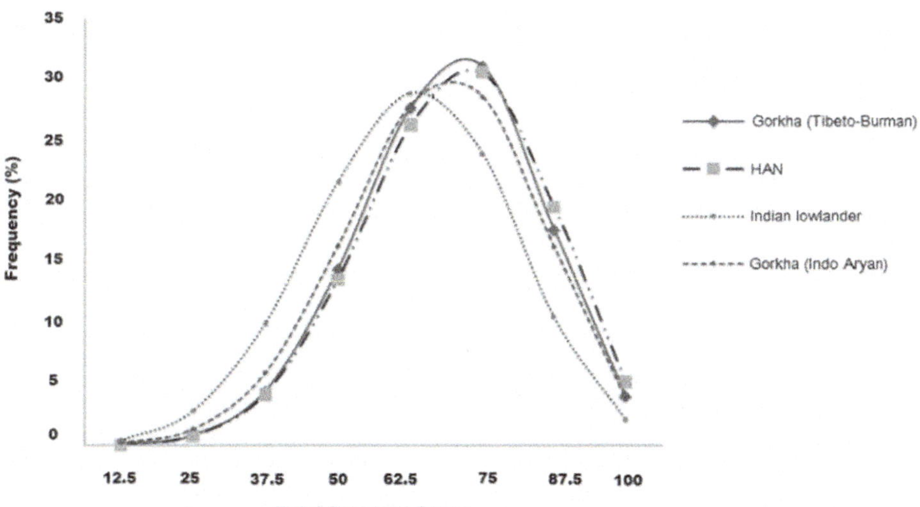

Fig. 2 Frequency distribution of total genotype scores (TGS) derived from dataset of 100,000 randomly generated individuals of Indian lowlanders (IA), high-altitude native (TB), Gorkhas (IA) and Gorkhas (TB)

(although not significant after Bonferroni correction, $p < 0.00250$), could be attributed to their evolutionary adaptation. The observed genotypic frequency of *ACE I/D* in Tamangs was in agreement with frequency distribution reported from inhabitants of Kotyang, majority of whom were Tamangs [30]. Tamangs are indigenous inhabitants of the western Himalayan regions and one of the major Tibeto-Burman speaking communities who trace their ancestry to Tibet and further back to Mongolia (*Tamang people. World Public Library-eBooks*). Higher *I* allele frequency in Tamangs, similar to that found in Sherpas, suggests enhanced physical activity in the group. Predominance of homozygous *II* genotype and *I* allele of *ACE* in Gorkhas in the present study is in agreement with that observed in Gorkhas reported earlier, [10] majority of whom belonged to Indo-Aryan ethnicity. Predominance of *ACE I* allele in the Gorkhas suggests endurance and muscle efficiency [31, 32], the key determinants of performance and also associated with enhanced performance at high altitudes [31]. *ACE I* allele influences human physical performance and trainability [33, 34] and is also related to cardiorespiratory efficiency [35, 36]; although, contrary reports also exist showing no relationship between *ACE I/D* polymorphism and cardiorespiratory fitness [37].

ACTN3 gene is associated with performance and genotype across multiple cohorts of elite power athletes and also supported by gene knockout mouse model [38]. *Ter* (*X*) allele affects endurance ability of elite athletes while *Arg* (*R*) allele affects sprinting [13, 39]. It would be interesting to further investigate the polygenic potential of *ACTN3 RR* genotype (associated with sprinting) along with power-related muscle performance genes in this population. ACTN3 *Ter* (*X*) allele and the *TerTer* (*XX*) genotypes are significantly associated with certain groups of elite endurance athletes [14, 40]. The frequency distribution of *Ter (X)* allele in the male Gorkha soldiers is observed to be 0.394 with genotype frequency being 0.155 *XX* and 0.366 *RR*. Interestingly, the *XX* genotype frequency in the male Gorkha soldiers was observed to be lower than Gorkha and Indian lowlander soldiers belonging to Indo-Aryan linguistic phylum as well as Caucasians (Table 8). Similar to the frequency observed in male Gorkha soldiers (Tibeto-Burman), the *XX* genotype frequency has been reported to be ~0.170 in other Asian populations viz., HAN Chinese (CHB, Sino-Tibetan linguistic phylum) [41] and Japanese (HapMap Phase 3) while in Caucasians, the *XX* frequency is 0.22 (HapMap Phase 3). At the moment, we do not have an explanation for less *XX* genotype frequency in the Gorkha (Tibeto-Burman) population compared to Caucasian population; this appears to be a population-specific difference between Caucasian and Asian (Tibeto-Burman/Sino-Tibetan) population. The derived 577X allele has been shown to increase in frequency with distance from Africa, reaching the highest frequencies on the American continent [42].

Creatine kinase is an important enzyme in energy metabolism which catalyzes phosphorylation of creatine to phosphocreatine, an energy storage molecule and source of ATP [43]. Muscle-specific creatine kinase gene (*CKMM*) correlates with athletic performance and *CKMM AA* genotype is considered as one of the genetic markers associated with predisposition to endurance-related sports activity [17]. The *CKMM A* allele probably influences gene expression and results in a decrease in muscle isoform of creatine kinase activity in myocytes leading to enhanced activation of oxidative phosphorylation and endurance development [17]. The frequency of the *CKMM A* allele varies from 85% in the Chinese population [44] to 68% in white Americans [16] with Caucasoids having 65–71% [45]. In the male Gorkha soldiers, frequency of *CKMM A* allele was 80.34% and *AA* genotype 65.50% which was comparable to that observed in high-altitude natives from India. Interestingly, frequency of *AA* genotype was significantly higher in Gorkhas of Tibeto-Burman ethnicity as compared to Gorkhas of Indo-Aryan ethnicity. Higher frequency distribution of *Glu(G)*allele of *eNOS* compared to that of *Asp(T)* allele in the Gorkhas, similar to the frequencies observed in high-altitude natives, suggests adaptive advantage of *Glu(G)* allele through increased production of nitric oxide (NO). Higher frequency of *Glu(G)* allele has been reported in Sherpas [46] and Quechuas of Andean *altpino* [47]. Higher exhaled NO has also been observed in Tibetan and Bolivian Aymara population [48, 49].

Maximum oxygen uptake capacity (VO_{2max}), the maximal amount of oxygen per unit of time that can be delivered to the peripheral organs including the skeletal muscle (where it is used to sustain muscular contraction at peak exercise), is a bench mark measure of physical performance/work capacity [50]. It provides an index of functional reserve of the organ systems involved and limitation that can be encountered at peak exercise [51, 52]. In the present study, the overall VO_{2max} in the population was found to be 51.34 ± 7.22 ml kg^{-1} min^{-1} with Tamangs showing the highest maximal oxygen uptake compared to other subgroups ($p < 0.05$) (Table 4). Higher VO_{2max} is reflected in better performance in running, hill climbing and endurance work [53, 54]. VO_{2max} in the male Gorkha soldiers was higher as compared to the values reported from Indian general population [55–57] suggesting overall better endurance potential of Gorkhas (Tibeto-Burman) at the physiological level. We did not, however, observe statistically significant association between VO_{2max}, and the studied polymorphisms in the Gorkhas either individually with four genetic variants or when combined genotype profile of each individual was analysed in the 122 volunteers who participated in the assessment of VO_{2max} (Additional file 3: Table S3 and Additional file 4: Table S4). It is probable that the small cohort of individuals for VO_{2max} may be limiting the interpretation of the result or it may also be probable that VO_{2max} is indeed not associated with the studied polymorphisms. Rankinen and co-workers [58] analysed elite endurance athletes with VO_{2max} values over 83 ml kg^{-1} and found no trend for excess *I* allele or low number of *DD* homozygotes of *ACE*. A genomic scan for maximal oxygen uptake in Caucasian families of the HERITAGE Family study reported many potential candidate gene loci on many chromosomal regions, but no linkage was observed on chromosome 17 on the *ACE* locus [59]. It appears logical to suggest that the study of influence of genotypes on the VO_{2max} should be conducted in an increased cohort of healthy individuals for genetic association to be more evident. In addition to maximal rate of oxygen uptake, at least two other endurance phenotypes (economy of movement and lactate/ventilator threshold) also contribute to endurance performance phenotype (time taken to travel a given distance) as seen in elite competition [11]. A fourth phenotype, namely oxygen uptake kinetics, may also be discretely related. These phenotypes are yet to be associated with specific genetic polymorphisms in a healthy adult population. Unbiased genome-wide approaches have been used in search for genomic region, transcripts and DNA variants linked or associated with endurance performance related trait [60–63]. Bouchard et al. [60] studied association of 324,611 SNPs with the response of VO_{2max} to endurance training in 473 Whites from HERITAGE. None of the SNPs reached genome-wide significance even though there were several SNPs moderately associated with VO_{2max} trainability [60]. A meta-analysis of genome-wide association study of two cohorts of elite endurance athletes and controls revealed only one statistically significant marker (*rs558129* at *GALNTL6* locus, $p = 0.0002$), and no panel of genomic variation common to the elite candidate athletic group was identified [64].

Human physical capability is influenced by many environmental and genetic factors, and it is generally accepted that physical performance phenotypes are highly polygenic [65, 66]. Potential for elite human physical performance is limited by the similarity of polygenic profiles with 99% of people differing by no more than seven genotypes from the typical profile [11]. The predicted mean TGS for favourable endurance profile in endurance elite athletes was significantly higher (70.2 ± 15.6) compared to general Spanish population (60.70 ± 12.21) and about 3000 individuals out of a total population of ~41 million people were predicted to have theoretically optimal polygenic profile (TGS = 100) for seven candidate genes [27]. In the simulated population of Gorkhas in the present study, mean TGS obtained was 69.01 ± 15.40 for favourable endurance. It was interesting to note that 4% of the population (15 individuals out of 374) exhibited an optimal TGS (100) for endurance with another 16% of the population (60 individuals out of 374) showing a TGS of ~87. Compared to Gorkhas, only 2 and 10% of Indian lowlanders had TGS 100 and TGS 87, respectively. Analysis of TGS 100 and TGS 87.5 between Gorkha (Tibeto-Burman) and Indian lowlanders, using 3×2 contingency table (www.vassarstats.net/newcs.html), demonstrated significant difference between the cohorts ($p < 0.0001$) suggesting an overall more favourable polygenic endurance profile in Gorkha population. With 4% of the male Gorkha soldiers (who are otherwise drawn from the general population) having the optimal endurance profile, this would mean that nearly 1.7 million, out of an estimated 43 million (31 million of Nepalese from Nepal and about 12 million Nepalese domiciled in India, Nepal Census 2011) would have the optimal endurance profile. Even if new candidate polymorphisms are scored, probability of presence of individuals with optimal genotypes for endurance still remains large in this population. The Gorkhas are thus genetically endowed with the endurance phenotypes; they have the genetic advantage with higher co-occurrence of *ACE II/ACTN3 XX/CKMM AA/eNOS GG* in the population. Genetic endowment coupled with high-intensity training which considerably increases maximal oxygen uptake, of young adolescent Gorkhas will definitely bring performance improvement in many sporting events. It may not be farfetched to postulate that such individuals can rewrite the world records. It is accepted that in addition to genetic potential and physical environment, a performance record is a function of economic and social opportunity. Individuals from small geographical area hold many world athletic records. Although genetic explanations is lacking, there are considerable regional and ethnic variations in typical frequencies of many genotypes e.g., frequency of *ACE II* is higher in some regions of Oceania than most of Europe while athletes of north and east African descent excel in endurance events and those of west African descent excel in sprint events [67]. Interestingly, 5% of high-altitude natives (Tibeto-Burman) also had TGS 100 and 19% had TGS 87 similar to the TGS frequency observed in Gorkhas (Tibeto-Burman). The observation presents a scope for us to state that Tibeto-Burman mountain population per se has higher TGS score linked to endurance genotype than the lowlander Indian population.

It may be argued that the soldiers used in the present study may not be representative of the entire Gorkha population as recruitment in Indian Army may be selective. For examining this issue, we compared the genotypic frequencies obtained from participants of Indian Army with those reported from general Indian population (Table 9). The genotypic frequency distribution in both the army and general population was not statistically different (except for *ACTN3*), substantiating the fact that the genotypic frequency distribution obtained from soldier population of the Indian Army is generally reflective of the frequency in general Indian population. As an extension of this observation, we state that the data obtained in the Gorkhas (Tibeto-Burman) in the present study reflects the general Gorkha population frequency.

Limitations

The present study, however, is not without limitation as only four endurance-associated polymorphisms were studied. These four polymorphisms were chosen because of definitive information about their association with endurance, exercise performance, muscle performance, generation of rapid forceful contraction, high values of VO_{2max} and endurance elite status and also for reason that frequency data for these polymorphisms were available in the Indian population for comparison and computation of TGS. Further studies

Table 9 Comparison of genotypic and allelic frequency distribution between participants of the Indian Army and general Indian population

			Indo-Aryan			Dravidian			General Population		
			Indian Army	General population		Indian Army	General population		Indian Army	General population	
SNP	Variants	Genotype			p^*			p^*			p^*
rs1799752	*ACE I/D*	*II*	0.25[a]	0.26[b]	0.71	0.29[a]	0.37[e]	0.18			
		ID	0.50[a]	0.54[b]		0.53[a]	0.42[e]				
		DD	0.24[a]	0.20[b]		0.18[a]	0.21[e]				
		Allele									
		I	0.51[a]	0.53[b]	0.55	0.56[a]	0.58[e]	0.64			
		D	0.49[a]	0.46[b]		0.44[a]	0.42[e]				
rs1815739	*ACTN3 Arg(R) 577Ter(X)*	*RR*	0.18[a]	0.16[c]	*0.04*	0.24[a]					
		RX	0.56[a]	0.45[c]		0.48[a]	NA	NA			
		XX	0.26[a]	0.39[c]		0.28[a]					
		Allele									
		R	0.46[a]	0.39[c]	*0.05*	0.48[a]					
		X	0.54[a]	0.61[c]		0.52[a]					
rs1799983	*eNOS Glu298Asp*	*GG*	0.64[i]	0.71[d]	0.12	0.73[i]	0.74[f]	0.45			
		GT	0.33[i]	0.27[d]		0.25[i]	0.26[f]				
		TT	0.01[i]	0.07[d]		0.01[i]	0.00[f]				
		Allele									
		G	0.81[i]	0.85[d]	0.90	0.86[i]	0.87[f]	0.76			
		T	0.18[i]	0.15[d]		0.14[i]	0.13[f]				
rs1042713	*ADRB2 Arg16Gly*	*GG*							0.31[g]	0.25[k]	0.49
		AG							0.53[g]	0.53[k]	
		AA							0.16[g]	0.22[k]	
		Allele									
		G							0.56[g]	0.52[k]	0.25
		A							0.43[g]	0.48[k]	
rs41317140	*REN C/T*	*CC*	0.62[j]	0.69[h]	0.35						
		CT	0.35[j]	0.31[h]							
		TT	0.02[j]	0.00[h]							
		Allele									
		C	0.80[j]	0.84[h]	0.29						
		T	0.20[j]	0.16[h]							

Data for CKMM is not available in Indian general population

NA data not available

*Significance for genotypic and allelic frequency is assumed when $p < 0.05$. The significant p values are italicized

[a][10]; [b][76]; [c][77]; [d][78]; [e][79]; [f][80]; [g][23]; [h][81]; [i]Present study; [j]unpublished; [k]values computed by clubbing the data from [82] and [83]

are required in larger cohorts and with additional endurance-related polymorphisms to evaluate the role of genetic variations in determining sports performance. It is also mentioned that in absence of objective data, we have used the extension of the observation seen in general Indian population and Indian army to state that the data obtained in the male Gorkha soldiers in the present study reflects the general Gorkha population frequency.

Implications

The findings of the present study imply that young talented adolescents from the high hill population, having polygenic endurance profiles linked with higher TGS could be selected and given appropriate training in endurance-related sports activities with prospects of competing in Olympics and other sports events held in high-altitude environment. Earlier studies have shown that whole body physiological variables related to O_2 consumption are influenced by the level of training of the individual [68–71]. It has been shown that long-term endurance training in a coordinated fashion impacts muscle epigenetics and affects thousands of methylation sites and genes associated with improvement in muscle function and health [72]. Appropriate training combined with favourable genetic profile will definitely be advantageous for achievement of elite athletic status by this sub-mountainous population.

Conclusions

The present study provides a novel perspective on endurance genetics based on polygenic profiling in the Gorkha population. The study reports for the first time the genotypic and allelic frequencies of four endurance-associated genetic markers in the male Gorkha soldiers (Tibeto-Burman). The study also highlights that nearly 4% of the Gorkha soldiers (Tibeto-Burman) exhibit an optimal total genotypic score (100) for endurance, indicating genetic potential of this population for achieving excellence in endurance-related elite sports activities.

Endnotes

[1]The Gorkhas derive their name from Guru Gorakhanath of eighth century. The shrine dedicated to Guru Gorakhnath was part of Gorkha Durbar built on a rocky crag in Nepal in 1639 from where the Gorkhas began their soldiering and where the ancient army called "Gurujiko Paltan" was raised. The 400-year-old shrine dedicated to Guru Gorkhnath was devastated in the massive earthquake that struck Nepal on 25 April 2015.

Additional files

Additional file 1: Table S1. One-way ANOVA (PostHocTukey test) of VO_{2max} in five subpopulation of male Gorkha soldiers (TB). (DOCX 22 kb)

Additional file 2: Table S2. Frequency of combined genotype distribution in male Gorkha soldiers. (DOC 106 kb)

Additional file 3: Table S3. Descriptive statistics and comparative analysis of maximal oxygen uptake ($VO_{2\ max}$ in ml kg^{-1} min^{-1}) between genotypes and groups. (DOC 36 kb)

Additional file 4: Table S4. Association analysis of combinatorial genotype profiles with maximal oxygen uptake (VO_{2max} in ml kg^{-1} min^{-1}). (DOC 36 kb)

Additional file 5: Table S5. Frequency distribution of total genotype score (TGS) from male Gorkha soldiers ($n = 374$). (a) Tabular information of TGS. (b) Graphical representation of TGS. (DOC 85 kb)

Additional file 6: Table S6. Total genotype score and percentage of frequency for all the possible combinations of four polymorphisms in male Gorkha soldiers. (DOC 89 kb)

Additional file 7: Table S7. Comparison of physiological characteristics and VO_{2max} in male Gorkha soldiers grouped according to total genotype score (TGS). (DOCX 32 kb)

Acknowledgements

Authors wish to thank the Army HQ SD branch, the Commanding Officers of the Units and the volunteers who participated in the study. Authors also thank Neha Thakur for the typing of the manuscript.

Funding

This work was supported by the Defence Research and Development Organization Grant No. S&T-09/DIP-251 (C6.0. SR) at the Defence Institute of Physiology and Allied Sciences.

Authors' contributions

SS conceived the study and coordinated and wrote the manuscript. SR, SaS, IS, LRV, TC and MSP collected the samples and participated in the physiological measurements. SM, KP and AT performed the genetic experiments and statistical analysis. All authors read and approved the final manuscript.

Competing interests

The authors, Seema Malhotra, Kiran Preet, Arvind Tomar, Shweta Rawat, Sayar Singh, Inderjeet Singh, L. Robert Varte, Tirthankar Chatterjee, M.S Pal and Soma Sarkar declare that they have no conflict of interest.

Author details

[1]Defence Institute of Physiology and Allied Sciences (DIPAS), Ministry of Defence. Government of India, Lucknow Road, Delhi 110054, India. [2]Defence Research and Development Establishment (DRDE). Ministry of Defence, Government of India, Jhansi Road, Gwalior 474002, Madhya Pradesh, India.

References

1. Caplan L. Bravest of the brave: representation of 'The Gorkha' in British military writings. Modern Asian Studies. 1991;25:571–97.
2. Chappell M. The Gurkhas. Oxford: Osprey Publishing; 1993.
3. Haaland G, Gurung P. Globalization of interaction systems and the culture in ethnicity: popular songs and the production of Nepali ethnoscapes in South-East Asia. Internat J Diversity Organisations Communities Nations. 2007;7:77–84.

4. Rai B. Gorkhas: The Warrior Race. 2nd ed. Delhi: Kalpaz Publications; 2009.
5. Garrido E, Rodas G, Javierre C, Segura R, Estruch A, Ventura JL. Cardiorespiratory response to exercise in elite Sherpa climbers transferred to sea level. Med Sci Sports Exerc. 1997;29:937–42.
6. Droma Y, Hanaoka M, Basnyat B, Arjyal A, Neupane P, Pandit A, et al. Adaptation to high altitude in Sherpas: association with the insertion/deletion polymorphism in the angiotensin-converting enzyme gene. Wilderness Environ Med. 2008;19:22–9.
7. Ahmetov II, Fedotovskaya ON. Sport genomics: current state of knowledge and future directions. Cell and Mol Exerc Physiol. 2012;1:1–24.
8. Ma F, Yang Y, Li X, Zhou F, Gao C, Li M, et al. The association of sport performance with ACE and ACTN3 genetic polymorphisms: a systematic review and meta-analysis. PLoS ONE. 2013;8:e54685.
9. Hennis PJ, O'Doherty AF, Levett DZH, Grocott MPW, Montgomery HM. Genetic factors associated with exercise performance in atmospheric hypoxia. Sports Med. 2015;45:745–61.
10. Bhagi S, Srivastava S, Sarkar S, Singh SB. Distribution of performance- related gene polymorphisms (ACTN3 R577X and ACE ID) in different ethnic groups of the Indian Army. J Basic Clin Physiol Pharmacol. 2013;24:225–34.
11. Williams AG, Folland JP. Similarity of polygenic profiles limits the potential for elite human physical performance. J Physiol. 2008;586:113–21.
12. MacArthur DG, North KN. ACTN3: a genetic influence on muscle function and athletic performance. Exerc Sport Sci Rev. 2007;35:30–4.
13. Alfred T, Ben-Shlomo Y, Cooper R, Hardy R, Cooper C, Deary IJ, et al. ACTN3 genotypes, athletic status and life course physical capability: meta-analysis of the published literature and findings from nine studies. Hum Mutat. 2011;32:1008–18.
14. Yang N, MacArthur DG, Gulbin JP, Hahn G, Beggs AH, Easteal S, et al. ACTN3 genotype is associated with human elite athletic performance. Am J Hum Genet. 2003;73:627–31.
15. Eynon N, Duarte JA, Oliveira J, Sagiv M, Yamin C, Meckel Y, et al. ACTN3 R577X polymorphism and Israeli top-level athletes. Int J Sports Med. 2009;30:695–8.
16. Rivera MA, Dionne FT, Wolfarth B, Chagnon M, Simoneau JA, Pérusse L, et al. Muscle-specific creatine kinase gene polymorphisms in elite endurance athletes and sedentary controls. Med Sci Sports Exerc. 1997;29:1444–7.
17. Fedotovskaya ON, Popov DV, Vinogradova OL, Akhmetov II. Association of muscle-specific creatine kinase (CKMM) gene polymorphism with physical performance of athletes. Human Physiol. 2012;38:89–93.
18. Sprouse C, Tosi LL, Gordish-Dressman H, Abdel-Ghani MS, Panchapakesan K, Niederberger B, et al. CK-MM polymorphism is associated with physical fitness test scores in military recruits. Mil Med. 2015;180:1001–5.
19. Wolfarth B, Rankinen T, Muhlbauer S, Ducke M, Rauramaa R, Boulay MR, et al. Endothelial nitric oxide synthase gene polymorphism and elite endurance athlete status: the Genathlete study. Scand J Med Sci Sports. 2008;18:485–90.
20. Rankinen T, Rice T, Pérusse L, Chagnon YC, Gagnon J, Leon AS, et al. NOS3 Glu298Asp genotype and blood pressure response to endurance training: the HERITAGE family study. Hypertension. 2000;36:885–9.
21. Green DJ, Maiorana A, O'Driscoll G, Taylor R. Effect of exercise training on endothelium-derived nitric oxide function in humans. J Physiol. 2004;561:1–25.
22. Ahsan A, Norboo T, Baig M, Qadar Pasha MA. Simultaneous selection of the wild type genotypes of the G894T and 4B/4A polymorphisms of NOS3 associate with high altitude adaptation. Ann Hum Genet. 2005;69:260–7.
23. Tomar A, Malhotra S, Sarkar S. Polymorphism profiling of nine high altitude relevant candidate gene loci in acclimatized sojourners and adapted natives. BMC Genet. 2015;16:112.
24. van Driem GL. Languages of the Himalayas: an ethnolinguistic handbook of the greater Himalayan region, containing an introduction to the symbiotic theory of language (2 vols). Leiden: Brill; 2001.
25. Ray US, Mukhopadhyaya S, Purkayastha SS, Asnani V, Tomer OS, Prashad R, et al. Effect of yogic exercises on physical and mental health of young fellowship course trainees. Ind J Physiol Pharmacol. 2001;45:37–53.
26. Lindpaintner K, Pfeffer MA, Kreutz R, Stampfer MJ, Grodstein F, LaMotte F, et al. A prospective evaluation of an angiotensin-converting-enzyme gene polymorphism and the risk of ischemic heart disease. N Engl J Med. 1995;332:706–11.
27. Ruiz JR, Gomez-Gallego F, Santiago C, Gonzalez-Freire M, Verde Z, Foster C, et al. Is there an optimum endurance polygenic profile? J Physiol. 2009;587:1527–34.
28. Valière N, Berthier P, Mouchiroud D, Pontier D. Gemini: software for testing the effects of genotyping errors and multitubes approach for individual identification. Mol Ecol Notes. 2002;2:83–6.
29. Hughes DC, Day SH, Ahmetov II, Williams AG. Genetics of muscle strength and power: polygenic profile similarity limits skeletal muscle performance. J Sports Sci. 2011;29:1425–34.
30. Umemura S, Kawasaki T, Ishigami T, Fujita T, Hibi K, Kawasaki M, et al. Angiotensin-converting enzyme gene polymorphism in Nepal. J Hum Hypertens. 1998;12:527–31.
31. Montgomery HE, Marshall R, Hemingway H, Myerson S, Clarkson P, Dollery C, et al. Human gene for physical performance. Nature. 1998;393:221–2.
32. Puthucheary Z, Skipworth JR, Rawal J, Loosemore M, Van Someren K, Montgomery HE. The ACE gene and human performance: 12 years on. Sports Med. 2011;41:433–48.
33. Bray MS, Hagberg JM, Pérusse L, Rankinen T, Roth SM, Wolfarth B, et al. The human gene map for performance and health-related fitness phenotypes: the 2006-2007 update. Med Sci Sports Exerc. 2009;41:35–73.
34. Bouchard C. Genomic predictors of trainability. Exp Physiol. 2012;97:347–52.
35. Cambien F, Poirier O, Lecerf L, Evans A, Cambou JP, Arveiler D, et al. Deletion polymorphism in the gene for angiotensin-converting enzyme is a potent risk factor for myocardial infarction. Nature. 1992;359:641–4.
36. Tiret L, Kee F, Poirier O, Nicaud V, Lecerf L, Evans A, et al. Deletion polymorphism in angiotensin-converting enzyme gene associated with parental history of myocardial infarction. Lancet. 1993;341:991–2.
37. Verlengia R, Rebelo AC, Crisp AH, Kunz VC, Dos Santos Carneiro Cordeiro MA, Hirata MH, et al. Lack of association between ACE indel polymorphism and cardiorespiratory fitness in physically active and sedentary young women. Asian J Sports Med. 2014;5:e22768.
38. Eynon N, Hanson ED, Lucia A, Houweling PJ, Garton F, North KN, et al. Genes for elite power and sprint performance: ACTN3 leads the way. Sports Med. 2013;43:803–17.
39. Druzhevskaya AM, Ahmetov II, Astratenkov IV, Rogozkin VA. Association of the ACTN3 R577X polymorphism with power athlete status in Russians. Eur J Appl Physiol. 2008;103:631–4.
40. Yang N, MacArthur DG, Wolde B, Onywera VO, Boit MK, Lau SY, et al. The ACTN3 R577X polymorphism in East and West African athletes. Med Sci Sports Exerc. 2007;39:1985–8.
41. Shang X, Zhang F, Zhang L, Huang C. ACTN3 R577X polymorphism and performance phenotypes in young Chinese male soldiers. J Sports Sci. 2012; 30:255–60.
42. Amorim CE, Acuna-Alonzo V, Salzano FM, Bortolini MC, Hunemeier T. Differing evolutionary histories of the ACTN3*R577X polymorphism among the major human geographic groups. PLoS ONE. 2015;10, e0115449.
43. Yamashita K, Yoshioka T. Profiles of creatine kinase isoenzyme compositions in single muscle fibres of different types. J Muscle Res Cell Motil. 1991;12:37–44.
44. Zhou DQ, Hu Y, Liu G, Wu J, Gong L. An A/G polymorphism in muscle-specific creatine kinase gene in Han population in northern China. Yi Chuan. 2005;27:535–8.
45. Heled Y, Bloom MS, Wu TJ, Stephens Q, Deuster PA. CK-MM and ACE genotypes and physiological prediction of the creatine kinase response to exercise. J Appl Physiol. 2007;103:504–10.
46. Droma Y, Hanaoka M, Basnyat B, Arjyal A, Neupane P, Pandit A, et al. Genetic contribution of the endothelial nitric oxide synthase gene to high altitude adaptation in sherpas. High Alt Med Biol. 2006;7:209–20.
47. Wang P, Ha AY, Kidd KK, Koehle MS, Rupert JL. A variant of the endothelial nitric oxide synthase gene (NOS3) associated with AMS susceptibility is less common in the Quechua, a high altitude native population. High Alt Med Biol. 2010;11:27–30.
48. Erzurum SC, Ghosh S, Janocha AJ, Xu W, Bauer S, Bryan NS, et al. Higher blood flow and circulating NO products offset high-altitude hypoxia among Tibetans. Proc Natl Acad Sci U S A. 2007;104:17593–8.
49. Beall CM, Laskowski D, Strohl KP, Soria R, Villena M, Vargas E, et al. Pulmonary nitric oxide in mountain dwellers. Nature. 2001;414:411–2.
50. Di Prampero PE. Factors limiting maximal performance in humans. Eur J Appl Physiol. 2003;90:420–9.
51. Roca J, Rabinovich R. Clinical excercise testing. In: lung function testing. Eur Resp Mon. 2005;31:146–65.

52. Richardson RS. Oxygen transport and utilization: an integration of the muscle systems. Adv Physiol Educ. 2003;27:183–91.
53. Dua GL, Sen Gupta J. A study of physical work capacity of sea level residents on prolonged stay at high altitude and comparison with high altitude native residents. Ind J Physiol Pharmacol. 1980;24:15–24.
54. Gupta JS, Dua GL, Srinivasulu N, Malhortra MS. Changes in exercise heart rate in lowlanders after prolonged stay at high altitude (4000 m). Aviat Space Environ Med. 1975;46:907–10.
55. Bandyopadhyay A, Bandyopadhyay P. Cardiorespiratory fitness in college students of Uttar Pradesh, India. J Exerc Sci Physiotherapy. 2007;3:44–7.
56. Nabi T, Rafiq N, Qayoom O. Assessment of cardiovascular fitness [VO2 max] among medical students by Queens College step test. Int J Biomed Adv Res. 2015;6:418–21.
57. Dhara S, Chatterjee K. A study of VO2 max in relation with body mass index (BMI) of physical education students. Res J Physic Edu Sci. 2015;3:9–12.
58. Rankinen T, Bernd W, Simoneau JA, Maier-Lenz D, Rauramaa R, Rivera M, et al. No association between the angiotensin-converting enzyme ID polymorphism and elite endurance athlete status. J Appl Physiol. 2000;88:1571–5.
59. Bouchard C, Rankinen T, Chagnon YC, Rice T, Pérusse L, Gagnon J, et al. Genomic scan for maximal oxygen uptake and its response to training in the HERITAGE Family Study. J Appl Physiol. 2000;88:551–9.
60. Bouchard C, Sarzynski MA, Rice TK, Kraus WE, Church TS, Sung YJ, et al. Genomic predictors of the maximal O(2) uptake response to standardized exercise training programs. J Appl Physiol (1985). 2011;110:1160–70.
61. Rankinen T, Sung YJ, Sarzynski MA, Rice TK, Rao DC, Bouchard C. Heritability of submaximal exercise heart rate response to exercise training is accounted for by nine SNPs. J Appl Physiol (1985). 2012;112:892–7.
62. Timmons JA, Knudsen S, Rankinen T, Koch LG, Sarzynski M, Jensen T, et al. Using molecular classification to predict gains in maximal aerobic capacity following endurance exercise training in humans. J Appl Physiol (1985). 2010;108:1487–96.
63. Argyropoulos G, Stutz AM, Ilnytska O, Rice T, Teran-Garcia M, Rao DC, et al. KIF5B gene sequence variation and response of cardiac stroke volume to regular exercise. Physiol Genomics. 2009;36:79–88.
64. Rankinen T, Fuku N, Wolfarth B, Wang G, Sarzynski MA, Alexeev DG, et al. No evidence of a common DNA variant profile specific to world class endurance athletes. PLoS ONE. 2016;11, e0147330.
65. Rankinen T, Bray MS, Hagberg JM, Perusse L, Roth SM, Wolfarth B, et al. The human gene map for performance and health-related fitness phenotypes: the 2005 update. Med Sci Sports Exerc. 2006;38:1863–88.
66. Spurway N. Top-down studies of genetic contribution to differences in physical capacity. In: Spurway N, Wackerhage H, editors. Genetics and Molecular Biology of Muscle Adaptation. London: Churchill Livingstone, Elsevier; 2006. p. 25–59.
67. Kyle CV, Abbott W, Young RP, Nijmeijer B, Simmons D, Braatvedt GD. Angiotensin-1-converting enzyme and angiotensinogen gene polymorphisms in Maori and Pacific Island people in New Zealand. Intern Med J. 2001;31:116–8.
68. Bassett DR, Howley ET. Limiting factors for maximum oxygen uptake and determinants of endurance performance. Med Sci Sports Exerc. 2000;32:70–84.
69. Meyer T, Lucía A, Earnest CP, et al. A conceptual framework for performance diagnosis and training prescription from submaximal gas exchange parameters theory and application. Int J Sports Med. 2005;26 Suppl 1:S38–48.
70. Saunders PU, Pyne DB, Telford RD, et al. Factors affecting running economy in trained distance runners. Sports Med. 2000;34:465–85.
71. Myburgh KH. What makes an endurance athlete world-class? Not simply a physiological conundrum. Comp Biochem Phys A. 2003;136:171–1.
72. Lindholm ME, Marabita F, Gomez-Cabrero D, Rundqvist H, Ekström TJ, Tegnér J, Sundberg CJ. An integrative analysis reveals coordinated reprogramming of the epigenome and the transcriptome in human skeletal muscle after training. Epigenetics. 2014;12:1557–69.
73. Yang YZ, Wang YP, Guan W, Du Y, Ga Q, Ge RL. No relation between ACE-I/D polymorphism and high altitude pulmonary edema in the Han Chinese. Zhongguo Ying Yong Sheng Li Xue Za Zhi. 2013;29:508–11. 517.
74. Higaki J, Baba S, Katsuya T, Sato N, Ishikawa K, Mannami T, et al. Deletion allele of angiotensin-converting enzyme gene increases risk of essential hypertension in Japanese men: The Suita Study. Circulation. 2000;101:2060–5.
75. Pannu H, Kim DH, Seaman CR, Van Ginhoven G, Shete S, Milewicz DM. Lack of an association between the angiotensin-converting enzyme insertion/deletion polymorphism and intracranialaneurysms in a Caucasian population in the United States. J Neurosurg. 2005;103:92–6.
76. Badaruddoza and Sudhir N. No evidence for association between ACE gene insertion (I)/deletion (D) polymorphism and hypertension in north Indian Punjabi population. Int J Hum Genet. 2012;12:179–85.
77. Kothari ST, Chheda P, Chawla S, Chatterjee L, Chaudhry SK, Das BR. ACTN3 R577X polymorphism in asian Indian athletes. Int J Hum Genet. 2011;11:149–53.
78. Srivastava K, Biswas UK, Narang R, Varghese JJ, Das N. Prevalence of eNOS Glu298Asp polymorphism in healthy volunteers from a region of northern India. Community Genet. 2005;8:180–3.
79. Deeba F, Jamil K, Rabbani S, Waheed MA, Rao H. Association of angiotensin converting enzyme gene I/D polymorphism with vitiligo in South Indian population. Int J Med Med Sci. 2009;1:9–12.
80. Nishevitha NS, Angeline T, Jeyaraj N. Endothelial nitric oxide synthase (eNOS) Glu298-> Asp polymorphism (G894T) among south Indians. Indian J Med Res. 2009;129:68–71.
81. Purkait P, Suthar PC, Purohit VK, Naidu JM, Sarkar BN. Renin-angiotensin-aldosterone system gene polymorphisms in Type 2 diabetic patients among the Mewari population of Rajasthan. Int J Biol Med Res. 2013;4:3128–34.
82. Shah NJ, Vinod Kumar S, Gurusamy U, Annan Sudarsan AK, Shewade DGJ. Effect of ADRB2 (adrenergic receptor β2) gene polymorphisms on the occurrence of asthma and on the response to nebulized salbutamol in South Indian patients with bronchial asthma. Asthma. 2015;52:755–62.
83. Kumar A, Tripathi M, Srivastava MV, Vivekanandhan S, Prasad K. Relationship between polymorphisms in beta-2 adrenergic receptor gene and ischemic stroke in North Indian Population: a hospital based case control study. BMC Res Notes. 2014;7:396.

5

Efficacy of wearing compression garments during post-exercise period after two repeated bouts of strenuous exercise: a randomized crossover design in healthy, active males

Kazushige Goto[1,2*], Sahiro Mizuno[2] and Ayaka Mori[2]

Abstract

Background: The efficacy of wearing [a] compression garment (CG) between repeated bouts of exercise within a same day has not been fully understood. The present study determined the effect of wearing a CG after strenuous exercise sessions (consisting of sprint exercise, resistance exercise, drop jump) twice a day on exercise performance, muscle damage, and inflammatory responses.

Methods: Eleven physically active males (age, 22.7 ± 0.9 years; height, 175.7 ± 6.7 cm; body mass, 73.6 ± 10.2 kg; BMI, 23.8 ± 2.7 kg/m^2) performed two trials (a randomized crossover design), consisting of the trial with either wearing a whole-body CG during post-exercise period (CG trial) or the trial with wearing a normal garment without specific pressure (CON trial). Two exercise sessions were conducted in the morning (09:00–10:00, Ex1) and afternoon (14:00–15:00, Ex2). Immediately after completing 60 min of each exercise, the subjects in the CG trial changed into a whole-body CG. Time-course changes in exercise performance (bench press power, jump performances, repeated sprint ability), blood variables (lactate, glucose, myoglobin, creatine kinase, interleukin-6, leptin), and scores of subjective feeling (fatigue, muscle soreness) were compared between the CG and CON trials before Ex1 (8:40), immediately before Ex2 (14:00, 4 h after Ex1), 4 h after Ex2 (19:00), and 24 h after the onset of Ex1 (9:00).

(Continued on next page)

* Correspondence: kagoto@fc.ritsumei.ac.jp
[1]Faculty of Sport and Health Sciences, Ritsumeikan University, 1-1-1, Nojihigashi, Kusatsu, Shiga 525-8577, Japan
[2]Graduate School of Sport and Health Science, Ritsumeikan University, Kusatsu, Shiga 525-8574, Japan

(Continued from previous page)

Results: Two bouts of exercise significantly decreased performances of counter movement jump (main effect for time: $P = 0.04$, $F = 3.75$, partial $\eta^2 = 0.27$) and rebound jump (main effect for time: $P = 0.00$, $F = 12.22$, partial $\eta^2 = 0.55$), while no significant difference was observed between the two trials (interaction: $P = 0.10$, $F = 1.96$, partial $\eta^2 = 0.16$ for counter movement jump, $P = 0.93$, $F = 0.01$, partial $\eta^2 = 0.001$ for rebound jump). Repeated sprint ability (power output during 10 × 6 s maximal sprint, 30-s rest periods between sprints) did not differ significantly between the two trials at any time points. Power output during bench press exercise was not significantly different between the two trials (interaction: $P = 0.46$, $F = 0.99$, partial $\eta^2 = 0.09$ for Ex1, $P = 0.74$, $F = 0.38$, partial $\eta^2 = 0.04$ for Ex2, $P = 0.22$, $F = 1.54$, partial $\eta^2 = 0.13$ for 24 h after the onset of Ex1). Serum myoglobin, creatine kinase, leptin, and plasma interleukin-6 were not significantly different between the two trials (interaction: $P = 0.16$, $F = 2.23$, partial $\eta^2 = 0.18$ for myoglobin; $P = 0.39$, $F = 0.81$, partial $\eta^2 = 0.08$ for creatine kinase; $P = 0.28$, $F = 1.30$, partial $\eta^2 = 0.13$ for leptin; $P = 0.34$, $F = 1.05$, partial $\eta^2 = 0.12$ for interleukin-6). Muscle soreness at 24 h during post-exercise period was significantly lower in the CG trial than in the CON trial for pectoralis major muscle ($P = 0.04$), while the value was inversely lower in the CON trial for hamstring ($P = 0.047$).

Conclusions: Wearing a whole-body CG during the post-exercise period after two bouts of strenuous exercise sessions separated with 4 h of rest did not promote recovery of muscle function for lower limb muscles nor did it attenuate exercise-induced muscle damage in physically active males.

Keywords: Post-exercise treatment, Fatigue, Exercise-induced muscle damage, Muscle function

Key points

- Wearing a whole-body compression garment during the post-exercise period did not markedly affect recovery of muscular strength.
- Indirect muscle damage markers in blood (e.g., serum myoglobin, creatine kinase) were not influenced by wearing a compression garment during the post-exercise period.
- It was likely that the use of compression garments during the post-exercise period may have had some favorable effect on recovery of power output for upper body muscles.

Background

Since athletes commonly perform intensive physical training or competitions on consecutive days, facilitation of recovery process is important to maximize competitive success and to prevent excessive fatigue [1]. Several strategies are currently employed on sports fields to aid the recovery process, including massage [2], active recovery [3], water immersion [2], contrast bathing [4], and hyperbaric oxygen supply [5]. In addition, the use of compression garments (CG) during post-exercise period has been recently increasing attention as a novel option to promote muscular strength recovery and to attenuate exercise-induced muscle damage [6–8].

Although some evidences exist for beneficial effects of wearing a CG during exercise [9–12], majority of previous studies failed to support the performance-enhancing effect of the use of a CG during exercise [8, 13–19]. In a latest review [20], CG did not reveal positive effects on running performance, maximal and submaximal oxygen uptake, or the performance of strength-related tasks after running. In addition, MacRae et al. [8] suggested that the use of CG may have had some help for certain aspects of jump performance in some situations [9]. However, only limited evidence [12] showed the beneficial effects of CG on the performance of other exercise types (e.g., pedaling exercise, running). Alternatively, improvement of recovery by wearing a CG during post-exercise period is more apparent [6, 7, 10, 21–24]. Kraemer et al. [7] demonstrated that wearing a whole-body CG for 24 h after resistance training caused rapid recovery of power output for the bench press throw and attenuated muscle soreness with lower creatine kinase (CK) concentration on the following morning. Jakeman et al. [6, 22] reported that the recovery of jump performance following 100 plyometric drop jumps was significantly improved when the subjects wore a CG during post-exercise period. Furthermore, we have previously reported that recovery of muscular strength for upper limb muscles was significantly improved during early phase (3–8 h) of post-resistance exercise period by wearing whole-body CG. However, for the lower limb muscle, a significantly faster recovery of muscular strength occurred at 24 h after exercise [24]. In a previous study using endurance exercise, wearing CG for 24 h after 30 min of downhill running promoted significantly recovery of counter movement jump height [25]. Potential factor for promoted recovery by CG during post-exercise period is suggested to be reductions of venous blood pooling and subsequent swelling in muscles [26]. In addition, Born et al. [27] pointed out that the use of CG during post-exercise may assist performance recovery.

Athletes are often required to conduct strenuous exercise or competition twice a day, separated with several hours (12 h <) of rest. However, the influence of wearing CG between the repeated bouts of exercise within a same day has not been fully understood. Duffield et al. [26] reported that combined treatment of cold water immersion (15 min at 10 °C) and wearing CG (during 3 h) after the tennis specific drill and match play sessions promoted recovery of counter movement jump (CMJ) height at the beginning of subsequent match play. However, due to the recovery enhancing effect by cold water immersion [28–30], the impact of the use of CG itself has not been identified.

Therefore, the purpose of the present study was to determine effect of the CG during post-exercise period after two repeated bouts of exercise (including repeated sprint exercise, resistance exercise, drop jump) on exercise performance (e.g., power output during bench press exercise, jump height, rebound jump index), muscle damage, and inflammatory responses. We hypothesized that the use of CG during post-exercise period after the two repeated bouts of exercise would promote recovery of muscle function.

Methods

Subjects

Eleven men (mean ± SD: age, 22.7 ± 0.9 years; height, 175.7 ± 6.7 cm; body weight, 73.6 ± 10.2 kg; BMI, 23.8 ± 2.7 kg/m^2) participated in the present study. None of them was taking part in any regular training program at the start of the experiment (with exercising recreationally once per week). However, all subjects had several years of experience performing strenuous resistance training. The inclusion criteria for subject selection were experience with strenuous resistance training at least a year, no habit of wearing CG in daily sport activities. The subjects were informed about the purpose of the study and the experimental procedures, and they provided a written informed consent. The present study was approved by the Ethics Committee for Human Experiments at Ritsumeikan University, Japan, in accordance with the Helsinki Declaration.

Experimental overview

The present study was performed with a randomized crossover design. The subjects visited the laboratory four times throughout the experimental period. On the first visit, all subjects provided a written informed consent. On the second visit, one-repetition maximum (1RM) for four exercises was measured to determine the weights to be used for each exercise on the experimental days. The subjects also conducted a familiarization session of exercise protocol, consisting of 10 × 6 s all-out sprint separated with 30-s rest between the sprints under 7.5% of each body weight, 10 × 3 sets resistance exercise for four exercises, and 5 × 10 drop jumps (50 jumps in total).

On the third and fourth visits, the subjects completed two experimental trials, either with the use of a CG (CG trial) or without the use of a CG (CON trial) during post-exercise period after performing two repeated bouts of exercise, separated with 4 h of rest (Ex1: 9:00–10:00, Ex2: 14:00–15:00). The CG and CON trials were conducted in a random order separated by a month. Immediately after completing 60 min of each exercise, the subjects in the CG trial changed into a whole-body CG (Recharge; Under Armour, Baltimore, MD) [7, 24]. The pressure levels applied for the present CG were previously reported [25], 11.5 ± 0.6 hPa for thigh and 17.6 ± 1.8 hPa for calf. In the CON trial, the subjects wore a non-CG, identical type of sports wear without specific compression. The appropriate size of the CG for each subject was chosen on the basis of the garment's instruction manual and involved measurements of the height, chest, waist, and ankle circumferences. The subjects wore the prescribed garments throughout the whole recovery period (4 h after Ex1 and approximately 18 h after Ex2), except during two repeated bouts of exercise (60 min for each exercise), during measurements of exercise performances, blood drawing, and showering at night. Time courses of changes in upper and lower body muscular strength and power, blood metabolites, hormone and cytokine levels, and scores of muscle soreness and fatigue were monitored during 24 h after the onset of Ex1 (Fig. 1).

On the experimental days, all subjects stayed at the same facility located in the university. They spent time by reading books, listening music, or watching DVD. They were allowed to consume water ad libitum. The subjects were given identical lunch (12:00) and dinner (19:00) in both trials. The sleep duration on exercise days was controlled from 23:00 to 07:00.

Strenuous exercise session

Exercise consisted of three different exercises to mimic regular training for improving fitness levels among team sport athletes, including repeated sprint exercise, resistance exercise, and drop jump. We selected this protocol because all exercises are commonly used for daily training on sport fields. For the repeated sprint exercise, the subjects completed 10 × 6 s all-out sprint separated with 30 s rest between the sprints using an electromagnetically braked cycle ergometer (Power Max VIII; Konami Corporation, Tokyo, Japan). The resistance of pedaling was set at 7.5% of each body weight. Resistance exercise consisted of four exercises: three exercises for upper body muscles (chest press, lat pull down, shoulder press) and an exercise for lower limb muscles (bilateral leg press) using weight stack machines (Life Fitness, Ltd.,

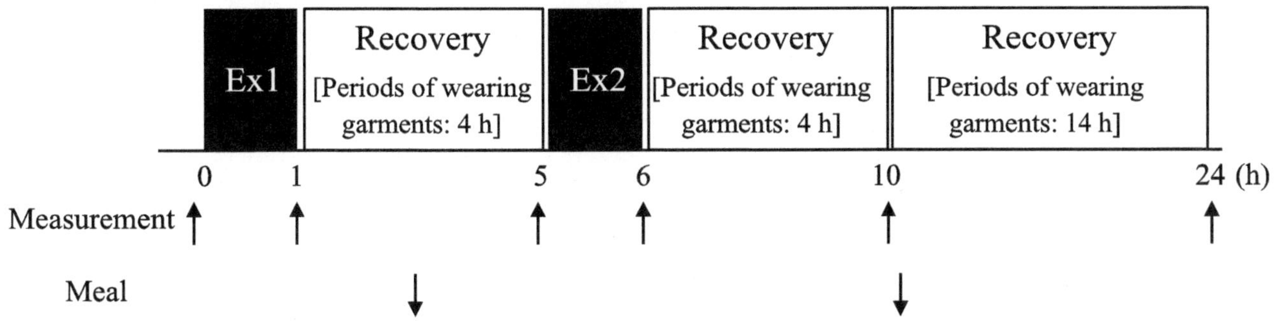

Fig. 1 Timeline of measurements and meal consumption. All subjects performed two bouts of exercise sessions (Ex1, Ex2) with wearing normal garment, while they kept wearing either CG (CG trial) or normal garment (CON trial) during the recovery period

Tokyo, Japan). Each exercise involved 10 repetitions, with five sets for chest press and lat pull down and three sets for shoulder press and bilateral leg press. The resistance was set as 75% of 1RM for each exercise. The subjects rested for 2 min between sets and exercises. Before the training session in each trial, the subjects performed warm-up sets comprising 10 repetitions at 50% of the 1RM and stretching of the major muscle groups targeted by the exercises. For drop jump, the subjects completed 5 × 10 drop jumps (50 jumps in total) from a height of 40 cm. All jumps were performed with placing hands on hips. After landing, they are requested to pause at a squatting position, with hand on hips and knees flexed to approximately 90° and subsequently conducted vertical jump with maximal effort [6, 22]. Each exercise session including repeated sprint exercise, resistance exercise, and drop jump lasted 60 min. The exercise session was repeated twice in the morning (9:00–10:00, Ex1) and afternoon (14:00-15:00, Ex2) under supervision by laboratory staff.

Measurements

Before Ex1 (8:40), immediately after Ex1 (10:00), immediately before Ex2 (14:00, 4 h after Ex1), 4 h after Ex2 (19:00), and 24 h after the onset of Ex1 (9:00), maximal power for bench press, jump performance, blood variables, scores of fatigue, and muscle soreness were evaluated. The repeated sprint ability was also evaluated three times: during Ex1, during Ex2, and at 24 h during post-exercise period (Fig. 1).

Evaluation of repeated sprint ability

To evaluate repeated sprint ability, the subjects performed repeated sprint exercise, comprising 10 × 6 s all-out sprint with a 30-s rest period between sprints. Before the exercise, the subjects completed a standardized warm-up on an electromagnetically braked cycle ergometer (Power Max VIII; Konami Corporation, Tokyo, Japan). The applied load for the repeated sprint test was equivalent to 7.5% of the subjects' body weight. The mean power outputs during each set of sprint were recorded by a computer (Edge E420, Lenovo, Beijing, China) every 0.1 s using specially designed software (Konami, Tokyo, Japan). The power output decrement (%) was calculated by percentage reduction of power output over the 10 sprints.

Strength measurement

For the indication of muscular power output for upper and lower limb muscles, bench press power output and jump performances were evaluated. Power output for bench press power output during concentric phase (elevating phase) was determined using an accelerometer (Myotest SPORT, Myotest SA, Sion, Switzerland) connective to a bench press bar [25]. After the beep, the subjects completed bench press exercise during concentric (elevating) phase as fast as possible. The weight of the exercise was set equivalent to 40% of 1RM, and mean power output (MPO) during the elevating phase was calculated. The measurement was repeated three times, and the maximal value was adopted.

Jump performance was evaluated using two types of jump tests. For the CMJ test, the subjects performed a maximal vertical jump on a platform (CT-916, Takei Scientific Instruments Co. Ltd., Niigata, Japan) that was connected to a personal computer. Subjects were instructed to perform a maximal jump while placing hands on the lumbar division to eliminate upper limb effects. The vertical jump flight time was recorded. From the flight time, the CMJ height was calculated using the formula [(Jump height (m) = 1/8 (flight time)^2 × (the gravity constant)]. The rebound jump (RJ) test was then performed to evaluate stretch shortening ability for lower limb muscles. The subjects were instructed five repeated maximal jumps on a platform with minimum contact time, and the jump height, contact time, and RJ index (jump height/contact time) were calculated [6]. From the obtained results from the five jumps, the average value among three values except the highest and lowest values was adopted for further analysis.

Blood variables

Venous blood samples were obtained from an antecubital vein before Ex1, immediately after Ex1, immediately before Ex2 (4 h after Ex1), 4 h after Ex2, and 24 h after the onset of Ex1 to determine blood glucose and lactate concentrations. Serum creatine kinase (CK), myoglobin (Mb), leptin, and plasma interleukin-6 (IL-6) concentrations were also evaluated before Ex1 and at 24 h after the onset of Ex1. Serum and plasma samples were obtained by centrifuging for 10 min and were stored at −80 °C until analysis. Serum CK and Mb concentrations were measured at a clinical laboratory (SRL Inc., Tokyo, Japan). The intra-assay CVs were 3.4% for CK and 6.0% for Mb measurements. Serum leptin and plasma IL-6 concentrations were measured with enzyme-linked immunosorbent assay (ELISA) using kits from R&D Systems (Minneapolis, MN, USA). The intra-assay CV was 9.5% for leptin and 8.2% for IL-6, respectively.

The blood glucose and lactate concentrations were measured immediately after blood collection using an automatic glucose analyzer (Free Style, Nipro Corporation, Osaka, Japan) and lactate analyzer (Lactate Pro2; Arkray Inc. Kyoto, Japan), respectively.

Scores of fatigue and muscle soreness

Scores of subjective fatigue and vitality were evaluated six times (before Ex1, immediately after Ex1, before Ex2, immediately after Ex2, 4 h after Ex2, 24 h after the onset of Ex1) using a 100-mm visual analogue scale (VAS), where 0 mm represented "no fatigue (or "filled vitality") at all" and 100 mm represented "unbearable fatigue (or "no vitality at all")" [21]. At 24 h after the onset of Ex1, muscle soreness was assessed using a 100-mm VAS, where 0 mm represented "no pain at all" and 100 mm represented "unbearable pain". The subjects were asked to rate the feeling experienced by making the line.

Statistical analysis

Data are expressed as means ± standard deviation (SD). For comparisons of time-course changes in exercise performance, blood variables, and subjective feeling of fatigue, a two-way analysis of variance (ANOVA) with repeated measures was initially applied. When the ANOVA revealed a significant interaction or main effect, a Tukey-Kramer test was performed for post hoc analyses. For comparison of scores of subjective feeling evaluated at 24 h after the onset of Ex1, a paired *t* test was applied. For all tests, $P < 0.05$ was considered significant.

Results

Figure 2 presents time course of change in MPO during bench press. No significant interaction ($P = 0.65$, $F = 0.67$, partial $\eta^2 = 0.06$) or main effect for trial ($P = 0.14$, $F = 2.63$, partial $\eta^2 = 0.21$) was observed, and there was a significant main effect for time ($P = 0.00$, $F = 24.60$, partial $\eta^2 = 0.71$). In the CON trial, the MPO during bench

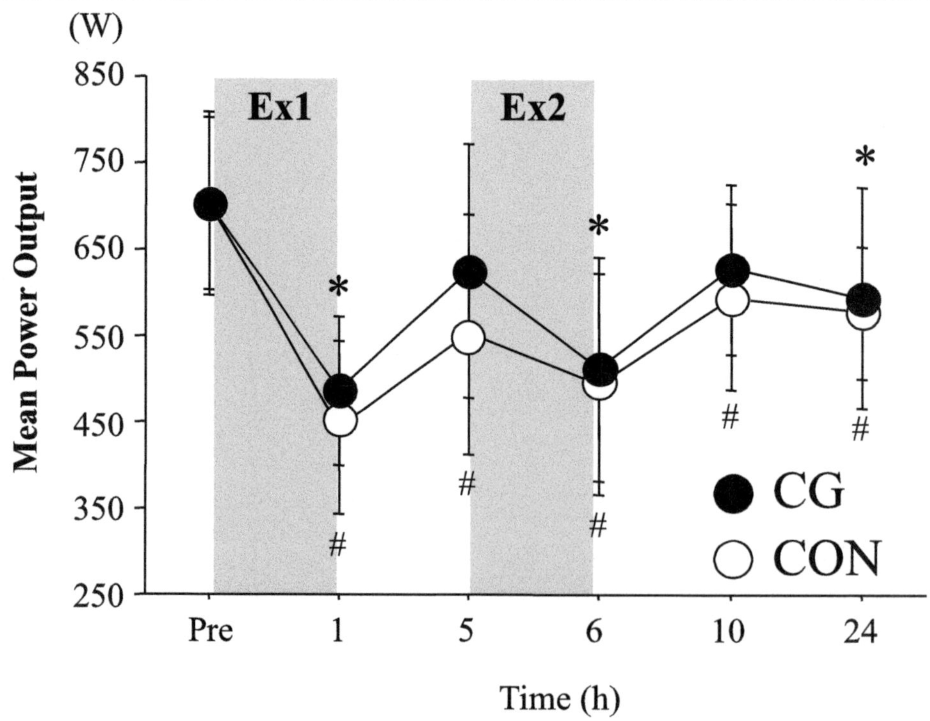

Fig. 2 Mean power output for bench press exercise. *Shaded boxes* indicate duration of exercises. Values are means ± SD. *$P < 0.05$ vs. Pre (CG); #$P < 0.05$ vs. Pre (CON)

press remained significantly lower from baseline value (Pre) at all time points during post-exercise period. However, in the CG trial, there was no significant difference from baseline value at 5 h (4 h after Ex1) and 10 h (4 h after Ex2) for the MPO. When the peak power output during the elevating phase of bench press exercise was compared, the CON trial showed significantly lower values from baseline value (Pre) at all points during post-exercise period (main effect for time: $P = 0.00$, $F = 22.86$, partial $\eta^2 = 0.70$). However, in the CG trial, there was no significant difference from the baseline value at 5 h (4 h after Ex1) and 10 h (4 h after Ex2), which were similar results from those for MPO.

Figure 3 presents time course of change in jump performance for CMJ and RJ. Exercise significantly reduced CMJ height during post-exercise period (main effect for time: $P = 0.04$, $F = 3.75$, partial $\eta^2 = 0.27$), with no significant interaction between trial and time ($P = 0.10$, $F = 1.96$, partial $\eta^2 = 0.16$). There was a significant main effect of time for all variables for RJ (RJ height: $P = 0.02$, $F = 4.17$, partial $\eta^2 = 0.29$, contract time: $P = 0.00$, $F = 13.37$, $\eta^2 = 0.57$, index: $P = 0.00$, $F = 12.22$, partial $\eta^2 = 0.55$). However, no significant interaction (RJ height: $P = 0.66$, $F = 0.40$, $\eta^2 = 0.04$, contract time: $P = 0.42$, $F = 0.93$, partial $\eta^2 = 0.09$, index: $P = 0.17$, $F = 1.65$, partial $\eta^2 = 0.14$) or main effect for trial (RJ height: $P = 0.24$, $F = 1.58$, partial $\eta^2 = 0.14$, contract time: $P = 0.34$, $F = 0.99$, partial $\eta^2 = 0.09$, index: $P = 0.93$, $F = 0.01$, partial $\eta^2 = 0.001$) was observed for any variables.

Figure 4 presents time course of changes in power output during repeated sprint test during Ex1 and Ex2 and at 24 h during the post-exercise period. Power output during repeated sprint test markedly decreased with progress of number of sprints (main effect for set: $P = 0.00$, $F = 93.7$, partial $\eta^2 = 0.90$ for Ex1, $P = 0.00$, $F = 81.1$, partial $\eta^2 = 0.89$ for Ex2, $P = 0.00$, $F = 27.6$, partial $\eta^2 = 0.73$ for 24 h). However, no significant interaction (trial × sprint) or main effect for trial was observed during Ex1 (interaction: $P = 0.46$, $F = 0.99$, partial $\eta^2 = 0.09$, main effect for trial: $P = 0.72$, $F = 0.14$, partial $\eta^2 = 0.01$), during Ex2 (interaction: $P = 0.74$, $F = 0.38$, partial $\eta^2 = 0.04$, main effect for trial: $P = 0.42$, $F = 0.70$, partial $\eta^2 = 0.07$), or at 24 h (interaction: $P = 0.22$, $F = 1.54$, partial $\eta^2 = 0.13$, main effect for trial: $P = 0.65$, $F = 0.22$, partial $\eta^2 = 0.73$) during the post-exercise period. Furthermore, power output decrement did not differ significantly between the two trials during Ex1, during Ex2, or at 24 h during post-exercise period ($P > 0.05$).

Blood lactate concentrations were markedly increased after Ex1 and Ex2 (main effect for time: $P = 0.00$, $F = 73.5$, partial $\eta^2 = 0.88$). However, there responses were similar between the CG and CON trials, and no significant difference between the trials was not observed at any time points (interaction: $P = 0.38$, $F = 0.93$, partial η^2

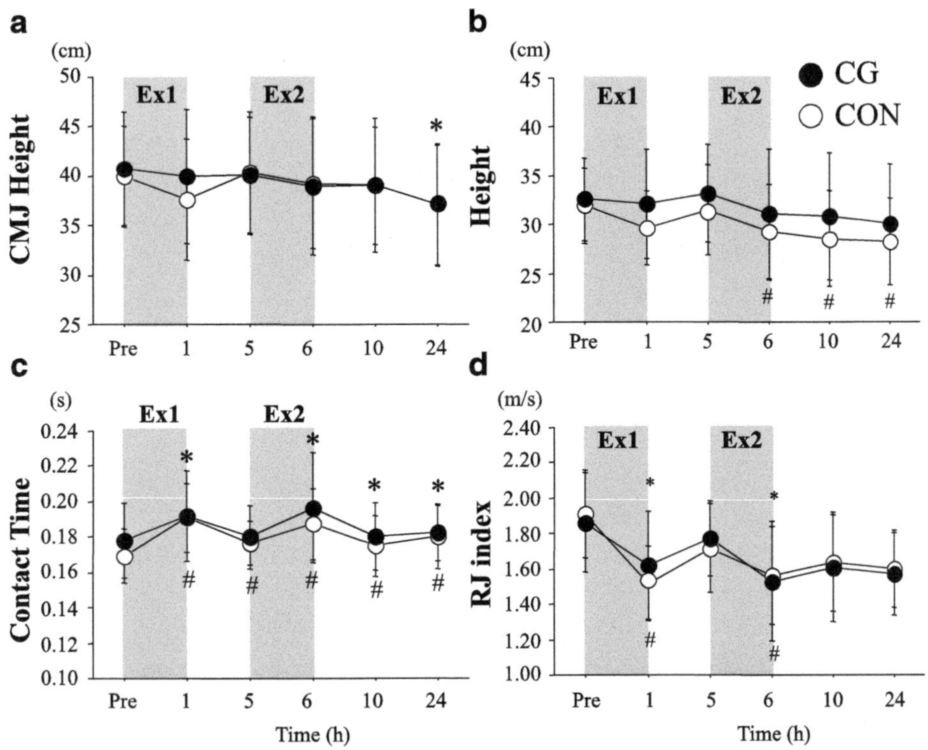

Fig. 3 Results of CMJ (**a**) and RJ (**b**–**d**). Height of CMJ (**a**) and height (**b**), contact time (**c**), and index (**d**) during RJ are presented here. *Shaded boxes* indicate duration of exercises. Values are means ± SD. **P* < 0.05 vs. Pre (CG); #*P* < 0.05 vs. Pre (CON)

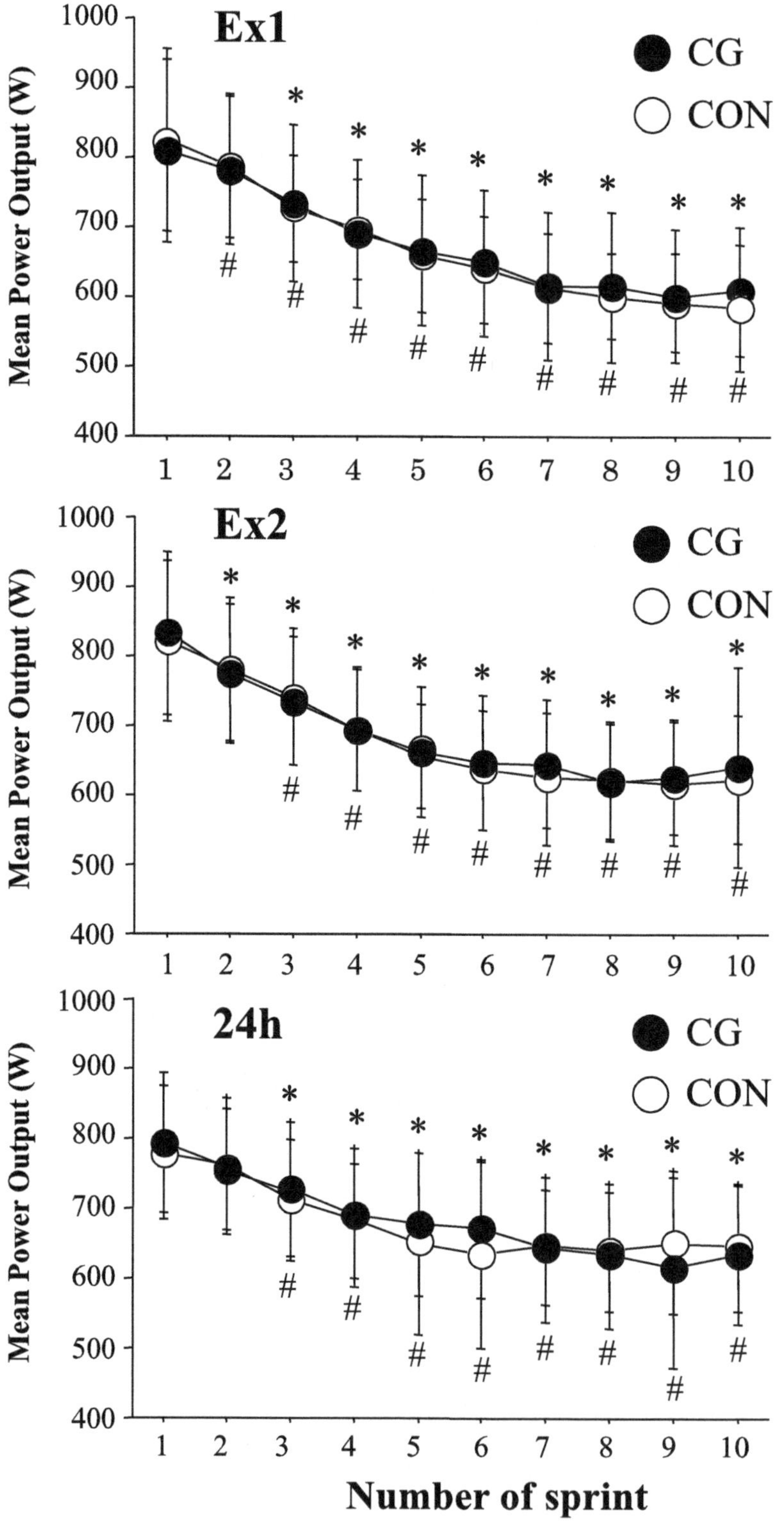

Fig. 4 Power output during repeated sprint test. Values are means ± SD. *$P < 0.05$ vs. the value in the first sprint (CG); #$P < 0.05$ vs. the value in the first sprint (CON)

= 0.09). Similarly, exercise increased significantly blood glucose concentration (main effect for time: $P = 0.00$, $F = 19.2$, partial $\eta^2 = 0.66$), with no significant difference between the two trials (interaction: $P = 0.18$, $F = 1.61$, partial $\eta^2 = 0.14$, main effect for trial: $P = 0.40$, $F = 0.76$, partial $\eta^2 = 0.07$).

Table 1 presents changes in blood variables before exercise and at 24 h of post-exercise period. Before the exercise, there was no significant difference for any blood variables between the two trials. Serum Mb concentration did not change significantly after exercise ($P = 0.16$, $F = 2.23$, partial $\eta^2 = 0.18$), with no significant difference between the trials (interaction: $P = 0.32$, $F = 1.09$, partial $\eta^2 = 0.10$). Serum CK concentration significantly increased at 24 h during post-exercise period (main effect for time: $P = 0.046$, $F = 5.17$, partial $\eta^2 = 0.34$), and no significant interaction (trial × time) or main effect for trial was observed (interaction: $P = 0.39$, $F = 0.81$, partial $\eta^2 = 0.08$, main effect for trial: $P = 0.26$, $F = 1.45$, partial $\eta^2 = 0.13$). Plasma IL-6 and serum leptin concentrations did not change significantly at 24 h during post-exercise period (interaction: $P = 0.34$, $F = 1.05$, partial $\eta^2 = 0.12$ for plasma IL-6, $P = 0.28$, $F = 1.30$, partial $\eta^2 = 0.13$ for serum leptin).

The score of subjective muscle soreness at 24 h during post-exercise period was significantly lower in the CG trial than in the CON trial for pectoral major muscle [CG: 33 ± 21 mm, CON: 48 ± 25 mm, $P = 0.04$, d = 0.65], while the value was inversely lower in the CON trial than in the CG trial for hamstring [CG: 43 ± 24 mm, CON: 34 ± 26 mm, $P = 0.047$, d = 0.36]. There was no significant difference in scores of subjective muscle soreness for biceps branch, triceps brachii, or quadriceps femoris. Exercise significantly increased score of subjective fatigue (main effect for time: $P = 0.00$, $F = 64.26$, partial $\eta^2 = 0.87$). However, time course of change in subjective fatigue was not significantly different between the two trials during post-exercise period (interaction: $P = 0.52$, $F = 0.85$, partial $\eta^2 = 0.08$, main effect for trial: $P = 0.75$, $F = 0.11$, partial $\eta^2 = 0.01$).

Table 1 Changes in blood variables

		Pre			24 h		
Myoglobin (ng/mL)	CG	35	±	9	64	±	28*
	CON	32	±	6	56	±	36*
Creatine kinase (U/L)	CG	161	±	114	602	±	427*
	CON	110	±	34	544	±	286*
IL-6 (pg/mL)	CG	0.16	±	0.18	0.14	±	0.12
	CON	0.10	±	0.05	0.11	±	0.06
Leptin (ng/mL)	CG	1.4	±	1.7	1.3	±	1.8
	CON	1.5	±	1.8	1.1	±	1.5

Values are means ± SD
*Significantly different from Pre ($P < 0.05$)

Discussion

In the present study, we have determined influence of wearing CG during post-exercise period on changes in exercise performance and exercise-induced muscle damage markers in response to two repeated bouts of training sessions separated with 4 h of rest period. Consequently, time-course changes in exercise performances for lower limb muscles or muscle damage markers in blood were similar between CG and CON trials. For the upper body muscles, no significant interaction (trial × time) or main effect for trial was found for MPO during bench press exercise. However, the use of CG revealed faster recovery of the MPO 4 h after the first bout (Ex1) and second bout (Ex2) of exercise sessions ($P > 0.05$ vs. baseline value), whereas in the CON trial, the MPO remained significantly lower throughout 24 h of post-exercise period.

The height of CMJ and performance variables for RJ did not differ significantly between CG and CON trials over 24 h of post-exercise period. Moreover, no significant difference in repeated sprint ability was observed between the two trials at any time points. These results differ from the findings from earlier studies in which wearing CG during post-exercise period promoted recovery of CMJ height [6, 22], MVC [6, 24], maximal isokinetic strength for lower limb muscles [22], and maximal power output during 5 min of pedaling [10]. In the present study, all subjects started wearing the CG from immediately after completing first bout of exercise (Ex1), and we have tested whether the recovery of muscle function was improved even during the early phase (4 h) of post-exercise period. In a previous study by Jakemen et al. [6], the subjects wore the CG for 12 h after 100 drop jumps. Consequently, recovery of performances for squat jump and CMJ was significantly improved by wearing CG at 24 h, but not at 1 h during post-exercise period. We have previously observed that wearing CG during post-exercise period facilitated significantly recovery of MVC for lower limb muscles at 24 h after resistance exercise. However, improved recovery of MVC was not observed at 1, 3, 5, and 8 h after the exercise [24]. Therefore, 4 h of wearing CG after the first exercise session may be insufficient to assist recovery of muscle function for lower limb muscles. Moreover, repeated sprint ability did not differ significantly between the two trials during Ex2 (at 4 h after completing Ex1) or at 24 h during post-exercise period. Because exercise-induced muscle damage impairs repeated sprint ability and sprint running performance [31], the use of CG during post-exercise period was expected to attenuate impairment of repeated sprint ability. The absence of improved repeated spring ability in the CG trial was inconsistent with a report [23] that showed increased performance for repeated sprint performance (10 × 40 m run) by wearing CG during 24 h of post-exercise period in rugby players. However, in the present study, repeated sprint ability during Ex2 and at 24 h during post-exercise period did not differ significantly from the value during Ex1 (baseline value) in either trial, suggesting that the exercise-induced decrement of power output was not evident during post-exercise period.

The MPO during bench press exercise significantly decreased immediately after Ex1 and Ex2 in both trials. However, in the CG trial, the MPO was recovered to baseline value following wearing CG for 4 h after both Ex1 and Ex2, while the values at the same time points remained significantly lower from baseline value in the CON trial. Influence of wearing CG on recovery of muscle function for upper body muscles has not been fully elucidated, but bench press throw power was significantly higher at 24 h after resistance exercise when the subjects wore the whole-body CG during post-exercise period. In contrast, promoted recovery of muscle function was not observed for lower limb muscles [7]. We have also shown that recovery of 1RM for chest press was significantly improved at 3, 5, and 8 h after the resistance exercise by wearing whole-body CG during post-exercise period [24]. Although somewhat inconsistent results exist [32], it is likely that wearing whole-body CG elicits recovery for upper body muscle function rather than for lower body muscles. However, in the present study, the recovery enhancing effect for upper body muscle function by wearing CG was smaller compared with two previous studies using resistance exercise protocols [7, 24]. The different outcome may be explained by difference in number of resistance exercise employed (four to six exercises in the previous studies vs. three exercises in the present study).

According to a recent systematic review and meta-analysis by Hill et al. [33], the use of CG after damaging exercise had a moderate effect in reducing the severity of muscle soreness and CK elevation and promoting recovery of muscle strength and power. In fact, 66% of the subjects analyzed (205 subjects in total from different studies) experienced reduced elevation of CK concentration. Similarly, Kraemer et al. [7] revealed that serum CK concentration at 24 h after resistance exercise was significantly lower after wearing whole-body CG during post-exercise period than the value after wearing non-compression garment. The score of muscle soreness for pectoral major muscle was significantly lower in the CG trial at 24 h during post-exercise period. Although mechanism for reduced muscle damage markers by wearing CG is still speculative, applied pressure by the garments generates an external pressure gradient that attenuates changes in osmotic pressure and reduces the space available for swelling and hematoma to occur [23]. A reduction of osmotic pressure with attenuating swelling may provide impaired inflammatory action and experience of soreness. In contrast, there were no significant differences between the two trials at 24 h during post-exercise period for serum CK, Mb, leptin, and plasma IL-6 concentrations. This result is not surprising, because the finding corresponds to previous reports presenting no influence of CG during post-exercise period on muscle damage markers in blood (e.g., CK, Mb, IL-6, C-reactive protein) [24, 34, 35].

Some limitations in the present study need to be considered carefully. In the present study, a psychological effect cannot be excluded because it is difficult to use CG in completely blinded conditions. However, we did not display detailed information of the prescribed CG, including expected outcomes and hypothesis. Furthermore, blood variables in the present study reflect physiological responses for both upper and lower body muscles, and we cannot clarify the differences in muscle damage and inflammatory responses between upper body and lower body muscles. Finally, we were not able to measure the pressure levels applied for the present subjects, although we have previously determined the pressure levels of the same CG among different subjects [25]. Therefore, it is possible that inter-individual differences of pressure levels and/or insufficient levels of pressure may have masked efficacy of the CG.

From practical viewpoints, the present findings may provide information regarding post-exercise treatment to promote recovery of maximal power output during training schedule with strenuous training sessions twice a day. The facilitation of recovery of muscular power output will be important to improve quality of subsequent training session, and wearing the CG during post-exercise period may have had some positive effects on recovery. Further researches are required to determine the efficacy of combined effects of CG and other traditional treatments (e.g., cold water immersion) on recovery of exercise performance in competitive athletes.

Conclusions

In conclusion, wearing whole-body CG during post-exercise period after two bouts of exercise sessions separated with 4 h of rest period did not promote recovery of muscle function for lower limb muscles or did not affect exercise-induced muscle damage markers in blood among physically active males. However, it was likely that the use of CG during post-exercise period may have had some favorable effect on recovery of power output and severity of muscle soreness for upper body muscles.

Abbreviations

1RM: One-repetition maximum; ANOVA: Analysis of variance; CG trial: Trial with wearing compression garment during post-exercise period; CK: Creatine kinase; CMJ: Counter movement jump; CON trial: Trial without wearing compression garment during post-exercise period; ELISA: Enzyme-linked immunosorbent assay; IL-6: Interleukin-6; Mb: Myoglobin; MPO: Mean power output; RJ: Rebound jump; SD: Standard deviation; VAS: Visual analogue scale

Acknowledgements
The present study was supported by a Grant-in-Aid for Scientific Research from the Japan Society for the Promotion of Science. We would like to thank all of the subjects who participated in the study.

Funding
This study is funded by the Japan Society for the Promotion of Science.

Authors' contributions
KG contributed to the study design, data collection, analysis, and manuscript writing. SM contributed to the data collection, analysis, and manuscript writing. AM contributed to the study design, data collection, and analysis. All authors read and approved the final manuscript.

Competing interests
There is no conflict of interest to be declared by any of the authors.

References
1. Bahnert A, Norton K, Lock P. Association between post-game recovery protocols, physical and perceived recovery, and performance in elite Australian Football League players. J Sci Med Sport Elsevier. 2013;16:151–6.
2. Viitasalo JT, Niemelä K, Kaappola R, Korjus T, Levola M, Mononen HV, et al. Warm underwater water-jet massage improves recovery from intense physical exercise. Eur J Appl Physiol Occup Physiol. 1995;71:431–8.
3. Suzuki M, Umeda T, Nakaji S, Shimoyama T, Mashiko T, Sugawara K. Effect of incorporating low intensity exercise into the recovery period after a rugby match. Br J Sports Med. 2004;38:436–40.
4. Gill ND, Beaven CM, Cook C. Effectiveness of post-match recovery strategies in rugby players. Br J Sports Med. 2006;40:260–3.
5. Barnett A. Using recovery modalities between training sessions in elite athletes: does it help? Sports Med. 2006;36:781–96.
6. Jakeman JR, Byrne C, Eston RG. Lower limb compression garment improves recovery from exercise-induced muscle damage in young, active females. Eur J Appl Physiol. 2010;109:1137–44.
7. Kraemer WJ, Flanagan SD, Comstock BA, Fragala MS, Earp JE, Dunn-Lewis C, et al. Effects of a whole body compression garment on markers of recovery after a heavy resistance workout in men and women. J Strength Cond Res. 2010;24:804–14.
8. MacRae BA, Cotter JD, Laing RM. Compression garments and exercise: garment considerations, physiology and performance. Sports Med. 2011;41: 815–43.
9. Berry MJ, McMurray RG. Effects of graduated compression stockings on blood lactate following an exhaustive bout of exercise. Am J Phys Med. 1987;66:121–32.
10. Chatard JC, Atlaoui D, Farjanel J, Louisy F, Rastel D, Guézennec CY. Elastic stockings, performance and leg pain recovery in 63-year-old sportsmen. Eur J Appl Physiol. 2004;93:347–52.
11. Bringard A, Perrey S, Belluye N. Aerobic energy cost and sensation responses during submaximal running exercise–positive effects of wearing compression tights. Int J Sports Med. 2006;27:373–8.
12. Scanlan AT, Dascombe BJ, Reaburn PRJ, Osborne M. The effects of wearing lower-body compression garments during endurance cycling. Int J Sports Physiol Perform. 2008;3:424–38.
13. Ali A, Creasy RH, Edge JA. Physiological effects of wearing graduated compression stockings during running. Eur J Appl Physiol. 2010;109:1017–25.
14. Duffield R, Cannon J, King M. The effects of compression garments on recovery of muscle performance following high-intensity sprint and plyometric exercise. J Sci Med Sport. 2010;13:136–40.
15. Dascombe BJ, Hoare TK, Sear JA, Reaburn PR, Scanlan AT. The effects of wearing undersized lower-body compression garments on endurance running performance. Int J Sports Physiol Perform. 2011;6:160–73.
16. Faulkner JA, Gleadon D, McLaren J, Jakeman JR. Effect of lower-limb compression clothing on 400-m sprint performance. J Strength Cond Res. 2013;27:669–76.
17. Del Coso J, Areces F, Salinero JJ, González-Millán C, Abián-Vicén J, Soriano L, et al. Compression stockings do not improve muscular performance during a half-ironman triathlon race. Eur J Appl Physiol. 2014;114:587–95.
18. Sperlich B, Born D-P, Zinner C, Hauser A, Holmberg H-C. Does upper-body compression improve 3 × 3-min double-poling sprint performance? Int J Sports Physiol Perform. 2014;9:48–57.
19. Beliard S, Chauveau M, Moscatiello T, Cros F, Ecarnot F, Becker F. Compression garments and exercise: no influence of pressure applied. J Sports Sci Med. 2015;14:75–83.
20. Engel FA, Holmberg H-C, Sperlich B. Is There Evidence that Runners can Benefit from Wearing Compression Clothing? Sports Med. 2016;46:1939–52.
21. Kraemer WJ, Bush JA, Wickham RB, Denegar CR, Gómez AL, Gotshalk LA, et al. Influence of compression therapy on symptoms following soft tissue injury from maximal eccentric exercise. J Orthop Sports Phys Ther. 2001;31: 282–90.
22. Jakeman JR, Byrne C, Eston RG. Efficacy of lower limb compression and combined treatment of manual massage and lower limb compression on symptoms of exercise-induced muscle damage in women. J Strength Cond Res. 2010;24:3157–65.
23. Hamlin MJ, Mitchell CJ, Ward FD, Draper N, Shearman JP, Kimber NE. Effect of compression garments on short-term recovery of repeated sprint and 3-Km running performance in Rugby Union players. J Strength Cond Res. 2012;26:2975–82.
24. Goto K, Morishima T. Compression garment promotes muscular strength recovery after resistance exercise. Med Sci Sports Exerc. 2014;46:2265–70.
25. Mizuno S, Morii I, Tsuchiya Y, Goto K. Wearing compression garment after endurance exercise promotes recovery of exercise performance. Int J Sports Med. 2016;37:870–7.
26. Duffield R, Murphy A, Kellett A, Reid M. Recovery from repeated on-court tennis sessions: combining cold-water immersion, compression, and sleep recovery interventions. Int J Sports Physiol Perform. 2014;9:273–82.
27. Born D-P, Sperlich B, Holmberg H-C. Bringing light into the dark: effects of compression clothing on performance and recovery. Int J Sports Physiol Perform. 2013;8:4–18.
28. Yanagisawa O, Niitsu M, Yoshioka H, Goto K, Kudo H, Itai Y. The use of magnetic resonance imaging to evaluate the effects of cooling on skeletal muscle after strenuous exercise. Eur J Appl Physiol. 2003;89:53–62.
29. Bailey DM, Erith SJ, Griffin PJ, Dowson A, Brewer DS, Gant N, et al. Influence of cold-water immersion on indices of muscle damage following prolonged intermittent shuttle running. J Sports Sci. 2007;25:1163–70.
30. Vaile J, Halson S, Gill N, Dawson B. Effect of cold water immersion on repeat cycling performance and thermoregulation in the heat. J Sports Sci. 2008; 26:431–40.
31. Twist C, Eston R. The effects of exercise-induced muscle damage on maximal intensity intermittent exercise performance. Eur J Appl Physiol. 2005;94:652–8.
32. Duffield R, Edge J, Merrells R, Hawke E, Barnes M, Simcock D, et al. The effects of compression garments on intermittent exercise performance and recovery on consecutive days. Int J Sports Physiol Perform. 2008;3:454–68.
33. Hill J, Howatson G, van Someren K, Leeder J, Pedlar C. Compression garments and recovery from exercise-induced muscle damage: a meta-analysis. Br J Sports Med. 2014;48:1340–6.
34. Pruscino CL, Halson S, Hargreaves M. Effects of compression garments on recovery following intermittent exercise. Eur J Appl Physiol. 2013;113:1585–96.
35. Hill JA, Howatson G, van Someren KA, Walshe I, Pedlar CR. Influence of compression garments on recovery after marathon running. J Strength Cond Res. 2014;28:2228–35.

Observational Review and Analysis of Concussion: a Method for Conducting a Standardized Video Analysis of Concussion in Rugby League

Andrew J. Gardner[1,2*], Christopher R. Levi[1,2] and Grant L. Iverson[3,4,5]

Abstract

Background: Several professional contact and collision sports have recently introduced the use of sideline video review for club medical staff to help identify and manage concussions. As such, reviewing video footage on the sideline has become increasingly relied upon to assist with improving the identification of possible injury. However, as yet, a standardized method for reviewing such video footage in rugby league has not been published. The aim of this study is to evaluate whether independent raters reliably agreed on the injury characterization when using a standardized observational instrument to record video footage of National Rugby League (NRL) concussions.

Methods: Video footage of 25 concussions were randomly selected from a pool of 80 medically diagnosed concussions from the 2013–2014 NRL seasons. Four raters (two naïve and two expert) independently viewed video footage of 25 NRL concussions and completed the Observational Review and Analysis of Concussion form for the purpose of this inter-rater reliability study. The inter-rater reliability was calculated using Cohen's kappa (κ) and intra-class correlation (ICC) statistics. The two naïve raters and the two expert raters were compared with one another separately.

Results: A considerable number of components for the naïve and expert raters had almost perfect agreement (κ or ICC value ≥ 0.9), 9 of 22 (41%) components for naïve raters and 21 of 22 (95%) components for expert raters. For the concussion signs, however, the majority of the rating agreement was moderate (κ value 0.6–0.79); both the naïve and expert raters had 4 of 6 (67%) concussion signs with moderate agreement. The most difficult concussion sign to achieve agreement on was blank or vacant stare, which had weak (κ value 0.4–0.59) agreement for both naïve and expert raters.

Conclusions: There appears to be value in expert raters, but less value for naive raters, in using the new Observational Review and Analysis of Concussion (ORAC) Form. The ORAC Form has high inter-rater agreement for most data elements, and it can be used by expert raters evaluating video footage of possible concussion in the NRL.

Keywords: Concussion, Video analysis, Injury management

Key Points

- Identifying concussion from the sideline during a match is challenging, but with the use of video out-of-view or fleeting signs may be captured and a player can be removed from play.
- Having a reliable form for coding and analysing concussion can be a useful adjunct to the sideline clinical management strategy of the athletic trainer and team physician.

We present the first objective and reliable coding form for rugby league to capture the game situation, the mechanism of injury, and possible signs of concussion.

* Correspondence: andrew.gardner@neurogard.com.au
[1]Centre for Stroke and Brain Injury, School of Medicine and Public Health, University of Newcastle, Callaghan, New South Wales, Australia
[2]Hunter New England Local Health District Sports Concussion Program, John Hunter Hospital, Newcastle, New South Wales, Australia
Full list of author information is available at the end of the article

Background

Rugby league is a high-intensity collision sport [23]. The game is played continuously in two 40-min halves, and game-play involves two teams of 13 on-field players and four interchange players who may be switched in and out of the game. The published incidence rates of concussion in rugby league vary [12]; at the National Rugby League (NRL) level, medically diagnosed concussions in three clubs from the 2013 season revealed an incidence rate of 14.8 concussions per 1000 player match hours [15], while a rate of 28.3 concussion per 1000 player match hours were reported from one NRL club over a 15-year (1998–2012) period [41]. The incidence of use of the concussion interchange rule (CIR) was 24.0 (95% CI 20.7–27.9) uses of the CIR per 1000 NRL player match hours [14] and 44.9 (95% CI 38.5–52.3) uses of the CIR per 1000 National Youth Competition player match hours [15].

One method that has becoming increasingly relied upon to assist with improving the identification of possible concussion has been the review of video footage on the sideline. The use of video for reviewing a concussion may identify signs of injury that may have been blocked from view or otherwise missed by medical staff. A number of professional contact and collision sports have recently introduced the use of sideline video review for club medical staff to help identify and manage concussions [29]. A number of studies of video footage have been conducted in a variety of sports, for example, rugby league [13–15], rugby union [25], and Australian Rules Football [9, 29, 30]. Other sports, such as boxing [37], soccer [1], taekwondo [24], ice hockey [6, 10, 18, 19], and lacrosse [28], have also reported on the use of video footage for understanding the circumstances and mechanisms of injury unique to their sports. A risk prediction model among National Hockey League (NHL) players reported that both visual signs of concussion and information pertaining to mechanisms of injury improved a clinician's ability to identify athletes who should be removed from play and evaluated [6]. Specifically, the study indicated that suspected loss of consciousness, motor incoordination or balance problems, being in a fight, having an initial hit from another player's shoulder, and having a secondary hit on the ice were all associated with increased risk of subsequent concussion diagnosis.

Sport-specific coding criteria of concussion for game situational factors and injury mechanisms have been developed for hockey (e.g., the 'Heads-Up Checklist' [20]), but these criteria do not generalize to other sports like rugby union or rugby league. Video criteria and coding forms require validation in each individual sport [29, 30]. In a more recent NHL study examining the predictive ability of visual signs of concussion, loss of consciousness, motor incoordination, and blank/vacant look had a positive association with concussion diagnosis, whereas slow to get up and clutching of the head, despite occurring frequently, had low positive predictive values [10].

Several video studies have examined signs of concussion, together with player characteristics, injury characteristics, and match situational factors, in professional rugby league [13–15]. In 2014, video reviews of injury have been implemented in the NRL to help medical staff and promote player health and safety. The aim of this study was to present a standardized observational recording form and to determine whether independent raters agreed on the antecedent events, mechanisms of injury, and concussion signs when using the form to code digital video records of concussions in the NRL.

Methods

Participants

This study was conducted in the national professional rugby league competition in Australia during the 2013 and 2014 seasons. All medically diagnosed concussion events during 2013 and 2014 NRL seasons were available to be included in this study.

Procedure

For this study, 25 medically diagnosed concussions were randomly selected from the 2013 to 2014 NRL seasons' video library ($n = 80$). The video library included only excerpts of the incidents for each case, not the entire game. The duration of the game footage recorded for each of the 25 cases selected from the library and used in this study ranged from 138 to 473 s. Four raters (two 'expert' and two 'naïve') independently reviewed the video footage of the 25 NRL concussion events. The naïve raters were novices of the sport. They had limited to no knowledge or experience with rugby league match play and no experience identifying and managing concussion. The expert raters were defined as individuals with experience in rugby league match play and expertise in concussion management at the professional (NRL) level. Both expert raters had at least one NRL season of experience working on the sideline for an NRL club with the responsibility of identifying and assessing athletes suspected of having sustained a concussion.

The medically diagnosed NRL concussion library was gathered from three teams during the 2013 season ($n = 20$ concussions) [13], and all teams during the 2014 NRL season ($n = 60$ concussions). The Concussion in Sport Group consensus definition of concussion was used by all clubs involved in this study [32]. Raters viewed the match digital records of 25 concussions using the Quicktime Multimedia Player V.7.7.5. Each rater completed all components of the form for each of the 25 concussion events. The raters were permitted to view the incident as many times as required and in any playback speed as deemed necessary to complete all categories of the form. All participants provided informed consent. This study was conducted in accordance with the standards of the ethics outlined in the Declaration of Helsinki. Approval of this study was provided by the University of Newcastle Human Ethics Committee.

Instruments

A rating form was created to provide a simple but standardized framework for coding and analysing video footage of the situations and consequences of concussion events in rugby league. The form was developed by a neuropsychologist with extensive experience in the sport and concussion management and was based on work conducted previously in ice hockey in North America, and a similar, but not identical, approach to validating the form was used for the validation of the 'Heads-Up Checklist' [20]. The form was adapted to include specific information to rugby league. Concussion signs that have been previously examined in video review studies in rugby league were included [13–15]. The form consists of various sections related to the player and game characteristics (e.g., ball carrier versus tackler, tackle height, type of play, etc.), the anatomical region of contact, the injury location on the field of play, the injured player's on-field management, and six possible concussion signs (see Fig. 1).

Statistical Analysis

The results from the two naïve raters and the expert raters were considered separately. The intra-class correlation (ICC) was used to determine the level of agreement between the two naïve raters and the two expert raters for interval and ratio variables (i.e. 'number of players in tackle' and 'time taken to leave'). Inter-rater reliability analyses using Cohen's kappa (κ) statistics [17] were used to determine the level of agreement between the two naïve raters and the two expert raters for all other (nominal) variables. Unlike the total percent agreement, Cohen's kappa considers the proportional agreement that could occur simply by chance. The κ coefficients are calculated by considering the proportion of rater agreement and the expected proportion [17]. Using the interpretations of κ described by McHugh [34], κ agreement was categorized as almost perfect (>.90), strong (.80–.90), moderate (.60–.79), weak (.40–.59), minimal (.21–.39) and none (0–.20). All analyses were performed using IBM SPSS Statistics V.23.0 [21] and used two-sided tests for significance at the 0.05 level, with 95% confidence intervals (CIs).

Results

The inter-rater reliabilities for the various components of the rating form for both the naïve and expert raters are

Observational Review and Analysis of Concussion (ORAC) Form

Time in Game: __:__min Score: __-__ **Day** or **Night** match (please circle)? Tackle No?: ____

Injured player: ☐ Ball Carrier ☐ Tackler ☐ Other: ____ **Playing Position:** ____

Tackle Height? ☐ High (torso or higher) ☐ Low (hip height or lower)

Foul Play? Was a penalty awarded? ☐ Yes ☐ No ☐ Unsure

Was the offending player placed on report? ☐ Yes ☐ No ☐ Unsure

Type of play?

☐ Hit up ☐ Kick return ☐ Kicking ☐ Contesting possession of the ball

☐ Backline move ☐ Line Break

Initial contact (from the striking player to the player who was struck)?

☐ Shoulder ☐ Upper arm ☐ Forearm/wrist/hand ☐ Elbow ☐ Head/face

☐ Torso/chest ☐ Hip ☐ Thigh/upper leg ☐ Knee

☐ Lower leg/foot/boot ☐ Playing surface ☐ other: ____

☐ **N/A - Secondary contact (from the striking player to the player who was struck, if applicable)?**

☐ Shoulder ☐ Upper arm ☐ Forearm/wrist/hand ☐ Elbow ☐ Head/face

☐ Torso/chest ☐ Hip ☐ Thigh/upper leg ☐ Knee

☐ Lower leg/foot/boot ☐ Playing surface ☐ other: ____.

☐ **N/A - Tertiary contact (from the striking player to the player who was struck, if applicable)?**

☐ Shoulder ☐ Upper arm ☐ Forearm/wrist/hand ☐ Elbow ☐ Head/face

☐ Torso/chest ☐ Hip ☐ Thigh/upper leg ☐ Knee

☐ Lower leg/foot/boot ☐ Playing surface ☐ other: ____.

Region of Contact

☐ Head/Face ☐ Neck ☐ Chest/Torso ☐ Back ☐ Inconclusive

Location of impact

☐ Anterior ☐ Posterior ☐ Lateral ☐ Dorsal (top of head) ☐ Inconclusive

Number of players involved in the tackle: ____

Anticipation of the impact by player who was struck? ☐ Yes ☐ No ☐ Unsure

On-field Medical Attention? ☐ Yes ☐ No ☐ Unsure

Removed from Play? ☐ Yes ☐ No ☐ Unsure

How Did the Player Leave the Field?

☐ Left Field of Play Unassisted ☐ Walked off assisted by Trainer(s) ☐ Stretcher

☐ Medicab ☐ Unsure / no video footage / inconclusive ☐ Other: ____

Location on the Field (Place an X on the field where the incident took place & an arrow for the direction of play)

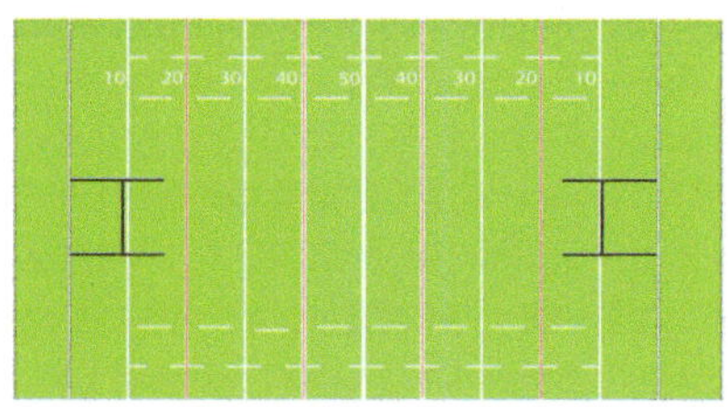

Time taken to leave the field of play? ____ **seconds.**

If removed from play, did the player return to play later in the same game? ☐ Yes ☐ No

Concussive Signs on Video (please refer to *concussion signs* definitions at the bottom of this page)

(i) Did the player clutch or shake their head? ☐ Yes ☐ No ☐ Insufficient video footage to decide

(ii) Was the player slow to get up? ☐ Yes ☐ No ☐ Insufficient video footage to decide

(iii) Did the player have wobbly legs? ☐ Yes ☐ No ☐ Insufficient video or player did not return to their feet.

(iv) Evidence of a blank/vacant stare? ☐ Yes ☐ No ☐ Insufficient video footage to decide

(v) Evidence of unresponsiveness? ☐ Yes ☐ No ☐ Insufficient video footage to decide

* *Length of time the player remained motionless on the playing surface:* ____ secs.

(vi) Evidence of a post-impact seizure? ☐ Yes ☐ No ☐ Insufficient video footage to decide

Fig. 1 The Observational Review and Analysis of Concussion (ORAC) Form

presented in Table 1. For the naïve raters, 6 of 20 (30%) components of the form, and 5 of 6 (83%) concussions signs, had κ values between .60 and .79 ('moderate' agreement), while 2 of 2 (100%) interval/ratio variables of the form had very good ICC. According to the interpretations of κ described by McHugh [34], 8 of 22 components were categorized as 'almost perfect'; 3 components were classified as 'strong'; 2 components were classified as 'weak'; 2 components were classified as 'minimal'; and one of the components (playing position) was not classified. For the concussion signs, the naïve raters had no signs that had 'almost perfect' or 'strong' agreement; 5 (83%) signs were classified as 'moderate' and 1 (17%) sign was classified as 'weak'.

For the expert raters, 19 of 20 (95%) components of the form had κ values of between .90–1.00 ('almost perfect' agreement) and one (5%) had moderate agreement. The expert raters had perfect ICC for 2 of 2 (100%) interval/ratio variables. For the concussion signs, the expert raters had 1 of 6 (17%) of concussions signs with κ values between .80–.90 ('strong' agreement); 4 (67%) of were classified as 'moderate'; and 1 (17%) was classified as 'weak' agreement. No signs classified by either the naïve or expert raters had a 'minimal' or 'none' level of agreement.

There were nine components that were all rated with 'almost perfect' agreement by both the naïve and the expert raters (game time, score, whether the concussed player was a ball carrier or a tackler, the number of players involved in the tackle, whether the offending player was placed on report by a match official, the initial contact, the region of contact, whether the player was removed from play, and how the player left the field). The level of agreement between the expert raters and between the naïve raters was also very consistent for the tackle height and whether the injury occurred as a result of foul play (i.e., the offending player was penalized). The naïve raters had a 'strong' level of agreement for these components. The naïve raters had a moderate level of agreement on whether the game was played during the night or day, the tackle number in the set, the anatomical location of the impact, and the location of the field where the concussion took place, whereas all of these components had an 'almost perfect' level of agreement between the two expert raters. The expert raters also achieved an 'almost perfect' level of agreement on the secondary contact, whether the concussed player had anticipated the impact that caused the injury, and the time taken to leave the field of play. However, the naïve raters only had a 'minimal' level of agreement on these components. For type of play, and whether or not the player returned to play, the naïve raters had a 'weak' agreement on these components compared to the 'almost perfect' agreement by the expert raters. Whether or not there was secondary contact was the most difficult component to agree upon; the expert raters' level of agreement was 'moderate' for this component, and the naive raters' level of agreement was 'minimal' (see Table 1).

Regarding concussion signs, slow to get up had the best level of agreement between expert and naïve raters of all possible concussion signs (strong and moderate agreement, respectively), whereas a blank or vacant stare had the worst agreement (both rater groups had a 'weak' level of agreement). Clutch or shake head, gait ataxia (or having wobbly legs), unresponsiveness, and post-impact seizure-like features had moderate agreement for both expert and naïve raters.

Discussion

Rugby League is a full contact collision sport that has high concussion incidence rates [13–15]. The in-game management and decision-making process surrounding concussion is a challenge. Video review is increasingly being used as one method for improving this in-game decision-making process for medical staff, although a standardized approach to the use of such information had not been published. Although there is a large body of research examining on-field markers of concussion and their association with outcome [2–5, 7, 8, 11, 16, 22, 26, 27, 31, 33, 35, 36, 38–40, 42–46], very few of these studies have been focused on possible signs of concussion at the time of injury (versus collected later as part of a questionnaire or interview with the athlete). This study presents a standardized observational form and examines intra-rater and inter-rater agreement on the antecedent events, mechanisms of injury, and concussion signs. Overall, the results of this study suggest that a certain level of knowledge about the game is required to complete the form components accurately. Expert rates achieved an 'almost perfect' level of agreement on 21/22 (95%) of components compared to only 9/22 (41%) components for the naïve raters.

In a similar study conducted with the 'Heads-Up Checklist' for National Hockey League (NHL) concussions, the naïve raters also had worse agreement across components pertaining to the antecedent events and mechanism of injury compared to the expert raters. Of the 15 components in version 1 of the Heads-Up Checklist, naïve raters 7 (47%) had weak or minimal agreement, compared to only 1 of the 15 (7%) components for the expert raters [20]. For the Heads-Up Checklist, the acceleration of the head (which was not considered a component or review item in our form) was the single component with the worst agreement across naïve and expert raters. Rating secondary contact was also challenging in the hockey study as it was in the current study. The location of the playing surface where the concussion

Table 1 Inter-rater reliability (κ, ICC) for naïve and expert raters for each component of the form

	Expert raters (κ)	McHugh [34] κ Agreement Classification	Naïve raters (κ)	McHugh [34] κ Agreement Classification
Component				
Game time	1.00	Perfect	1.00	Perfect
Score	1.00	Perfect	0.95	Perfect
Day/night game	1.00	Perfect	0.70	Moderate
Tackle number	1.00	Perfect	0.75	Moderate
Ball carrier vs. tackler	1.00	Perfect	0.92	Perfect
Playing position	1.00	Perfect	NR	N/A
Tackle height	1.00	Perfect	0.86	Strong
Foul play	0.90	Perfect	0.89	Strong
Offending player on report	0.90	Perfect	1.00	Perfect
Type of play	1.00	Perfect	0.56	Weak
Initial contact	0.90	Perfect	0.90	Perfect
Secondary contact	0.71	Moderate	0.27	Minimal
Region of contact	1.00	Perfect	1.00	Perfect
Location of impact	1.00	Perfect	0.70	Moderate
Anticipation of impact	0.70	Perfect	0.37	Minimal
On-field medical attention	1.00	Perfect	0.65	Moderate
Removal from play	1.00	Perfect	1.00	Perfect
How did the player leave	1.00	Perfect	1.00	Perfect
Location of the field	1.00	Perfect	0.79	Moderate
Did they return to play	1.00	Perfect	0.43	Weak
	Expert raters (ICC)		**Naïve raters (ICC) (95% CIs)**	
Number of players in tackle	1.00		0.87 (0.68–0.95)	
Time taken to leave	1.00		0.99 (0.97–1.00)	
	Expert raters (κ) (95% CIs)	**McHugh [34] κ Agreement Classification**	**Naïve raters (κ) (95% CIs)**	**McHugh [34] κ Agreement Classification**
Concussion signs				
Clutch or shake head	0.73 (0.46–0.93)	Moderate	0.63 (0.36–0.87)	Moderate
Slow to get up	0.83 (0.15–1.00)	Moderate	0.52 (0.09–1.00)	Strong
Gait ataxia	0.73 (0.47–0.94)	Moderate	0.60 (0.58–0.61)	Moderate
Blank/vacant stare	0.50 (0.23–0.76)	Weak	0.44 (0.15–0.71)	Weak
Unresponsiveness	0.78 (0.56–1.00)	Moderate	0.70 (0.45–0.93)	Moderate
Post-impact seizure	0.65 (N/A)	Moderate	0.53 (0.04–0.90)	Moderate

McHugh κ Agreement Classification: almost perfect (>.90), strong (.80–.90), moderate (.60–.79), weak (.40–.59), minimal (.21–.39), and none (0–.20)
CIs confidence intervals, *ICC* intra-class correlation, κ kappa, *N/A* not applicable, *NR* not recorded

occurred and the time in the game when the concussion occurred were the two components with the strongest agreement by naïve and expert raters for the hockey study [20]. For the current study, the time in the game was rated well. However, the location on the field did not have a high agreement for the naïve raters. The discrepancy between naïve raters for the hockey study compared to this rugby league study may have occurred for at least three reasons. First, we divided the playing surface in our study into 12 different components and the hockey study used fewer zones. Second, the hockey study designated offensive ends and defensive ends, whereas the rugby league study required the raters to record the direction of the play, and some of the disagreement between the naïve raters for the location on the field was due to the indication of the direction of the play. Finally, the hockey study used naïve raters who where more familiar with their sport (i.e., 'individuals with limited experience who might have played or coached [ice] hockey at a competitive level'), whereas our naïve raters were complete novices, who had limited to no experience even watching the sport as fans and certainly no experience identifying concussions.

In the current study, there were a number of variables that appear to rely on knowledge, understanding, and experience with rugby league match play (i.e., the expert raters outperformed the naïve raters). For example, there were large differences between the coding by expert and naïve raters of variables such as secondary contact and anticipation of impact. There was also a large difference between the coding by expert and naïve raters on whether the player returned to play. This variable required the raters to watch the remainder of a game (following the injury) to determine if the injured athlete subsequently returned to the field of play. Interchanges can occur during play or during a stoppage in play, and they are not always announced on the broadcaster footage. It appears that the naïve raters were not as savvy in identifying the return to play of an interchanged athlete and/or did not identify the athlete as being re-involved in match play following their return to the field of play.

As with our previous video reviews of concussion signs [14, 15], we once again found that determining whether a concussed player had a blank or vacant stare was difficult to agree upon. We had weak agreement between naïve (0.44, 95% CI = 0.15–0.71) and expert (0.50, 95% CI = 0.23–0.76) raters in this study, and our previous work has also revealed difficulty with agreement between raters (i.e., 0.36 (95% CI = 0.29 to 0.43) [14] and 0.62 (95% CI = 0.37 to 0.88) [15]). In a recent Australian Football League (AFL) video review, inter-rater reliability for the blank/vacant stare on first review was reported to be 0.24 (95% CI = 0.04 to 0.41) and minimal improvements were observed on second review [0.26 (95% CI = 0.07 to 0.43)]. The intra-rater reliability in the AFL study was somewhat better for the two raters over the two rating sessions [i.e. 0.63 (95% CI = 0.50 to 0.74) and 0.36 (95% CI = 0.18 to 0.51)]. The concussion sign 'blank/vacant stare' was reported to have 9% sensitivity, 100% specificity, 100% positive predictive value and 58% negative predictive value in the sample of AFL concussions [29]. When the quality of the video (including the zoom capacity to see the players face) is limited, attempting to code the presence or absence of a blank or vacant stare from video is challenging [15]. This supports the notion that good-quality video from multiple camera angles are crucial for effective video surveillance of injuries [30]. In the current study, however, this was not a limitation, suggesting that it is also important to have clear definitions, including the inclusion and exclusion criteria for coding concussion signs [30]. In a recent series of video reviews of concussions from the AFL [9, 29, 30], Makdissi and Davis indicated that video review may be an avenue that facilitates the assessment of the mechanism and impact of injury and allows for the identification of brief early signs of concussion [29]. The authors suggest that video analysis may be a useful adjunct to the sideline assessment of possible concussion [29] and that the implementation of a flowchart may improve the timely assessment of concussion [9].

We recently completed a study on the frequency (or base rates) of concussion signs in NRL match play (Gardner et al., under review). That study reviewed every game ($n = 201$) from the 2014 NRL season, which included 127,062 tackles, and found unresponsiveness occurred 52 times [24 (46%) were diagnosed with a concussion], slow to get up occurred 2240 times [60 (3%) were diagnosed with a concussion], clutching or shaking the head occurred 361 times [38 (11%) were diagnosed with a concussion], gait ataxia occurred 102 times [35 (34%) were diagnosed with a concussion], blank or vacant stare occurred 98 times [45 (46%) were diagnosed with a concussion], and a post-impact posturing or seizure occurred 4 times [3 (75%) were diagnosed with a concussion]. The unresponsiveness sign had 40% sensitivity, 91% specificity, 46% positive predictive value, and 89% negative predictive value. The slow to get up sign had 100% sensitivity, 50% specificity, 27% positive predictive value, and 100% negative predictive value. Clutching or shaking the head had 63% sensitivity, 46% specificity, 18% positive predictive value, and 87% negative predictive value. Gait ataxia had 58% sensitivity, 79% specificity, 34% positive predictive value, and 91% negative predictive value. Blank or vacant stare had 75% sensitivity, 84% specificity, 46% positive predictive value, and 95% negative predictive value. Post-impact seizure had 5% sensitivity, 100% specificity, 75% positive predictive value, and 85% negative predictive value in the 2014 NRL season (Gardner et al., under review).

One of the unusual and unexpected findings of this study was the discrepancy observed between the naïve raters in coding variables that were conceivably thought to be obvious (e.g., game time, score, day/night game). The naïve raters did not always have 100% agreement. Because rugby league is a continuous sport, it is common for the game to continue despite an injury, and therefore, the game clock also does not stop. As such, an injury can occur well before the game and the game clock is stopped. The discrepancies in the 'time in game' variable are explained by this issue; one of the naïve reviewers recorded the time correctly (i.e., when the injury occurred), whereas the other naïve rater often recorded the time when the game clock was stopped. In terms of the 'game score' variable, it is possible that the naïve raters were unfamiliar with teams, and therefore, errors were made in coding the score of each team. For the 'day/night game' variable, there were a number of games that were played during twilight, as well as the footage of some of those cases being zoomed in, and the wide view did not make the day/night difference obvious to the naïve raters who do not watch NRL games.

Video review appears to be a useful adjunct to traditional methods for making in-game decisions pertaining to the identification of potential concussion (and an athlete subsequently being removed from play). However, to better understand and quantify the value of this process, future research should be conducted under time limits and/or during a game to replicate the real-world/practical pressure, neither of which was replicated in this study. Future studies might focus on whether agreement between experts improves under 'ideal circumstances' (i.e. as many reviews as required without time limitations) versus 'real-world circumstances' (i.e. a quick decision required to identify a possible injury and immediately remove the athlete from play).

The current study has several limitations. Firstly, clubs used their own personnel and methods for identifying possible injuries on the field and diagnosing concussions on the sideline, which presumably makes the final specific criteria for a 'medically diagnosed concussion' variable across clubs. The current study does not generalize to the real-world use of in-game video analysis because the study was not conducted under the time pressure associated with in-game decision-making. Further, the sample size is small, and only two naïve and two expert reviewers were used. Whether the current results hold true for more cases and a greater number of raters is unknown.

Conclusions

The present study suggests that determining the presence or absence of a blank or vacant stare is challenging for both naïve and expert raters to rate reliably, but that showing unresponsiveness (i.e. possible LOC), clutching or shaking of the head, a post-impact seizure, or being slow to get up are more reliably rated signs. However, in this study, there was no variability in the clinical outcome measure, as our sample came from a pool of individuals who were all medically diagnosed with a concussion. Therefore, the predictive value of any one component or concussion sign, or a combination of these items, is unknown and may be the focus of future research. Given the variability of in-game decision-making in professional rugby league [13–15], we sought to provide validation of a standardized approach for collecting information surrounding possible concussions to help inform the in-game decision-making process. Although the form was created for all levels of competition, it only had a good level of agreement among experienced raters. Therefore, it might only be useful for those teams or clubs that have experts available to them (i.e., the professional level). For lower levels of competition, the form may have less of a benefit, because the naïve raters had a low level of agreement on many components of the form. It is important to note, however, that the management of suspected concussion at these lower levels should always be conservative. If a concussion is suspected, then the athlete should be removed from play and not returned to play the same day [32]. At the professional level, data collected from this form may allow for a thorough understanding of the situational and contextual factors related to concussion, which may be used to strategize future interventions to reduce the risk of concussion at this level.

Acknowledgements
The authors would like to thank Mrs. Kathryn Gurr and Ms. Vanessa Case (University of Newcastle, School of Medicine and Public Health) for completing the video review as the nominated naïve raters and Dr. Jinho Lee (School of Human Movement and Nutrition Sciences, University of Queensland) for completing the review as an expert rater.

Funding
The funding was provided by Hunter Medical Research Institute (HMRI) supported by Anne Greaves.

Financial Disclosure
None.

Authors' Contributions
AG conceived the design of the study, designed the data collection tool, collected the video footage, liaised with the other raters to complete the data collection and monitored the data collection, managed the study database, conducted the statistical analysis, and drafted, revised, and finalized the manuscript. He had the final veto on the submission. CL assisted with the design of the study and provided the editorial comment to the drafts of the manuscript prepared for the submission. GI assisted with the design of the study, assisted with the statistical analysis of the data, provided expert editorial comment for all the drafts of the manuscript, and had the final veto on the submission. All authors read and approved the final manuscript.

Competing Interests
Andrew Gardner is an early career fellow with the National Health and Medical Research Council (NHMRC) and is supported by the School of Medicine and Public Health, University of Newcastle, and the Priority Research Centre for Stroke and Brain Injury, School of Medicine and Public Health, University of Newcastle. He has a clinical practice in neuropsychology involving individuals who have sustained sport-related concussion (including current and former athletes). He has operated as a contracted concussion consultant to the Australian Rugby Union (ARU) from July 2016. He has received travel funding

from the Australian Football League (AFL) to present at the Concussion in Football Conference in 2013 and 2017. The previous grant funding includes the NSW Sporting Injuries Committee, the Brain Foundation (Australia), and the Hunter Medical Research Institute (HMRI), supported by Jennie Thomas. He is currently funded through the HMRI, supported by Anne Greaves, and the University of Newcastle's Priority Research Centre for Stroke and Brain Injury. Christopher Levi declares that he has no conflict of interest. Grant Iverson has been reimbursed by the government, professional scientific bodies, and commercial organizations for discussing or presenting research relating to mild TBI and sport-related concussion at meetings, scientific conferences, and symposiums. He has a clinical and consulting practice in forensic neuropsychology involving individuals who have sustained mild TBIs (including athletes). He has received research funding from several test publishing companies, including ImPACT Applications, Inc., CNS Vital Signs, and Psychological Assessment Resources (PAR, Inc.). He received past salary support from the Harvard Integrated Program to Protect and Improve the Health of National Football League Players Association Members. He acknowledges unrestricted philanthropic support from the Mooney-Reed Charitable Foundation and ImPACT Applications, Inc.

Author details

[1]Centre for Stroke and Brain Injury, School of Medicine and Public Health, University of Newcastle, Callaghan, New South Wales, Australia. [2]Hunter New England Local Health District Sports Concussion Program, John Hunter Hospital, Newcastle, New South Wales, Australia. [3]Department of Physical Medicine and Rehabilitation, Harvard Medical School, Spaulding Rehabilitation Hospital, Boston, MA, USA. [4]MassGeneral Hospital for Children™ Sport Concussion Program, Boston, MA, USA. [5]Home Base, A Red Sox Foundation and Massachusetts General Hospital Program, Boston, MA, USA.

References

1. Andersen TE, Larsen Ø, Tenga A, Engebretsen L, Bahr R. Football incident analysis: a new video based method to describe injury mechanisms in professional football. Br J Sports Med. 2003;37:226–32.
2. Asplund CA, McKeag DB, Olsen CH. Sport-related concussion: factors associated with prolonged return to play. Clin J Sport Med. 2004;14:339–43.
3. Baker JG, Leddy JJ, Darling SR, Rieger BP, Mashtare TL, Sharma T, Willer BS. Factors associated with problems for adolescents returning to the classroom after sport-related concussion. Clin Pediatr (Phila). 2015;54:961–8.
4. Barlow M, Schlabach D, Peiffer J, Cook C. Differences in change scores and the predictive validity of three commonly used measures following concussion in the middle school and high school aged population. Int J Sports Phys Ther. 2011;6:150–7.
5. Berz K, Divine J, Foss KB, Heyl R, Ford KR, Myer GD. Sex-specific differences in the severity of symptoms and recovery rate following sports-related concussion in young athletes. Physician Sport Med. 2013;41:58–63.
6. Bruce JM, Echemendia RJ, Meeuwisse W, Hutchison MG, Aubry M, Comper P. Development of a risk prediction model among professional hockey players with visible signs of concussion. Br J Sports Med. 2017; bjsports-2016-097091
7. Chermann JF, Klouche S, Savigny A, Lefevre N, Herman S, Bohu Y. Return to rugby after brain concussion: a prospective study in 35 high level rugby players. Asian J Sports Med. 2014;5:e24042.
8. Collins MW, Iverson GL, Lovell MR, McKeag DB, Norwig J, Maroon J. On-field predictors of neuropsychological and symptom deficit following sports-related concussion. Clin J Sport Med. 2003;13:222–9.
9. Davis G, Makdissi M. Use of video to facilitate sideline concussion diagnosis and management decision-making. J Sci Med Sport. 2016; online first.
10. Echemendia RJ, Bruce JM, Meeuwisse W, Hutchison MG, Comper P, Aubry M. Can visible signs predict concussion diagnosis in the National Hockey League? Br J Sports Med. 2017; bjsports-2016-097090.
11. Ellis MJ, Ritchie LJ, Koltek M, Hosain S, Cordingley D, Chu S, Selci E, Leiter J, Russell K. Psychiatric outcome after pediatric sports-related concussion. J Neurosurg Pediatr. 2015;16:709–18.
12. Gardner A, Iverson GL, Levi CR, Schofield PW, Kay-Lambkin F, Kohler RMN, Stanwell P. A systematic review of concussion in rugby league. Br J Sports Med. 2015;49:495–8.
13. Gardner AJ, Iverson GL, Quinn TN, Makdissi M, Levi CR, Shultz SR, Wright DK, Stanwell P. A preliminary video analysis of concussion in the National Rugby League. Brain Inj. 2015;29:1182–5.
14. Gardner AJ, Iverson GL, Stanwell P, Ellis J, Levi CR. A video analysis of use of the new "Concussion Interchange Rule" in the National Rugby League. Int J Sports Med. 2016;37(4):267–3.
15. Gardner AJ, Kohler RMN, Levi CR, Iverson GL. Usefulness of video review of possible concussions in National Youth Rugby League. Int J Sports Med. 2016; in press.
16. Guskiewicz KM, McCrea M, Marshall SW, Cantu RC, Randolph C, Barr W, Onate JA, Kelly JP. Cumulative effects associated with recurrent concussion in collegiate football players: the NCAA concussion study. JAMA. 2003;290:2549–55.
17. Hallgren KA. Computing inter-rater reliability for observational data: an overview and tutorial. Tutor Quant Methods Psychol. 2012;8:23–34.
18. Hutchison MG, Comper P, Meeuwisse WH, Echemendia RJ. A systematic video analysis of National Hockey League (NHL) concussions, part I: who, when, where and what? Br J Sports Med. 2015;49(8):547–51.
19. Hutchison MG, Comper P, Meeuwisse WH, Echemendia RJ. A systematic video analysis of National Hockey League (NHL) concussions, part II: how concussions occur in the NHL. Br J Sports Med. 2015;49(8):552–5.
20. Hutchison MG, Comper P, Meeuwisse WH, Echemendia RJ. An observational method to code concussions in the National Hockey League (NHL): the heads-up checklist. Br J Sports Med. 2014;48:125–9.
21. IBM Corp. IBM SPSS Statistics for Macintosh, Version 22.0. Armonk, NY: IBM Corp. 2013.
22. Kerr ZY, DeFreese JD, Marshall SW. Current physical and mental health of former collegiate athletes. Orthop J Sport Med. 2014;2:1–9.
23. King DA, Hume PA, Milburn PD, Guttenbeil D. Match and training injuries in rugby league: a review of published studies. Sport Med. 2010;40:163–78.
24. Koh JO, Watkinson EJ, Yoon Y-J. Video analysis of head blows leading to concussion in competition Taekwondo. Brain Inj. 2004;18:1287–96.
25. Kohler R, Makdissi M, McDonald W, Partridge B, Gardner AJ. A preliminary video review of in-game head injury incidents (HII) and use of the head injury assessment (HIA) from the 2015 super rugby season. Br J Sports Med. 2017;51:A78–A79.
26. Lau B, Lovell MR, Collins MW, Pardini J. Neurocognitive and symptom predictors of recovery in high school athletes. Clin J Sport Med. 2009;19:216–21.
27. Lau BC, Kontos AP, Collins MW, Mucha A, Lovell MR. Which on-field signs/symptoms predict protracted recovery from sport-related concussion among high school football players? Am J Sports Med. 2011;39:2311–8.
28. Lincoln AE, Caswell SV, Almquist JL, Dunn RE, Hinton RY. Video incident analysis of concussions in boys' high school lacrosse. Am J Sports Med. 2013;41:756–61.
29. Makdissi M, Davis G. The reliability and validity of video analysis for the assessment of the clinical signs of concussion in Australian football. J Sci Med Sport. 2016; online first.
30. Makdissi M, Davis G. Using video analysis for concussion surveillance in Australian football. J Sci Med Sport. 2016; online first.
31. McCrea M, Kelly JP, Randolph C, Cisler R, Berger L. Immediate neurocognitive effects of concussion. Neurosurgery. 2002;50:1032–40.
32. McCrory P, Meeuwisse WH, Aubry M, Cantu B, Dvorák J, Echemendia RJ, Engebretsen L, Johnston K, Kutcher JS, Raftery M, Sills A, Benson BW, Davis GA, Ellenbogen RG, Guskiewicz K, Herring SA, Iverson GL, Jordan BD, Kissick J, McCrea M, McIntosh AS, Maddocks D, Makdissi M, Purcell L, Putukian M, Schneider K, Tator CH, Turner M. Consensus statement on concussion in sport: the 4th International Conference on Concussion in Sport held in Zurich, November 2012. Br J Sports Med. 2013;47:250–8.
33. McDevitt J, Tierney RT, Phillips J, Gaughan JP, Torg JS, Krynetskiy E. Association between GRIN2A promoter polymorphism and recovery from concussion. Brain Inj. 2015;29:1674–81.
34. McHugh ML. Interrater reliability: the kappa statistic. Biochem Med. 2012;22:276–82.
35. Meehan WP, Mannix RC, Stracciolini A, Elbin RJ, Collins MW. Symptom severity predicts prolonged recovery after sport-related concussion, but age and amnesia do not. J Pediatr. 2013;163:721–5.
36. Meehan WP, Monuteaux MC. Early symptom burden predicts recovery after sport-related concussion. Nerurology. 2014;83:2204–10.
37. Miele VJ, Bailes JE. Objectifying when to halt a boxing match: a video analysis of fatalities. Neurosurgery. 2007; 60: 307-15-6.

38. Moor HM, Eisenhauer RC, Killian KD, Proudfoot N, Henriques AA, Congeni JA, Reneker JC. The relationship between adherence behaviors and recovery time in adolescents after a sports-related concussion: an observational study. Int J Sports Phys Ther. 2015;10:225–33.
39. Morgan CD, Zuckerman SL, Lee YM, King L, Beaird S, Sills AK, Solomon GS. Predictors of postconcussion syndrome after sports-related concussion in young athletes: a matched case-control study. J Neurosurgery Pediatr. 2015;15:589–98.
40. Nelson LD, Guskiewicz KM, Marshall SW, Hammeke T, Barr W, Randolph C, McCrea MA. Multiple self-reported concussions are more prevalent in athletes with ADHD and learning disability. Clin J Sport Med. 2016;26:120–7.
41. Savage J, Hooke C, Orchard J, Parkinson R. The incidence of concussion in a professional Australian rugby league team, 1998–2012. J Sports Med. 2013; online first.
42. Terwilliger VK, Pratson L, Vaughan CG, Gioia GA. Additional post-concussion impact exposure may affect recovery in adolescent athletes. J Neurotrauma. 2016;33:761–5.
43. Vargas G, Rabinowitz A, Meyer J, Arnett PA. Predictors and prevalence of postconcussion depression symptoms in collegiate athletes. J Athl Train. 2015;50:250–5.
44. Zuckerman SL, Apple RP, Odom MJ, Lee YM, Solomon GS, Sills AK. Effect of sex on symptoms and return to baseline in sport-related concussion. J Neurosurg Pediatr. 2014;13:72–81.
45. Zuckerman SL, Solomon GS, Forbes JA, Haase RF, Sills AK, Lovell MR. Response to acute concussive injury in soccer players: is gender a modifying factor? J Neurosurg Pediatr. 2012;10:504–10.
46. Zuckerman SL, Yengo-Kahn AM, Buckley TA, Solomon GS, Sills AK, Kerr ZY. Predictors of postconcussion syndrome in collegiate student-athletes. Neurosurg Focus. 2016;40:E13.

Staphylococcus Aureus Carriage in French Athletes at Risk of CA-MRSA Infection: a Prospective, Cross-sectional Study

E. Couvé-Deacon[1,2,3], D. Postil[4], O. Barraud[1,2,3], C. Duchiron[4], D. Chainier[1,2,3], A. Labrunie[5], N. Pestourie[3], P.M. Preux[5], B. François[1,2,4] and M.C. Ploy[1,2,3*]

Abstract

Background: *Staphylococcus aureus* (SA) is a leading cause of infectious diseases in sports teams. In recent decades, community-associated SA (CA-SA) strains have emerged worldwide and have been responsible for outbreaks in sports teams. There are very few data on the prevalence of these strains in France, and none on the carriage among athletes.

Methods: We conducted a cross-sectional study to determine the SA carriage proportion among athletes practicing sports at risk for CA-SA infection in a French county, and determined the methicillin-resistant and/or CA-SA proportion. We also analyzed SA carriage according to risks factors and studied the SA clonality in a sample of our population.

Results: We included 300 athletes; SA carriage proportion was 61% (n = 183) and one was MRSA carrier (0.33%). The MRSA strain belonged to the clonal complex ST5. None of the strain produced Panton Valentine Leucocidin, and we did not find clonal distribution within the teams. Interestingly, we found a high throat-only carriage (n = 57), 31.1% of the SA carriers.

Conclusion: We found a high SA carriage with a local epidemiology quite different than that reported in a similar population in the USA. Further studies on SA carriage should include throat sampling.

Trial registration: The approved protocol was registered on ClinicalTrial.gov, NCT01148485.

Keywords: *Staphylococcus aureus*, Community associated, Panton Valentine leukocidin, Nasal carriage, Throat carriage, Sports team

Keypoints

- The prevalence of *S. aureus* carriage in at-risk athletes was high but MRSA carriage was low and there was no community associated SA carriage.
- We found no clear evidence of clonal transmission. SA carriage out of outbreak period is probably complex, resulting of a balance between host susceptibility and endogenous flora with skin contact transmission within a sports team.
- Throat-only carriage represented a high percentage of the SA carriers which substantially inflated the nose carriage. Studies on SA carriage should include throat sampling for a better accuracy.
- Staphylococcal carriage prevention in this population could consist of simple hygiene measures promotion, known to efficiently halt SA transmission in sports teams.

* Correspondence: marie-cecile.ploy@unilim.fr
[1]University Limoges, UMR, 1092 Limoges, France
[2]INSERM, UMR, 1092 Limoges, France
Full list of author information is available at the end of the article

Background

Staphylococcus aureus (SA) is a leading cause of both community-acquired and healthcare-associated infections. Community-associated methicillin-resistant *S. aureus* (CA-MRSA) emerged worldwide during the last decade. CA-MRSA causes skin and soft-tissue infections such as multiple abscesses among healthy individuals, as well as life-threatening necrotizing pneumonia in children and young adults [1]. There is a strong epidemiological link between CA-MRSA causing deep primary skin infections and Panton-Valentine leukocidin (PVL). PVL-producing SA strains have a peculiar antibiotic susceptibility profile and are more susceptible to antimicrobials as compared to healthcare-associated MRSA [2]. The prevalence of CA-MRSA seems to be low but is increasing in Europe, although prevalence in clinical isolates vary according to the country from less than 0.5 to 15% across published studies [3].

Skin-to-skin contact and poor hygiene are risk factors for CA-MRSA outbreaks, and populations at risk of CA-MRSA infection include prisoners, military personnel, and sports teams [4]. Most studies of SA infections among athletes have been conducted in the USA, and also in the UK, Germany, and Japan [5, 6]. In the USA, CA-MRSA infections among athletes have become very frequent, the most at-risk sports being those involving physical contact, such as American football, rugby, and wrestling [5, 6]. CA-MRSA infections have also been linked to sports involving less physical contact but shared equipment, such as fencing, martial arts, cross-country running, volleyball, basketball, football, baseball, and weight-lifting [5]. Other sport-related SA infection risk factors include a high body mass index, use of equipment resulting in skin abrasion, and poor personal hygiene (sharing of personal items, failure to protect skin lesions) [6].

The anterior nasal cavities are the most common SA carriage site with the oropharynx (10–50%), but skin carriage is also frequent, especially on the hands (27–90%), perineum (22–60%), and axilla (8–19%), the intestinal tract, vagina, and skin lesions are also common carriage sites [7]. Nasal carriage has been associated in literature with a higher incidence of SA infections [7]. Twenty to 25% of healthy volunteers were reported to be permanent nasal carriers, 60% intermittent carriers and 20% permanent non-carriers [8]. In the US general population, 1.3% were nasal MRSA carriers, compared to 5.4% of athletes and individuals in daily contact with MRSA carriers [9, 10].

In France, the reported SA nasal carriage rates were about one third of the general population. However, unlike the USA, there are very few data on the prevalence of CA-MRSA in France, and none on carriage among athletes at risk of CA-MRSA infection. The aim of this study was to determine the SA carriage proportion among athletes practicing physical contact sports in a French county, and the proportion and ST types of isolates resistant to methicillin and/or producing the PVL. We also analyzed SA carriage according to the sport, hygiene habits, and medical history.

Methods

Study Design

We conducted a cross-sectional study of a representative sample of athletes in the French county of Limousin. We selected sports at risk of CA-MRSA infection, namely rugby, wrestling, basketball, volleyball, handball, fencing, martial arts, football, weight-lifting and baseball.

Based on the reported SA nasal carriage of 27 to 37.2% in the general population but with previous rate reported around 35% in the literature (15, 29), we determined that the required population size for an expected SA carriage proportion of 35%, a precision of 8%, and a type 1 risk of 5% was 150 subjects, calculated using Nquery Advisor 7.0 (Statistical Solutions, Saugus, MA, USA). The estimated sample size anticipated a missing data rate of 10%. We used cluster sampling—the cluster being a sports team—that included all registered teams practicing the targeted sports in Limousin. The teams were randomly selected. All subjects in a selected team were eligible for enrollment. As cluster sampling doubles the required population size, we included 300 subjects.

The study, as biomedical research, was authorized by the French competent authorities and the local ethics committee (CPP). The study was carried out exactly as described in the approved protocol (Clinicaltrials.gov, NCT01148485). The study was proposed to the randomly selected sport teams. When we obtained the team agreement, an appointment during a training session was decided. During the training session, participation was proposed to all present athletes. After information and obtainment of the signed consent of the athletes, the study sampling was done.

Inclusion and Exclusion Criteria

The inclusion criteria were age over 18 years, registration in a Limousin sport club, and practice of at least one of the selected sports. Exclusion criteria were inability to complete the study questionnaire or if sampling was not possible. Each participant signed informed consent forms and samples were collected during regular training sessions.

The athletes completed a questionnaire on demographic characteristics, sport practice, personal hygiene, and medical history.

Microbiological Procedures

Swab samples of the nose, throat, groin and skin lesions (defined as excoriation, erosion or crust of the skin) were transported to the microbiological laboratory at ambient temperature, seeded on *S. aureus* specific chromogenic media (chromID™ *S. aureus*, bioMerieux, Lyon, France) and incubated for 48 h at 37 °C in an aerobic atmosphere. SA was identified on the basis of colony aspect, Gram staining, and catalase, and coagulase production (Pastorex®, Fumouze, Levallois-Perret, France).

The antibiotic susceptibility profile of isolates was determined as recommended in the guidelines of the Antibiogram Committee of the French Microbiology Society

(CA-SFM). Methicillin susceptibility was studied with cefoxitin disks. When this failed to categorize the isolate as susceptible or resistant, the *mecA* gene (encoding methicillin resistance) was sought by real-time PCR with specific primers, the method was adapted from a previously published protocol [11]. The PVL-encoding gene was also sought by PCR in all SA isolates, as previously described [12]. MRSA strains were characterized by Multi-Locus Sequence Typing, Enright et al. method [13]. MLST is based on the sequencing of seven housekeeping genes, defining an allelic profile corresponding to a Sequence Type (ST). ST designations were those assigned by the MLST database (available from: URL: http://www.mlst.net).

An athlete was defined as a carrier if at least one strain of *S. aureus* was isolated from at least one of his or her samples, and as an MRSA carrier if at least one SA strain resistant to methicillin was detected in at least one sample.

ERIC PCR Strain Typing

We performed ERIC PCR for strain molecular typing [14] with the ERIC2 primer. To study clonal transmission within each team and between the different teams, we choose a sample of the strains isolated. Amplification products were separated by agarose gel electrophoresis in 2.0% agarose, and visualized by u.v. transillumination. The fingerprints obtained by ERIC–PCR were visually

Table 1 General Description of the Population

Label	Mean	Std Dev	Minimum	Maximum	Lower quartile	Median	Upper quartile
Age	30.40	10.10	18.02	86.77	22.76	27.97	35.69
Height	176.04	7.75	154.00	200.00	170.00	176.00	181.00
Weight	76.38	13.44	44.00	140.00	67.00	76.00	85.00
Body Mass Index	24.53	3.52	17.20	43.20	22.10	24.20	26.10
variable	Modality			Number of subjects		Percent	
Gender	M			247		82.33	
	F			53		17.67	
linked to healthcare system profession	NO			283		95.93	
	YES			12		4.07	
Sport competition level[a]	National			31		13.6	
	Pre-National			19		8.33	
	Region			142		62.28	
	Local			36		15.79	
Professional/amateur	Professional			8		2.67	
	Amateur			292		97.33	
Sport 27 teams	Martial art			45		15.00	
	Baseball			31		10.33	
	Basketball			19		6.33	
	Football			48		16.00	
	Weight-lifting			16		5.33	
	Handball			54		18.00	
	Wrestling			11		3.67	
	Rugby			56		18.67	
	Volleyball			20		6.67	
Championship	NO			58		19.53	
	YES			239		80.47	
Number of training session per week	Less than 1			21		7.02	
	1			66		22.07	
	2			141		47.16	
	2 and +			71		23.75	

[a]This variable does not include all the sports. Sports as martial arts, wrestling, and weight lifting are not included

compared. We classified strains in major clones (clone A, clone B, clone C...) that differ by two and more bands or minor clones profiles when there was only 1 or 2 bands difference (A1, A2, A3...).

Statistical Analysis

The study database was created with Oracle-based CLINSIGHT software (https://ecrf.clinsight.fr/nepha/), notably using the CS-DESIGNER module.

Statistical analysis used SAS V9.2 software (SAS Institute Cary, NC), and a p value <0.05 was considered to signify statistical significance. Quantitative variables are described as the mean ± standard deviation (SD) or the median and interquartile interval. Qualitative variables are described as numbers, percentages, and 95% confidence intervals.

Carriage proportions were compared according the sport and risk factor by using the chi^2 test or Fisher's exact test, depending on the theoretical number. To adjust the results, we performed a multivariate logistic regression. We selected the explanatory variables with a p value under 0.25. The selected variables were then computed to obtain the final model, with the variable to explain being the presence or absence of SA strain in the different samples.

Results

Population Characteristics

Between 11 January 2011 and 10 June 2011, we studied 300 athletes, comprising 247 men (82.3%) and 53 women (17.7%). Average age was 30.4 years (±10.1), average height 176.0 cm (±7.7), average weight 76.4 kg (±13.4), and the average body mass index 24.5 (±3.5). The athletes performed at local (12.0%, n = 36), regional (47.3%, n = 142), pre-national (6.3%, n = 19), or national level (10.3%, n = 31) and these level did not apply for 72 athletes due to their sport. Only one of the 27 studied teams was professional, representing 2.7% of the 300 athletes (Table 1).

SA and MRSA Carriage

Among the 300 athletes, 61.0% (n = 183) carried SA (95% confidence interval (95%CI) = [51.0; 70.0]). The proportion of MRSA carriage was 0.3% (n = 1) (95%CI = [0.0; 1.4]) overall and 0.5% (n = 1) (95%CI = [0.0; 1.7]) among SA carriers (n = 183). The MRSA strain belonged to the clonal complex ST5 and was isolated in the nose and skin lesion swabs of a handball player. None of the SA isolates produced PVL. We noticed a high variability of team SA carriage, from 0.0% in two karate teams (n = 10 and n = 3) to 100% in a wrestling team (n = 11) and a baseball team (n = 6). A rugby team had the largest number of members (n = 39) and presented a SA carriage of 74.4% (n = 29).

Interestingly, throat carriage was more frequent (n = 143, 47.7%) than nasal carriage (n = 111, 37.0%), and throat-only carriage was frequent (n = 57, 19.0%) in the population. We sampled 21 skin lesions, and skin lesion-only carriage was 1.7% (n = 5). Multiple sampling sites increased the chances of detecting SA carriage: nasal/throat sampling identified 93.4% of carriers, while nasal/throat/groin and nasal/throat/skin lesion sampling identified 97.3% of carriers.. SA carriage was detected only in the throat, nose or groin in respectively 31.1% (n = 57), 12.0% (n = 22), and 3.2% (n = 8) of SA carriers (n = 183) (Table 2).

Risk Factors for SA Carriage

A history of lengthy (>4 weeks) antibiotic therapy (p = 0.035), use of saunas (p = 0.093), weight-lifting facilities (p = 0.152), and a history of abscess in the previous year (p = 0.096) had a p value under 0.250 (Table 3) and were included in a multivariate logistic regression model. However, after a selection step of variables none of these four variables was significantly linked to SA carriage. No significant difference in SA carriage proportion was observed between the different sports (p = 0.422).

ERIC PCR SA Strain Typing

We selected teams to study SA clonality. We hypothesized that clone circulation within a team would be easier to

Table 2 SA Carriage According to the Sampling Sites

Location	Frequencies (% of carriers) (n = 183)
Nose	111 (60.6%)
Nose only	22 (12.0%)
Throat	143 (78.1%)
Throat only	57 (31.1%)
Groin	40 (21.8%)
Groin only	2 (3.2%)
Skin lesion	21 (11.5%)
Skin lesion only	5 (1.7%)
Nose and/or throat	171 (93.4%)
Nose and/or groin	121 (66.1%)
Nose and/or skin lesion	119 (65.0%)
Throat and/or groin	156 (85.2%)
Throat and/or skin lesion	151 (82.5%)
Groin and/or skin lesion	53 (29.0%)
Nose and/or throat and/or groin	178 (97.3%)
Nose and/or throat and/or skin lesion	178 (97.3%)
Nose and/or groin and/or skin lesion	127 (69.4%)
Throat and/or groin and/or skin lesion	161 (88.0%)
Nose and/or throat and/or groin and/or skin lesion	183 (100%)

Table 3 Risk Factors of the Athletes

A. Sport

Factor	SA Carriers/participants (%)	*p* value (test)
Baseball	18/31 (58.1%)	$p = 0.422$ (chi^2)
Basketball	13/19 (68.4%)	
Football	30/48 (62.5%)	
Weight-lifting	8/16 (50.0%)	
Handball	34/54 (63.0%)	
Rugby	39/56 (70.0%)	
Individual sports/martial arts (wrestling, judo, karate)	33/56 (58.9%)	
Volleyball	8/20 (40.0%)	

B. Hygiene

Factor	Modality	SA Carriers/participants (%)	*p* value (test)
Shared equipment	NO	39/61 (63.9%)	$p = 0.566$ (chi^2)
	YES	142/237 (59.9%)	
Shared healthcare materials	NO	149/240 (62.1%)	$p = 0.495$ (chi^2)
	YES	32/56 (57.1%)	
Shared personal effects	NO	108/176 (61.4%)	$p = 0.946$ (chi^2)
	YES	75/123 (61.0%)	
Skin damage during sport	Never	22/42 (52.4%)	$p = 0.574$ (Fisher)
	Rarely	57/94 (60.6%)	
	Sometimes	75/119 (63.0%)	
	Often	24/35 (68.6%)	
	Always	5/10 (50.0%)	
Sauna use	NO	176/285 (61.5%)	*$p = 0.093$ (chi^2)*
	YES	5/13 (38.5%)	
Use of training pool	NO	180/296 (60.8%)	$p = 1.000$ (Fisher)
	YES	1/2 (50.0%)	
Weights room use	NO	154/246 (62.6%)	*$p = 0.152$ (chi^2)*
	YES	27/52 (51.9%)	
Skin lesion disinfection	NO	77/132 (58.3%)	$p = 0.473$ (chi^2)
	YES	103/165 (62.4%)	
Protection of skin lesions	NO	119/198 (60.1%)	$p = 0.905$ (chi^2)
	YES	59/97 (60.8%)	
Protection of skin lesions during sport	NO	87/158 (61.4%)	$p = 0.767$ (chi^2)
	YES	83/139 (59.7%)	
Shower/bath frequency	Every other day	23/31 (74.2%)	$p = 0.267$ (chi^2)
	Once a day	126/211 (59.7%)	
	Several times a day	33/57 (57.9%)	

C. Medical history in the previous year

Factor	modality	SA Carriers/participants (%)	*p* value (test)
Hospitalization	NO	156/257 (60.7%)	$p = 0.795$ (chis^2)
	YES	27/43 (62.8%)	
Superficial skin lesions	NO	130/215 (60.5%)	$p = 0.763$ (chi^2)
	YES	53/85 (62.4%)	

Table 3 Risk Factors of the Athletes *(Continued)*

Skin abscess	NO	175/291 (60.1%)	*p = 0.096 (Fisher)*
	YES	8/9 (88.9%)	
Pneumonia	NO	181/297 (60.9%)	p = 1.000 (Fisher)
	YES	2/3 (66.7%)	
Antibiotic treatment	NO	158/256 (61.7%)	p = 0.447 (chi^2)
	YES	21/38 (55.3%)	
Long-term antibiotics	NO	182/294 (61.9%)	*p = 0.035 (Fisher)*
	YES	1/6 (16.7%)	
Chronic disease	NO	173/281 (61.6%)	p = 0.440 (chi^2)
	YES	10/19 (52.6%)	

$p < 0.25$ value are indicated in *italics*. Data is presented in three parts: A. SA carriage according to sport, B. SA carriage according to hygiene practice, C. SA carriage according to medical history in the previous year

detect in large team or team with the highest carriage. Fifty-nine isolates were typed. These isolates were obtained from 55 athletes in the 2 largest team rugby teams R012 (n = 39) and R031 (n = 17), with, respectively, 71.8 and 58.8% SA carriage and the two highest carriage teams, L001 (wrestling, n = 11) and B004 (baseball, n = 6) with a 100% SA carriage. We identified six major clones (clone A to clone F) and 11 minor clones profiles (Table 4). Clones A and B were found in all teams and clone F was found only in team L001. Altogether, the results did not show a clonal distribution of the SA between the teams. Furthermore, within each team, there was no evidence of a clonal transmission.

Discussion

We observed an overall *S. aureus* carriage proportion of 61% (95%CI: 51.0–70.0) among 300 French athletes. A previous European study showed a carriage rate in France of 21.1% (95%CI: 17.4–25.4) among 3870 healthy patients [15], but only the nose was sampled. The prevalence of SA carriage found here in our study is higher than that observed in the general population in other studies with multiple sampling sites [16–18]. This high SA carriage among athletes is not surprising, as SA transmission is facilitated by sharing of equipment and skin-to-skin contacts. In addition, athletes are known to have poor personal hygiene during sports, as reflected by reports of CA-MRSA outbreaks in sports teams [5, 6]. We report a high variability of team SA carriage, from 0.0% in a karate team to 100% in a wrestling team and a baseball team. Clonal transmission of SA within sports teams has already been demonstrated as well as the increase of SA isolates in the sweat of SA carriers during sport practice [19]. However, the typing of the strains did not show clear evidence of clonal transmission within the studied teams. Even though skin contact is known as the main transmission risk in SA outbreaks in sports team, the SA carriage out of outbreak period is probably more complex. Host susceptibility and endogenous flora are probably in balance with skin contact transmission within a sports team.

We observed a higher carriage in the throat (n = 143, 47.7%) than in the nose (n = 111, 37.0%), as recently reported in the general population worldwide [18, 20, 21]. Interestingly, throat only carriage represented 31.1% (n = 57) of our carriers (n = 183), and represented 19% of the total population (n = 300). Nose positivity accounted for 37% (111/300 subjects), which is comparable with many other studies on nasal SA carriage in the general population. However, when enriched with throat-only carriers, which are often not sought for in other studies, it added 57 cases, thus inflating the prevalence to close to 60% (168/300 subjects), which is much higher than most other studies. This raises the question as to what is the genuine rate of *S. aureus* carriage in the general population if throat swabbing would also be performed and highlights the fact that *S. aureus* does not only colonize the nose [16–18]. Due to this peculiar observation we could not really compare our high carriage proportion to other studies. This implies that a combination of throat and nose sampling should be used to detect SA carriage.

In the USA, CA-MRSA is endemic. However, only one publication reported no difference in CA-MRSA nasal carriage between college athletes (1.8%) and the general population (1.5%) [22]. Based on these reports, we expected to find a CA-MRSA carriage proportion of 1.0–2.0% among French athletes. However, in our study, none carried PVL producing MRSA.

One handball player carried a PVL-negative MRSA, in the nose and skin lesion, the strain belonged to the ST5, the second more frequent clonal complex isolated in France after ST8 [23]. In athletes, MRSA carriage differed according to the studies. A study reported that 23.1% (n = 44/190) of high-school football players in the USA had nasal colonization with methicillin-susceptible

Table 4 Distribution of the SA clones within the Selected Teams

Team	SA Team Carriage	Clone	Number of Strains
B004	100% (6/6)		
		A	2
		B	2
		D	1
		D1	1
L001[a]	100% (11/11)		
		A	1
		A1	1
		C	5
		C1	1
		C3	1
		D	2
		F	3
R012	71.8% (28/39)		
		A	5
		A1	6
		A3	1
		A4	1
		B	1
		B1	4
		C	2
		C2	2
		C4	1
		D	2
		E	2
		E1	1
R031[a]	58.8% (10/17)		
		A	2
		A2	1
		B	3
		B1	1
		C2	3
		E	1

[a]Some athletes carried several strains; thus, we report teams with a number of studied strains higher than the number of SA carriers

B004 was a baseball team, L001 was a wrestling team and R012 and R031 were rugby teams

SA, and none with MRSA [24]. On contrary, another study reported nose and skin MRSA carriage in 35.0% of 233 healthy athletes in the USA, and found that most isolates also harbored the PVL-encoding gene [16]. When our study started, most published data on MRSA carriage in the general and athlete populations came from the USA. A European study published during our study showed an MRSA carriage of 0.4% in the French general population [15], close to the 0.3% observed here in French athletes.

The link between SA carriage and outbreaks of skin and soft-tissue infections is not always clear. Outbreaks of PVL-positive MRSA infection have been reported in sports teams with high carriage of methicillin-susceptible SA (23.0 to 48.5%) but not significantly linked to CA-MRSA carriage [24–26]. In a 1-year surveillance study of MRSA nasal carriage among student athletes, colonization alone appeared insufficient to trigger outbreaks [24]. However, CA-SA infection outbreaks remain low in European athlete population compared to USA athlete population. The reported outbreaks are usually linked to poor hygiene practices and the implementation of simple hygiene measures can efficiently halt the transmission [27]. In our study, we did not find any PVL-positive MRSA carrier, nonetheless, the high SA carriage associated with skin contact during sport practice increases the risk of SA transmission between players [19] and therefore the risk of SA carriage and infection [7]. Previous study reported a higher risk of *S. aureus* carriage overtime in contact sports athletes and that efforts should focus to prevent transmission of *S. aureus* among these athletes [28]. Prevention of SA carriage and infection in that population could be achieved by simple hygiene measure promotion as skin wound disinfection and covering during practice, showering after practice and competition, using liquid soap rather than bar soap, washing clothes and equipment after practice, refraining from cosmetic body shaving, and discouraging athletes from sharing towels and personal hygiene items [29, 30]. Our data did not allow identifying risk factors for SA carriage. We found that long-term antibiotic therapy was associated with SA carriage, but this classical risk factor was no longer significant in multivariate analysis. As French data on SA carriage among athletes were lacking, we based our sample size on American data; we therefore overestimated the carriage proportion, which partly explains the lack of statistical power. Sample size was a major limitation to the study. Despite showing a high carriage, it was only out of 300 athletes. Finally, one interesting control would be to apply the same swabbing technique to a sample of the Limousin general population.

We sampled our athletes only once, mainly during the first half of the sports season. Two previous studies showed variations in MRSA carriage according to the athletic activity. In a one-year surveillance study of student football and lacrosse athletes, MRSA carriage ranged from 4.0 to 23.0%, with a peak during the period of maximal athletic activity [31]. Moreover, a 3-year surveillance study of CA-MRSA skin and soft-tissue infections in a collegiate football team, obtained evidence that variations in MRSA carriage might be related to the time of the competitive season or to outbreaks or isolated cases of CA-MRSA infection [32].

Conclusions

In our population of French athletes, we found a high SA carriage but a low MRSA carriage. Our local epidemiology was quite different than that reported in similar types of athletes in the USA, e.g., that the USA300 clone had not spread (yet) spread among our test population. We found a very high percentage of throat-only positive cultures, which substantially inflated the nasal carriage proportion. Further studies on *S. aureus* carriage should include throat sampling.

Staphylococcal carriage prevention in that population could consist in simple hygiene measures promotion, known to efficiently halt SA transmission in sports team.

Abbreviations

CA-MRSA: Community-associated methicillin-resistant *Staphylococcus aureus*; MLST: Multi locus sequence typing; MRSA: Methicillin-resistant *Staphylococcus aureus*; PVL: Panton Valentine leukocidin; SA: *Staphylococcus aureus*; ST: Sequence type

Acknowledgements

We thank Caroline Fenerol and Mathilde Saugeras for their assistance in patient inclusions and data collection, Julie Vignaud for her technical assistance and Marie Raymondeau for her help in data management. This study was sponsored by Limoges University hospital.

Funding

This study was supported by a grant from the Direction de la Recherche et Innovation de CHU de Limoges "2011" and Caisse Primaire d'Assurance Maladie de la Haute-Vienne.

Authors' Contributions

ECD designed the research, conducted it and compiled the data to produce the submitted manuscript. DP as Clinical Investigation Center delegate doctor conducted the research and revised the manuscript. OB was in charge of the medical validation of the microbiological analysis of the research and revised the manuscript. CD supervised and participated in the conduction of the research and revised the manuscript. DC was responsible for the technical aspect of the microbiological analysis, data entry, and revised the manuscript. AL was responsible of the data managing and analysis for the research and wrote part of the manucript. NP participated in the design of the study, data interpretation and the writing of the manuscript. PMP was in charge of the statistical methodology design, analysis validation, and revised the manuscript. BF as coordinator of the Clinical Investigation Center managed the conduction of the research and revised the manuscript. MCP as Principal Investigator of the research designed, conducted the research, and produced the submitted manuscript. Each author participated sufficiently in the work to take public responsibility for appropriate portions of the content; and agreed to be accountable for all aspects of the work in ensuring that questions related to the accuracy or integrity of any part of the work are appropriately investigated and resolved.

Competing Interests

Elodie Couvé-Deacon, Déborah Postil, Olivier Barraud, Cécile Duchiron, Delphine Chainier, Anaïs Labrunie, Nathalie Pestourie, Pierre-Marie Preux, Bruno François, and Marie-Cécile Ploy declare that they have no conflict of interest.

Author details

[1]University Limoges, UMR, 1092 Limoges, France. [2]INSERM, UMR, 1092 Limoges, France. [3]CHU Limoges, Laboratory of Bacteriology-Virology-Hygiene, 2 avenue Martin Luther King, 87042 Limoges, cedex, France. [4]INSERM, CIC-1435, F-87000 Limoges, France. [5]CHU Limoges, Centre d'Epidémiologie de Biostatistique et de Méthodologie de la Recherche, Limoges, France.

References

1. Dufour P, Gillet Y, Bes M, Lina G, Vandenesch F, Floret D, Etienne J, Richet H. Community-acquired methicillin-resistant *Staphylococcus aureus* infections in France: emergence of a single clone that produces Panton-Valentine leukocidin. Clin Infect Dis. 2002;35:819–24.
2. Otter JA, French GL. Community-associated meticillin-resistant *Staphylococcus aureus* strains as a cause of healthcare-associated infection. J Hosp Infect. 2011;79:189–93.
3. Otter JA, French GL. Molecular epidemiology of community-associated meticillin-resistant *Staphylococcus aureus* in Europe. Lancet Infect Dis. 2010; 10:227–39.
4. Tenover FC, Goering RV. Methicillin-resistant *Staphylococcus aureus* strain USA300: origin and epidemiology. J Antimicrob Chemother. 2009;64:441–6.
5. Cohen PR. The skin in the gym: a comprehensive review of the cutaneous manifestations of community-acquired methicillin-resistant *Staphylococcus aureus* infection in athletes. Clin Dermatol. 2008;26:16–26.
6. Grosset-Janin A, Nicolas X, Saraux A. Sport and infectious risk: a systematic review of the literature over 20 years. Med Mal Infect. 2012;42:533–44.
7. Wertheim HFL, Melles DC, Vos MC, van Leeuwen W, van Belkum A, Verbrugh HA, Nouwen JL. The role of nasal carriage in *Staphylococcus aureus* infections. Lancet Infect Dis. 2005;5:751–62.
8. Kluytmans J, van Belkum A, Verbrugh H. Nasal carriage of *Staphylococcus aureus*: epidemiology, underlying mechanisms, and associated risks. Clin Microbiol Rev. 1997;10:505–20.
9. Beam JW, Buckley B. Community-acquired methicillin-resistant *Staphylococcus aureus*: prevalence and risk factors. J Athl Train. 2006;41:337–40.
10. Salgado CD, Farr BM, Calfee DP. Community-acquired methicillin-resistant *Staphylococcus aureus*: a meta-analysis of prevalence and risk factors. Clin Infect Dis. 2003;36:131–9.
11. Lem P, Spiegelman J, Toye B, Ramotar K. Direct detection of mecA, nuc and 16S rRNA genes in BacT/Alert blood culture bottles. Diagn Microbiol Infect Dis. 2001;41:165–8.
12. Jarraud S, Mougel C, Thioulouse J, Lina G, Meugnier H, Forey F, Nesme X, Etienne J, Vandenesch F. Relationships between *Staphylococcus aureus* genetic background, virulence factors, agr groups (alleles), and human disease. Infect Immun. 2002;70:631–41.
13. Enright MC, Day NP, Davies CE, Peacock SJ, Spratt BG. Multilocus sequence typing for characterization of methicillin-resistant and methicillin-susceptible clones of *Staphylococcus aureus*. J Clin Microbiol. 2000;38:1008–15.
14. Vázquez-Sánchez D, López-Cabo M, Saá-Ibusquiza P, Rodríguez-Herrera JJ. Incidence and characterization of *Staphylococcus aureus* in fishery products marketed in Galicia (Northwest Spain). Int J Food Microbiol. 2012;157:286–96.
15. den Heijer CDJ, van Bijnen EME, Paget WJ, Pringle M, Goossens H, Bruggeman CA, Schellevis FG, Stobberingh EE. APRES Study Team. Prevalence and resistance of commensal *Staphylococcus aureus*, including meticillin-resistant *S. aureus*, in nine European countries: a cross-sectional study. Lancet Infect Dis. 2013;13:409–15.
16. Champion AE, Goodwin TA, Brolinson PG, Werre SR, Prater MR, Inzana TJ. Prevalence and characterization of methicillin-resistant *Staphylococcus aureus* isolates from healthy university student athletes. Ann Clin Microbiol Antimicrob. 2014;13:33.
17. Schechter-Perkins EM, Mitchell PM, Murray KA, Rubin-Smith JE, Weir S, Gupta K. Prevalence and predictors of nasal and extranasal staphylococcal colonization in patients presenting to the emergency department. Ann Emerg Med. 2011;57:492–9.
18. Sollid JU, Furberg AS, Hanssen AM, Johannessen M. *Staphylococcus aureus*: determinants of human carriage. Infect Genet Evol. 2014;21:531–41.
19. Suzuki K, Tagami K. Role of nasal *Staphylococcus aureus* carriage in transmission among contact athletes. Int J Sports Med. 2015;36:1186–91.

20. Fall C, Richard V, Dufougeray A, Biron A, Seck A, Laurent F, Breurec S. *Staphylococcus aureus* nasal and pharyngeal carriage in Senegal. Clin Microbiol Infect. 2014;20:O239–41.
21. Van Nguyen K, Zhang T, Thi Vu BN, Dao TT, Tran TK, Thi Nguyen DN, Thi Tran HK, Thi Nguyen CK, Fox A, Horby P, Wertheim H. *Staphylococcus aureus* nasopharyngeal carriage in rural and urban northern Vietnam. Trans R Soc Trop Med Hyg. 2014;108:783–90.
22. Rackham DM, Ray SM, Franks AS, Bielak KM, Pinn TM. Community-associated methicillin-resistant *Staphylococcus aureus* nasal carriage in a college student athlete population. Clin J Sport Med. 2010;20:185–8.
23. Dauwalder O, Lina G, Durand G, Bes M, Meugnier H, Jarlier V, Coignard B, Vandenesch F, Etienne J, Laurent F. Epidemiology of invasive methicillin-resistant *Staphylococcus aureus* clones collected in France in 2006 and 2007. J Clin Microbiol. 2008;46:3454–8.
24. Lear A, McCord G, Peiffer J, Watkins RR, Parikh A, Warrington S. Incidence of *Staphylococcus aureus* nasal colonization and soft tissue infection among high school football players. J Am Board Fam Med. 2011;24:429–35.
25. Begier EM, Frenette K, Barrett NL, Mshar P, Petit S, Boxrud DJ, Watkins-Colwell K, Wheeler S, Cebelinski EA, Glennen A, Nguyen D, Hadler JL, Connecticut Bioterrorism Field Epidemiology Response Team. A high-morbidity outbreak of methicillin-resistant *Staphylococcus aureus* among players on a college football team, facilitated by cosmetic body shaving and turf burns. Clin Infect Dis. 2004;39:1446–53.
26. Kazakova SV, Hageman JC, Matava M, Srinivasan A, Phelan L, Garfinkel B, Boo T, McAllister S, Anderson J, Jensen B, Dodson D, Lonsway D, McDougal LK, Arduino M, Fraser VJ, Killgore G, Tenover FC, Cody S, Jernigan DB. A clone of methicillin-resistant *Staphylococcus aureus* among professional football players. N Engl J Med. 2005;352:468–75.
27. Couvé-Deacon E, Tristan A, Pestourie N, Faure C, Doffoel-Hantz V, Garnier F, Laurent F, Lina G, Ploy M-C. Outbreak of Panton-Valentine leukocidin-associated methicillin-susceptible *Staphylococcus aureus* infection in a rugby team, France, 2010–2011. Emerg Infect Dis. 2016;22:96–9.
28. Jiménez-Truque N, Saye EJ, Soper N, Saville BR, Thomsen I, Edwards KM, Creech CB. Association between contact sports and colonization with *Staphylococcus aureus* in a prospective cohort of collegiate athletes. Sports Med. 2016; doi:10.1007/s40279-016-0618-6.
29. Levine H, Kayouf R, Rozhavski V, Sela T, Rajuan-Galor I, Ferber AT, Yona S, Gorochovski O, Halperin T, Hartal M. Neglect of skin wounds and the risk of becoming a *Staphylococcus aureus* nasal carrier: a cohort study. BMC Public Health. 2015;15:749.
30. Zinder SM, Basler RSW, Foley J, Scarlata C, Vasily DB. National Athletic Trainers' Association Position Statement: Skin Diseases. J Athl Train. 2010;45:411–28.
31. Creech CB, Saye E, McKenna BD, Johnson BG, Jimenez N, Talbot TR, Bossung T, Gregory A, Edwards KM. One-year surveillance of methicillin-resistant *Staphylococcus aureus* nasal colonization and skin and soft tissue infections in collegiate athletes. Arch Pediatr Adolesc Med. 2010;164:615–20.
32. Romano R, Lu D, Holtom P. Outbreak of community-acquired methicillin-resistant *Staphylococcus aureus* skin infections among a collegiate football team. J Athl Train. 2006;41:141–5.

8

Evidence of Concussion Signs in National Rugby League Match Play: a Video Review and Validation Study

Andrew J. Gardner[1,9*], David R. Howell[3,4,5], Christopher R. Levi[1,2] and Grant L. Iverson[6,7,8]

Abstract

Background: Many professional sports have introduced sideline video review to help recognise concussions. The reliability and validity of identifying clinical and observable signs of concussion using video analysis has not been extensively explored. This study examined the reliability and validity of clinical signs of concussion using video analysis in the National Rugby League (NRL).

Methods: All 201 professional NRL matches from the 2014 season were reviewed to document six signs of possible concussion (unresponsiveness, slow to get up, clutching/shaking head, gait ataxia, vacant stare, and seizure).

Results: A total of 127,062 tackles were reviewed. Getting up slowly was the most common observable sign (2240 times in the season, 1.8% of all tackles) but only 223 times where it appeared to be a possible concussion (0.2% of all tackles and 10.0% of the times it occurred). Additionally, clutching/shaking the head occurred 361 times (on 212 occasions this sign appeared to be due to a possible concussion), gait ataxia was observed 102 times, a vacant stare was noted 98 times, unresponsiveness 52 times, and a possible seizure 4 times. On 383 occasions, one or more of the observable signs were identified and deemed associated with a possible concussion. There were 175 incidences in which a player appeared to demonstrate two or more concussion signs, and 54 incidences where a player appeared to demonstrate three or more concussion signs. A total of 60 diagnosed concussions occurred, and the concussion interchange rule was activated 167 times. Intra-rater reliability (κ = 0.65–1.00) was moderate to perfect for all six video signs; however, the inter-rater reliability was not as strong (κ = 0.22–0.76). Most of the signs had relatively low sensitivity (0.18–0.75), but high specificity (0.85–1.00).

Conclusions: Using video replay, observable signs of concussion appear to be sensitive to concussion diagnoses when reviewing known injuries among professional rugby league players. When reviewing an entire season, however, certain signs occur very commonly and did not identify concussion. Thus, the implementation of video review in the NRL is challenging, but can provide a useful addition to sideline concussion identification and removal from play decisions.

Keywords: Concussion, Video analysis, Injury management, Return to play

* Correspondence: Andrew.Gardner@neurogard.com.au
[1]Centre for Stroke and Brain Injury, School of Medicine and Public Health, University of Newcastle, Callaghan, Australia
[9]Priority Research Centre for Stroke and Brain Injury, Level 5, McAuley Building, Calvary Mater Hospital, Waratah, NSW 2298, Australia
Full list of author information is available at the end of the article

Key Points

- The addition of video review to the assessment of concussion injury events may help improve consistency in the management of players, as well as assist in diagnostic decision-making in cases where signs may be transient and resolved by the time of the medical assessment.
- The signs of concussion appear to be quite sensitive to concussion when reviewing *known injuries*; however, when reviewing an entire season, some signs occur very commonly and usually do not reflect a concussive injury.
- Most signs of concussion had high specificity but low sensitivity when examining all tackles across a sporting season.

Background

Participation in many full contact and collision sports, such as rugby league, carries with it a risk of concussion [10]. In-game concussion diagnosis, however, remains a highly challenging task for the athletic trainer and sports medicine physician. On-field or sideline clinical assessments can be challenging due to the heterogeneous presentation of an athlete following a head impact, the non-specific nature of many of the clinical signs and symptoms of concussion [29], the absence of a reliable concussion biomarker [40], and the regularity with which some concussion signs emerge and evolve over time [31]. Recognising a potential concussion and removing an athlete from play is understood to be an important intervention for reducing the risk of a worse clinical outcome following injury [31]. However, it is acknowledged that in some instances, concussions may be missed from the sideline [25]. This may occur for a variety of reasons, but commonly the transient early physical signs may resolve before the player can be removed from play and assessed [25].

Some prior studies suggest that worse outcomes following concussion are associated with on-field signs and symptoms, such as loss of consciousness [28], amnesia [8, 28], mental status change for more than 5 min [8], and dizziness [23]. It is important to appreciate that the literature on the association between on-field signs and symptoms is mixed. For example, loss of consciousness has been associated with worse clinical outcomes in some [1, 4, 15, 28, 35, 39], but not in most studies [2, 3, 5, 8, 9, 16, 18, 22, 27, 30, 32, 36–38, 42, 43]. The vast majority of studies examining loss of consciousness base this finding on a questionnaire or interview completed with the athlete, not video review of the injury event for confirmation. Similarly, post-traumatic amnesia has been associated with worse clinical outcomes in some [15, 24, 28], but not in most studies [1–3, 8, 16, 18, 23, 27, 30, 34, 37, 38, 42]. Dizziness has been observed as an on-field symptom associated with a protracted recovery of greater than 21 days (6.34 time more likely) [23], but assessing dizziness is subjective and may or may not manifest as an objective sign (e.g., gait ataxia). Thus, video review may allow for the quantification of objective concussion signs, but not subjective symptoms.

In the sport of rugby league, the concussion incidence rates have been reported to vary widely depending on the level of competition [10]. In one study of three National Rugby League (NRL) clubs, a concussion incidence rate of 14.8 concussions per 1000 player match hours was reported [13], while a rate of 28.3 concussion per 1000 player match hours were reported from one NRL club over a 15-year (1998–2012) period [41].

The use of video footage on the sideline for reviewing a concussion has been introduced in a number of professional sports as a method to improve the recognition of a possible concussion that may be missed by on-field medical personnel [25]. Video studies have now been conducted in a variety of sports such as rugby league [11–13], rugby union [21], hockey [7], and Australian rules football [6, 25, 26]. In addition to the introduction of sideline video review, the governing body of the sport in Australia (the National Rugby League) implemented a new the "concussion interchange rule" (CIR). The CIR requires the mandatory removal of any player suspected of having sustained a concussion. The CIR allows a player to be removed from play for 15 min to be assessed by the club medical officer, including completing the Sports Concussion Assessment Tool third edition (SCAT-3). Following the assessment, if the player was not diagnosed with concussion, they are permitted to return to play without using an interchange. The incidence of use of the CIR was 24.0 (95% CI 20.7–27.9) uses of the CIR per 1000 NRL player match hours [12], and 44.9 (95% CI 38.5–52.3) uses of the CIR per 1000 National Youth Competition player match hours [13].

The primary aim of this study was to determine the rate of six objective concussion signs that occurred during the 2014 NRL season, as well as the sensitivity and the specificity of these signs to classify whether or not a diagnosed concussion resulted from the event. The secondary objective of this study was to analyse the intra- and inter-rater reliability of these signs using the video recordings of each incident that activated the CIR.

Methods

Participants

Participants for this study were the entire league of NRL players involved in match play during the 2014 season. Each team is comprised of a squad of approximately 25 players, and there are 16 teams in the league. There are 13 players on the field during the match.

Procedure

This study conducted a video analysis of every game during the 2014 National Rugby League (NRL) season. The full game video analysis for all games during the season was conducted retrospectively, at the conclusion of the season by the lead author. The video review was conducted independent of any club trainer or team medical staff. The video was used to examine all on-field signs. There was no prerequisite for recording the presence of a sign (e.g., contact with the head was not required). The lead researcher obtained information on the use of the CIR (i.e., the player's name and round in which the CIR was used). Each NRL team physician provided a list of players who had been diagnosed with concussion during the season. The club physician made the final diagnosis of concussion, based on conventional clinical examination techniques. For 162/167 (97%) uses of the CIR [12], and for all diagnosed concussions (n = 60), the Observational Review and Analysis of Concussion (ORAC) form [14] was used to record the game circumstances and details of the event as well as the presence or absence of six concussive signs (clutching or shaking head, slow to get up, gait ataxia, blank/vacant stare, unresponsiveness, and seizure). There were five uses of the CIR where the video of the incident was not located; none of these cases were diagnosed with a concussion. There were 162 (97%) cases where the CIR incident was identified, and 60 (100%) cases were medically diagnosed with a concussion. Two reviewers conducted the video analysis of these cases. To assess intra-rater reliability, one of the reviewers also completed a second review of 162 video clips of uses of the CIR, which included a review of all cases of medically diagnosed concussion.

All diagnosed concussions and 97% of the uses of the CIR were independently reviewed by two raters. The video raters were blinded to the club medical staff's documentation (i.e., they conducted their retrospective review of the video signs completely independently of the club medical staff). Both raters have experience in the identification of concussion on the sideline and with retrospective video review. The two raters determined whether any of six signs of concussion were present, absent, or indeterminable based on the available footage of the incident for every case. When there was disagreement between the two raters, both raters reviewed and discussed those cases in an effort to reach consensus. In the cases where consensus could not be achieved, ratings from an experienced third rater were used. Consent was obtained from all participants who used the CIR. This study was approved by the University of Newcastle Human Ethics Committee (H-2012-0344).

The ORAC form was created to provide a simple but standardised framework for coding and analysing video footage of the situations and consequences of concussion events in rugby league. The form was developed based on work conducted previously in ice hockey in North America [19], but was adapted to include specific information to rugby league. The form includes concussion signs that have been previously examined in video review studies in rugby league [11–13]. The form consists of various sections related to the player and game characteristics (e.g., ball carrier versus tackler, tackle height, type of play, etc.), the anatomical region of contact, the injury location on the field of play, the injured player's on-field management, and six concussive signs (defined in Table 1).

The full-match digital records of all 2014 NRL season matches (n = 210) were reviewed by a single rater (AG) using the Quicktime Multimedia Player V.7.7.5. The season prevalence of the six concussion signs were recorded by this rater. There was an important distinction made between observing a sign and instances where the sign 'looked like it was a concussion-related' sign, so there were two tallies made for each sign (i.e., an entire season tally of the sign regardless of the reasons for the player displaying that sign, and a season tally of the sign where

Table 1 Definition of video signs

Concussion sign	Definition
Clutch or shake head	The player holds his head or face in the palm of his hand or hands, or the player rubs or shakes his head in a manner that appears to demonstrate they are experiencing discomfort (i.e., not just wiping his face).
Slow to return to feet/play	Player took longer than usual to return to his feet (e.g., remained on the ground, got to his knees or to his haunches, and waited momentarily before standing), in the absence of another player holding him down.
Gait ataxia (wobbly legs)	Unable to stand steadily unaided or walk normally. Appears "clumsy". Upon standing and walking the player has unsteadiness, wobbly legs, balance problems, stumbles or falls over, drags his feet, or cannot walk straight independently.
Blank/vacant stare	The player is not visually focused on doctor/trainer when being spoken to, or assessed and asked to attend, and/or the player appears to be looking off into the distance. The player's face is expressionless.
Evidence of unresponsiveness	The player's body goes limp/floppy, the player loses control of muscles, the player *does not* protect (i.e., brace) himself when falling (e.g., ragdoll-like appearance). The player remains/lies motionless on the ground for a period of time longer than expected, or the player shows a lack of visible responsiveness to verbal stimuli.
Post-impact seizure	Tonic posturing—stiffening of limbs; or clonic movements—involuntary repetitive contraction and relaxation of the muscles, could include jerky movements, or shaking/convulsion of upper and/or lower limbs, or body.

the sign appeared to reflect a possible concussion). We operationally defined 'looked like a concussion' as all instances where there was an absence of another explanation for the sign. The digital records of events leading to the use of the CIR and medically diagnosed concussion were independently reviewed by two raters, on two separate occasions. The only circumstances that rendered a reported use of the CIR or concussion ineligible for inclusion were (i) any event where the video of the player was obstructed by other players or the match official(s) (n = 0), or (ii) where the incidence was unable to be located following a full-match review (n = 5 uses of the CIR; n = 0 diagnosed concussions). The ORAC form was used to code each application of the CIR and medically diagnosed concussion, in an identical methodology to previous studies in this setting [11–13]. See Fig. 1 for details.

Statistical Analysis

Descriptive analyses are presented as means (standard deviation) for continuous variables; categorical variables are presented as numbers included (n) or percentage of the total. Sensitivity, specificity, positive predictive value (PPV), and negative predictive value (NPV) were calculated for each of the six concussion signs using 2 × 2 contingency tables. The number of times a player demonstrated one or more of these signs that looked like a possible concussion sign (n = 383) during match play for the entire season was used as the denominator for calculating sensitivity, specificity, PPV, and NPV.

Intra- and inter-rater reliability analyses using Cohen's kappa (κ) statistics [17] were used for 162 (97%) cases where the CIR was used and for all of those cases that were medically diagnosed with concussion, to determine consistency among the two raters for each of the six individual signs. Unlike the total percent agreement, Cohen's kappa considers the proportional agreement that could occur simply by chance. The κ coefficients are calculated by considering the proportion of rater agreement and the expected proportion [17]. Using the interpretations of κ described by McHugh [33], κ agreement was categorised as almost perfect (>.90), strong (.80–.90), moderate (.60–.79), weak (.40–.59), minimal (.21–.39), and none (0–.20). All analyses were performed using IBM SPSS Statistics V.23.0 [20] and used two-sided tests for significance at the 0.05 level, with either 90 or 95% confidence intervals (CIs).

Results

During the 2014 season, the CIR was used on 167 occasions (97% [n = 162] were located and reviewed),

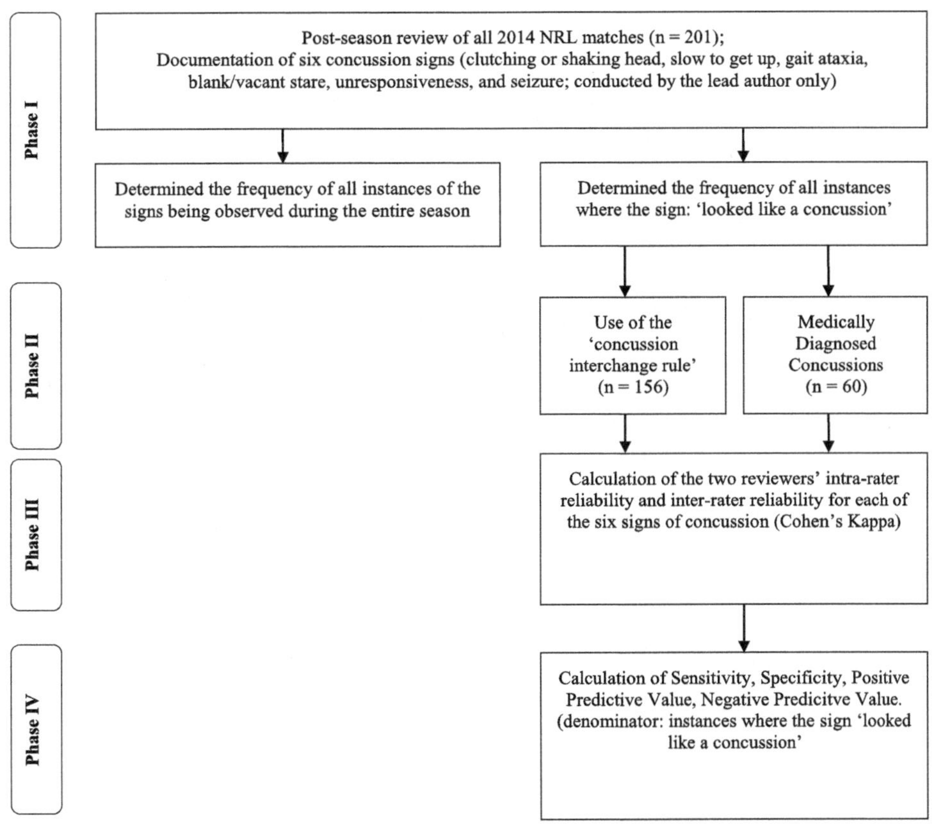

Fig. 1 Hierarchy of methods and procedures of video review process

and there were 60 medically diagnosed concussions. The incidence rate for concussion was 8.92 (95% CI = 6.96–11.43) per 1000 National Rugby League player match hours, or was approximately one concussion every 3.35 games. There were 127,062 tackles reviewed in the 201 matches, for an average of 632.1 tackles per match (Table 2). There was an important distinction made between observing a sign, and instances where the sign looked like it reflected a concussion. For example, in the 201 games reviewed, slow to get up was observed 2240 times but of those 2240 times on only 223 occasions slow to get up looked like it may have been a concussion-related sign (10.0%). Therefore, on 2017 occasions a player was slow to get up due to reasons other than a possible concussion. For example, the player stayed down to stay out of the way of play and avoid being penalised = 837, appeared to be fatigued = 706 or sustained another injury = 365; play had stopped = 78; or the opposition scored and the player stayed down = 31. The sign clutching or shaking head was observed 361 times and for 212 times the sign was considered possibly concussion-related (58.7%). Examples of when it was not considered concussion-related included when the player sustained a facial (non-nose) injury = 64 or a nose injury = 42, exhibited a disappointed or dismayed reaction to play = 27; wiped or shook off sweat from his head = 15, or appeared to have been poked in the eye = 1. All instances of observing unresponsiveness (n = 52), gait ataxia (n = 102), vacant stare (n = 98), and a post-impact seizure (n = 4) throughout the season were considered to be possibly concussion-related (Table 3).

Of the 223 instances of a player being slow to get up, 153 players were removed under the CIR (68.6%); return to play data was available for only 156/162 (96.3%) instances of the use of the CIR. Of those 153, 60 were medically diagnosed as having a concussion (39.2%), and all players who were medically diagnosed with concussion demonstrated the sign "slow to get up". The PPV and NPV for slow to get up were 0.27 and 1.00, respectively. Of the 212 instances of clutching or shaking head, 110 players were removed under the CIR (51.9%) and 38 were diagnosed with a concussion (34.5%). Of those who were diagnosed with concussion, players clutched or shook their heads 63.3% (38/60) of the time. The PPV and NPV for clutching or shaking head were 0.18 and 0.87, respectively. Of the 102 instances of gait ataxia, 87 players were removed under the CIR (85.3%) and 35 were diagnosed with concussion (40.2%). Gait ataxia was seen in 58.3% of players medically diagnosed with concussion. The PPV and NPV for gait ataxia were 0.34 and 0.91, respectively. Of the 98 instances of a blank or vacant stare, 93 players were removed under the CIR (94.9%) and 45 were diagnosed with concussion (48.4%). A blank or vacant stare was observed in 75.0% of players medically diagnosed with concussion. The PPV and NPV for blank or vacant stare were 0.46 and 0.95, respectively. Of the 52 instances in which a player appeared to have brief unresponsiveness following a tackle, 50 players were removed under the CIR (96.2%), of which 24 were diagnosed with a concussion (48%). Unresponsiveness on the field was observed in 40.0% (24/60) of players medically diagnosed with concussion. The PPV and NPV for unresponsiveness were 0.46 and 0.89, respectively. Of the 4 instances in which a player appeared to experience a post-impact seizure, 3 players were removed under the CIR (75.0%). All three players were medically diagnosed with a concussion (100%). There were three (5%) players who were medically diagnosed with concussion that showed signs of seizure-like activity. The PPV and NPV for seizure-like activity were 0.75 and 0.85, respectively (Table 4).

Table 2 Data summary of video analysis from the 2014 National Rugby League season

Variable	Total
Matches	201
Total number of tackles in the season	127,062
Average number of tackles per match	632.1
Average concussion interchange rule user per match	0.78
Concussion interchange rule (CIR) uses	167
Returned to play	80
No return to play	76
Diagnosed concussions	60
CIR, no return to play, and no concussion	16

Note: video footage for 5 cases of the use of the CIR could not be located and therefore were not coded for concussion signs
There were 6 CIR cases where return to play data is missing

One or more video signs of possible concussion were seen during 383 tackles (i.e., only 0.3% of the total number of tackles), most commonly demonstrating the characteristic "slow to get up" (Table 5). Considering five signs simultaneously (unresponsiveness, clutching/shaking head, gait ataxia, slow to get up, or blank/vacant stare), 34 (57%) of players medically diagnosed with concussion had three or more observable signs of concussion. There were a greater total number of signs observed in the concussed group compared to players that used the CIR and were cleared to return to play in the same game (Table 5). For the individual signs, those diagnosed with concussion were more likely to show evidence of unresponsiveness and a vacant stare. There was no difference between the number of observed signs between groups for clutching or shaking the head, or gait ataxia.

The players who were medically diagnosed with a concussion were significantly more likely (1.52 times) to exhibit unresponsiveness and a vacant stare (2.35 times) than players who were removed from play under the CIR, not diagnosed with a concussion, and were returned to

Table 3 Summary of the rates of concussion signs for the entire season, concussion-related signs, use of the CIR, and medically diagnosed concussions

Concussion sign	Entire season total	Possible concussion sign	Use of the CIR (*n* = 162)[a]	CIR missing data[a]	Medically Diagnosed concussion (*n* = 60)	Medically Diagnosed concussion missing data
Unresponsiveness	52	52	50	2	24	1
Slow to get up	2240	223	153	0	60	0
Clutching head	361	212	110	1	38	0
Gait ataxia	102	102	87	18	35	11
Vacant stare[b]	98	98	93	18	45	6
Possible seizure	4	4	3	0	3	0

Note: *CIR* concussion interchange rule
The "Entire Season Total" refers to every instance during the season that the sign was observed (whether it appeared to be a sign of concussion or not). The "Possible Concussion Sign" refers to the subset of the Entire Season Total in those instances where the sign was observed, and the sign appeared to be a possible concussion
[a]Video footage for 5 cases of the use of the CIR could not be located and therefore were not coded for concussion signs
[b]The frequency of missing data for the sign 'vacant stare' for the entire season total was not recorded

play. Clutching the head and gait ataxia were not significantly different signs between those who were and were not medically diagnosed with a concussion (see Table 1).

A sign that was always present in cases of diagnosed concussion was slow to get up (sensitivity = 100%), although it had low specificity (50%). A possible seizure was observed only four times during the season and on three occasions those athletes were medically diagnosed as having a concussion (3/60 diagnosed concussions; sensitivity = 5%, specificity = 100%). A blank or vacant stare had fairly high sensitivity and specificity (75% and 84%, respectively; see Table 4).

The intra-rater reliability of the video analysis of each sign of concussion was moderate to perfect, and perfect agreement was observed in three (clutch or shake head, slow to get up, and post-impact seizure) of the six signs. Moderate inter-rater reliability was observed in three of six of signs: clutch or shake head, slow to get up, and unresponsiveness (Table 6).

Discussion

To expand previous video analysis work in collision sports, this study explored the rate of six observable signs of concussion, as well as their sensitivity and specificity during match play of a National Rugby League season. The results of the current study revealed moderate to perfect intra-rater reliability or better for all video signs. For inter-rater reliability, clutching or shaking head, slow to get up, and unresponsiveness had moderate inter-rater reliability, whereas post-impact seizure had weak inter-rater reliability, and gait ataxia and blank or vacant stare had poor inter-rater reliability. These findings are relatively consistent with those reported from a video review study of concussion signs during Australia Football League (AFL) match play, which found that intra-rater reliability was generally better than inter-rater reliability, and blank or vacant stare was the sign with the lowest agreement [25].

Blank or vacant stare was the only sign that had reasonably high sensitivity (75%) and specificity (84%); all

Table 4 Rates, sensitivity, specificity, positive predictive value, and negative predictive value for concussion signs

Concussion sign	Sign present	Medically Dx concussion with sign	Sign absent	Medically Dx concussion without sign	Sign sens	95% CI	Sign spec	95% CI	PPV	95% CI	NPV	95% CI
Clutching or shaking head	212	38	171	22	0.63	0.51–0.75	0.46	0.44–0.48	0.18	0.14–0.21	0.87	0.83–0.91
Slow to get up	223	60	160	0	1.00	0.93–1.00	0.50	0.48–0.50	0.27	0.25–0.27	1.00	0.97–1.00
Gait ataxia	102	35	281	25	0.58	0.46–0.70	0.79	0.77–0.81	0.34	0.27–0.41	0.91	0.86–0.94
Blank or vacant stare	98	45	285	15	0.75	0.63–0.84	0.84	0.81–0.85	0.46	0.39–0.52	0.95	0.92–0.97
Unresponsiveness	52	24	331	36	0.40	0.29–0.50	0.91	0.89–0.93	0.46	0.34–0.58	0.89	0.87–0.91
Possible seizure	4	3	379	57	0.05	0.02–0.07	1.00	0.99–1.00	0.75	0.22–0.99	0.85	0.84–0.85

Note: All calculations were made using the number of times the sign was seen in concussed players, contrasted to the total number of times one or more signs (that appeared to represent a concussion) were seen (*n* = 383), for the entire season
≥ greater than or equal to, *CI* confidence interval, *Dx* diagnosed, *n* number, *NPV* negative predictive value, *PPV* positive predictive value, *Sens* sensitivity, *Spec* specificity

Table 5 Summary of video analysis findings for those situations in which the concussion interchange rule was used

Signs of concussion	Medically diagnosed concussion (*n* = 60)			No diagnosed concussion and no return to play[a] (*n* = 16)			Returned to play[a] (*n* = 80)			Diagnosed concussion vs. returned to play[a]		
	Present	Absent	Missing	Present	Absent	Missing	Present	Absent	Missing			
	% (*n*)	% (*n*)	% (*n*)	% (*n*)	% (*n*)	% (*n*)	% (*n*)	% (*n*)	% (*n*)	χ^2	*p*	RR (90% CI)
Unresponsiveness	40 (24)	58.3 (35)	1.7 (1)	43.8 (7)	56.3 (9)	0 (0)	23.8 (19)	75 (60)	1.3 (1)	4.35	.037	1.52 (1.06–2.10)
Slow to get up	100 (60)	0 (0)	0 (0)	100 (16)	0 (0)	0 (0)	96.3 (77)	3.7 (3)	0 (0)	Not applicable		
Clutching head	63.3 (38)	36.7 (22)	0 (0)	87.5 (14)	12.5 (2)	0 (0)	72.5 (58)	26.3 (21)	1.3 (1)	1.62	.203	0.77 (0.55–1.12)
Gait ataxia	58.3 (35)	23.3 (14)	18.3 (11)	62.5 (10)	37.5 (6)	0 (0)	52.5 (42)	38.8 (31)	8.8 (7)	2.43	.119	1.46 (0.94–2.38)
Vacant stare	75 (45)	15 (9)	10 (6)	62.5 (10)	37.5 (6)	0 (0)	47.5 (38)	37.5 (30)	15 (12)	10.43	.001	2.35 (1.40–4.30)
Possible seizure	5 (3)	95 (57)	0 (0)	0 (0)	100.0 (16)	0 (0)	0 (0)	100 (80)	0 (0)	Not applicable		
Total signs observed (*n*)	205	–	–	64	–	–	174	–	–	–	–	–

Note. Video footage for 5 cases of the use of the CIR could not be located and therefore were not coded for concussion signs; there were 6 CIR cases where return to play data is missing
[a]Return to play refers to return to play in the same game; *RR* risk ratio

other signs did not have both high sensitivity and specificity for a concussion diagnosis. Some of the signs had high sensitivity but low specificity, suggesting that those signs may be a useful marker in flagging a potential concussion, but not helpful in confirming the diagnosis. Therefore, medical personnel working in tandem on the sideline and with individuals reviewing video may be an appropriate strategy to achieve a sensitive and specific approach to concussion diagnosis. In a video review of concussion signs during match play in the Australian Football League (AFL), slow to get up had the highest sensitivity (87%), but low specificity (19%). All other video concussion signs examined in this prior study had high specificity but low sensitivity, such as blank and vacant look [specificity 100%, sensitivity 9%], motor incoordination [specificity 95%, sensitivity 29%], impact seizure [specificity 93%, sensitivity 7%], and rag doll appearance [specificity 91%, sensitivity 16%]). The highest PPV was found with the "blank and vacant look" (100%), and "motor incoordination" (81%) signs [25]. However, in the current study, we found that the highest PPV was for seizure (75%), while slow to get up (100%), blank or vacant stare (95%), and gait ataxia (91%) were the signs with the highest NPV.

The sign with the highest relative risk of diagnosed concussion was a blank or vacant stare (2.35 times more likely; 90% CI = 1.40–4.30), while unresponsiveness was 1.52 times more likely (90% CI = 1.06–2.10). Gait ataxia (1.46 times more likely; 90% CI = 0.94–2.38) and clutching or shaking head (0.77 times more likely; 90% CI = 0.55–1.12) were not statistically different. Blank or vacant stare appears to be a conceptually different sign to the other five. The detection of a blank or vacant stare tends to be through a secondary screening process, in that it is often only observed if, and when, a player is injured and the camera zooms in closely. It is also arguably the most subjective of the six signs and therefore vulnerable to greater variation between raters when classifying this sign. This notion is supported by the weaker inter-rater reliability of this sign not only in the current study but also in previous video review studies [12, 13, 25]. In our study, the low inter-rater reliability was due to one rater seeing the sign more often than the other, recording it as present, and then both raters ultimately agreeing that it was present. Observing a blank or vacant stare was rare in a recently published NHL video review study [7]. We do not know why the sign was so uncommon in that study compared to ours. It might be more difficult to see the sign through

Table 6 Intra-rater reliability and inter-rater reliability for the concussion signs

	Intra-rater (κ) (95% CIs)	McHugh [33] κ agreement classification	Inter-rater (κ) (95% CIs)	McHugh [33] κ agreement classification	Absolute disagreement (CIR cases, *n* = 162)
Clutch of shake head	1.00 (–,–)	Perfect	0.76 (0.60–0.91)	Moderate	43
Slow to get up	1.00 (–,–)	Perfect	0.64 (0.42–0.83)	Moderate	27
Gait ataxia	0.77 (0.63–0.90)	Moderate	0.37 (0.21–0.53)	Minimal	36
Blank/vacant stare	0.65 (0.44–0.84)	Moderate	0.22 (0.05–0.40)	Minimal	71
Unresponsiveness	0.84 (0.70–0.94)	Strong	0.75 (0.56–0.92)	Moderate	22
Post-impact seizure	1.00 (–,–)	Perfect	0.40 (0.00–0.72)	Weak	3

Note. *CIs* confidence intervals, κ Kappa McHugh, κ agreement was categorised as almost perfect (>.90), strong (.80–.90), moderate (.60–.79), weak (.40–.59), minimal (.21–.39), and none (0–.20)

a hockey helmet, and it might also be more difficult to see it based on camera angles when players are moving off the ice. Among the other signs, inter-rater reliability was the strongest for clutch or shake head, slow to get up, and unresponsiveness, each with a moderate agreement classification. These signs may be more easily seen during field-side evaluations; their intra-rater reliability was strong to perfect. In contrast, the minimal agreement between raters for gait ataxia or blank/vacant stare warrants caution with their use.

There were several limitations of the current study. In some instances, the available video footage was not sufficiently clear to code all signs (i.e., the view from the available camera angle was obscured, or a close up of the incident was not available). This 'missing data' was excluded from the analyses, which might have slightly improved the support for the utility of some of the visible signs. This was particularly true for the blank or vacant stare sign, where missing data on this sign was common. Despite being the most sensitive and specific sign for concussion diagnosis, blank or vacant stare had the worst inter-rater reliability (0.22, with 71 absolute disagreements between raters). For these reasons, if video review within professional sports are implemented, then access to high quality reviews with the capability of multi-angle and slow motion replays to allow for close ups would be optimal [25] and would reduce the likelihood of missing data. Although the video reviewer was blinded to the sideline assessment results and the medical diagnosis of concussion for this study, they were only partially blinded to the use of the CIR. Given that the process for enacting a use of this rule requires the trainer to provide a signal to the sideline, and the official on the sideline identifies the interchange with a green card, the video reviewer was able to identify many instances where the CIR was used. Another study limitation was that there were no concussions that were subsequently (beyond match day) diagnosed by the club medical and reported to the researchers, which is inconsistent with other video review studies that have reported a numbers of cases of post-game diagnosis of concussion [7]. A further limitation of the current study pertains to the generalizability of the current findings to other levels of rugby league. The current study was a post-game review of an adult, male, professional league, and as such the results may not necessarily be generalizable to in-match real-time analysis, or other levels of match play. Our use of an operational definition of exclusion to categorise the observed signs into 'plausible concussion signs' versus signs that were more likely attributable to other factors, was also a limitation in terms of its subjectivity and reproducibility for future work in video review of concussion signs. Finally, only one reviewer completed the coding of the entire game, for every game in the season; the inter-rater reliability of that type of coding is unknown.

Conclusions

A conservative approach to sideline concussion management would be to remove a player from play based on any evidence of possible concussion signs. This approach is encouraged as the best management strategy and in the best interest of the welfare of the player [31]. However, there is limited information available on the reliability and validity of identifying the objective signs of concussion when using video analysis, and indeed not all instances of observed concussion signs occur as a result of the player having sustained a concussion. The signs of concussion appear to be quite sensitive to concussion when reviewing known (i.e., medically diagnosed concussions) or suspected (i.e., players who have used the CIR) injury. When reviewing an entire season of match play, specific objective concussion signs such as slowness in getting up and clutching/shaking the head occurred commonly during professional rugby league match play, but did not typically reflect concussion occurrence. For these reasons, video injury surveillance can be difficult to interpret, but may provide a useful adjunct to the clinical assessment of potential concussion. With improved access to video replays, clear definitions and education regarding the observable signs, and improved communication between video observers and sideline medical personnel, the detection of concussion may improve.

Acknowledgements
The authors would like to thank Dr Jinho Lee (School of Human Movement and Nutrition Sciences, University of Queensland) for completing the video review of all uses of the CIR.

Funding
Funding was provided by Hunter Medical Research Institute (HMRI) supported by Anne Greaves.

Authors' contributions
AG conceived the design of the study, reviewed all game video, collected all of the study data, and drafted, revised, and finalised the manuscript. He had final veto on the submission. DH assisted with the design of the study, conducted the statistical analysis, provided expert editorial comment for all drafts of the manuscript, and had final veto on the submission. CL assisted with the design of the study and provided editorial comment to the final draft of the manuscript. GI assisted with the design of the study, assisted with the statistical analysis of the data, provided expert editorial comment for all drafts of the manuscript, and had final veto on the submission. All authors read and approved the final manuscript.

Competing interests
Andrew Gardner has a clinical practice in neuropsychology involving individuals who have sustained sport-related concussion (including current and former athletes). He has operated as a contracted concussion consultant to the Australian Rugby Union (ARU) from July 2016. He has received travel

funding from the Australian Football League (AFL) to present at the Concussion in Football Conference in 2013 and 2017. Previous grant funding includes the NSW Sporting Injuries Committee, the Brain Foundation (Australia), and the Hunter Medical Research Institute (HMRI), supported by Jennie Thomas. He is currently funded through the HMRI, supported by Anne Greaves, and the University of Newcastle's Priority Research Centre for Stroke and Brain Injury.
David Howell and Christopher Levi have no competing interests to declare. Grant Iverson has been reimbursed by the government, professional scientific bodies, and commercial organisations for discussing or presenting research relating to mild TBI and sport-related concussion at meetings, scientific conferences, and symposiums. He has a clinical and consulting practice in forensic neuropsychology involving individuals who have sustained mild TBIs (including athletes). He has received research funding from several test publishing companies, including ImPACT Applications, Inc., CNS Vital Signs, and Psychological Assessment Resources (PAR, Inc.). He acknowledges unrestricted philanthropic support from the Mooney-Reed Charitable Foundation and ImPACT Applications, Inc.

Author details

[1]Centre for Stroke and Brain Injury, School of Medicine and Public Health, University of Newcastle, Callaghan, Australia. [2]Hunter New England Local Health District Sports Concussion Program, John Hunter Hospital, Newcastle, New South Wales, Australia. [3]The Micheli Center for Sports Injury Prevention, Waltham, MA, USA. [4]Division of Sports Medicine, Department of Orthopaedics, Boston Children's Hospital, Boston, USA. [5]Brain Injury Center, Boston Children's Hospital, Boston, MA, USA. [6]Center for Health and Rehabilitation, Department of Physical Medicine and Rehabilitation, Harvard Medical School, 79/96 Thirteenth Street, Charlestown Navy Yard, Charlestown, MA, USA. [7]Spaulding Rehabilitation Hospital, Charlestown, USA. [8]MassGeneral Hospital for Children™ Sport Concussion Program, and Home Base, A Red Sox Foundation and Massachusetts General Hospital Program, Boston, MA, USA. [9]Priority Research Centre for Stroke and Brain Injury, Level 5, McAuley Building, Calvary Mater Hospital, Waratah, NSW 2298, Australia.

References

1. Asplund CA, McKeag DB, Olsen CH. Sport-related concussion: factors associated with prolonged return to play. Clin J Sport Med. 2004;14:339–43.
2. Bock S, Grim R, Barron TF, Wagenheim A, Hu YE, Hendell M, Deitch J, Deibert E. Factors associated with delayed recovery in athletes with concussion treated at a pediatric neurology concussion clinic. Childs Nerv Syst. 2015;31:2111–6.
3. Brown NJ, Mannix RC, O'Brien MJ, Gostine D, Collins MW, Meehan WP. Effect of cognitive activity level on duration of post-concussion symptoms. Pediatrics. 2014;133:e299–304.
4. Chermann JF, Klouche S, Savigny A, Lefevre N, Herman S, Bohu Y. Return to rugby after brain concussion: a prospective study in 35 high level rugby players. Asian J Sports Med. 2014;5:e24042.
5. Collins MW, Iverson GL, Lovell MR, McKeag DB, Norwig J, Maroon J. On-field predictors of neuropsychological and symptom deficit following sports-related concussion. Clin J Sport Med. 2003;13:222–9.
6. Davis G, Makdissi M. Use of video to facilitate sideline concussion diagnosis and management decision-making. J Sci Med Sport 2016; online first.
7. Echemendia RJ, Bruce JM, Meeuwisse W, Hutchison MG, Comper P, Aubry M. Can visible signs predict concussion diagnosis in the National Hockey League? Br J Sports Med 2017; bjsports-2016-097090.
8. Ellis MJ, Ritchie LJ, Koltek M, Hosain S, Cordingley D, Chu S, Selci E, Leiter J, Russell K. Psychiatric outcome after pediatric sports-related concussion. J Neurosurg Pediatr. 2015;16:709–18.
9. Erlanger D, Kaushik T, Cantu R, Barth JT, Broshek DK, Freeman JR, Webbe FM. Symptom-based assessment of the severity of a concussion. J Neurosurg. 2003;98:477–84.
10. Gardner A, Iverson GL, Levi CR, Schofield PW, Kay-Lambkin F, Kohler RMN, Stanwell P. A systematic review of concussion in rugby league. Br J Sports Med 2014; bjsports-2013-093102.
11. Gardner AJ, Iverson GL, Quinn TN, Makdissi M, Levi CR, Shultz SR, Wright DK, Stanwell P. A preliminary video analysis of concussion in the national rugby league. Brain Inj. 2015;29:1182–5.
12. Gardner AJ, Iverson GL, Stanwell P, Ellis J, Levi CR. A video analysis of use of the new "concussion interchange rule" in the national rugby league. Int J Sports Med. 2016;
13. Gardner AJ, RMN K, Levi CR, Iverson GL. Usefulness of video review of possible concussions in National Youth Rugby League. Int J Sports Med. 2016; in press
14. Gardner AJ, Levi CR, Iverson GL. Observational review and analysis of concussion: a method for conducting a standardised video analysis of concussion in rugby league. Sport Med - Open. 2017;3:26.
15. Guskiewicz KM, McCrea M, Marshall SW, Cantu RC, Randolph C, Barr W, Onate JA, Kelly JP. Cumulative effects associated with recurrent concussion in collegiate football players: the NCAA concussion study. JAMA. 2003;290: 2549–55.
16. Guskiewicz KM, Ross SE, Marshall SW. Postural stability and neuropsychological deficits after concussion in collegiate athletes. J Athl Train. 2001;36:263–73.
17. Hallgren KA. Computing inter-rater reliability for observational data: an overview and tutorial. Tutor Quant Methods Psychol. 2012;8:23–34.
18. Hinton-Bayre AD, Geffen G. Severity of sports-related concussion and neuropsychological test performance. Neurology. 2002;59:1068–70.
19. Hutchison MG, Comper P, Meeuwisse WH, Echemendia RJ. An observational method to code concussions in the National Hockey League (NHL): the heads-up checklist. Br J Sports Med. 2014;48:125–9.
20. IBM Corp . IBM SPSS statistics for Macintosh, version 22.0. Armonk: IBM Corp.
21. Kohler R, Makdissi M, McDonald W, Partridge B, Gardner AJ. A preliminary video review of in-game head injury incidents (HII) and use of the head injury assessment (HIA) from the 2015 super rugby season. Br J Sports Med. 2017;51:A78–9.
22. Lau B, Lovell MR, Collins MW, Pardini J. Neurocognitive and symptom predictors of recovery in high school athletes. Clin J Sport Med. 2009; 19:216–21.
23. Lau BC, Kontos AP, Collins MW, Mucha A, Lovell MR. Which on-field signs/symptoms predict protracted recovery from sport-related concussion among high school football players? Am J Sports Med. 2011;39:2311–8.
24. Lovell MR, Collins MW, Iverson GL, Field M, Maroon JC, Cantu R, Podell K, Powell JW, Belza M, Fu FH. Recovery from mild concussion in high school athletes. J Neurosurg. 2003;98:296–301.
25. Makdissi M, Davis G. The reliability and validity of video analysis for the assessment of the clinical signs of concussion in Australian football. J Sci Med Sport 2016; online first.
26. Makdissi M, Davis G. Using video analysis for concussion surveillance in Australian football. J Sci Med Sport 2016; online first.
27. Makdissi M, Davis G, Jordan B, Patricios J, Purcell L, Putukian M. Revisiting the modifiers: how should the evaluation and management of acute concussions differ in specific groups? Br J Sports Med. 2013;47:314–20.
28. McCrea M, Guskiewicz K, Randolph C, Barr WB, Hammeke TA, Marshall SW, Powell MR, Woo Ahn K, Wang Y, Kelly JP. Incidence, clinical course, and predictors of prolonged recovery time following sport-related concussion in high school and college athletes. J Int Neuropsychol Soc. 2013;19:22–33.
29. McCrea M, Iverson GL, Echemendia RJ, Makdissi M, Raftery M. Day of injury assessment of sport-related concussion. Br J Sports Med 2013; 47: 272–284 Available from: http://www.ncbi.nlm.nih.gov/pubmed/23479484.
30. McCrea M, Kelly JP, Randolph C, Cisler R, Berger L. Immediate Neurocognitive effects of concussion. Neurosurgery. 2002;50:1032–40.
31. McCrory P, Meeuwisse WH, Aubry M, Cantu B, Dvorák J, Echemendia RJ, Engebretsen L, Johnston K, Kutcher JS, Raftery M, Sills A, Benson BW, Davis GA, Ellenbogen RG, Guskiewicz K, Herring SA, Iverson GL, Jordan BD, Kissick J, McCrea M, McIntosh AS, Maddocks D, Makdissi M, Purcell L, Putukian M, Schneider K, Tator CH, Turner M. Consensus statement on concussion in sport: the 4th international conference on concussion in sport held in Zurich, November 2012. Br J Sports Med. 2013;47:250–8.
32. McDevitt J, Tierney RT, Phillips J, Gaughan JP, Torg JS, Krynetskiy E. Association between GRIN2A promoter polymorphism and recovery from concussion. Brain Inj. 2015;29:1674–81.
33. McHugh ML. Interrater reliability: the kappa statistic. Biochem Med. 2012;22: 276–82.
34. Meehan WP, Mannix RC, Stracciolini A, Elbin RJ, Collins MW. Symptom severity predicts prolonged recovery after sport-related concussion, but age and amnesia do not. J Pediatr. 2013;163:721–5.
35. Miller JH, Gill C, Kuhn EN, Rocque BG, Menendez JY, O'Neill JA, Agee BS,

Brown ST, Crowther M, Davis RD, Ferguson D, Johnston JM. Predictors of delayed recovery following pediatric sports-related concussion: a case-control study. J Neurosurg Pediatr. 2016;17:491–6.
36. Morgan CD, Zuckerman SL, Lee YM, King L, Beaird S, Sills AK, Solomon GS. Predictors of postconcussion syndrome after sports-related concussion in young athletes: a matched case-control study. J Neurosurgery Pediatr. 2015; 15:589–98.
37. Nelson LD, Guskiewicz KM, Marshall SW, Hammeke T, Barr W, Randolph C, McCrea MA. Multiple self-reported concussions are more prevalent in athletes with ADHD and learning disability. Clin J Sport Med. 2016;26:120–7.
38. Nelson LD, Tarima S, LaRoche AA, Hammeke TA, Barr WB, Guskiewicz K, Randolph C, McCrea MA. Preinjury somatization symptoms contribute to clinical recovery after sports-related concussion. Neurology. 2016;86:1856–63.
39. Pellman EJ, Viano DC, Casson IR, Arfken C, Powell J. Concussion in professional football: injuries involving 7 or more days out-part 5. Neurosurgery. 2004;55:1100–19.
40. Putukian M, Raftery M, Guskiewicz K, Herring S, Aubry M, Cantu RC, Molloy M. Onfield assessment of concussion in the adult athlete. Br J Sports Med. 2013;47:285–8.
41. Savage J, Hooke C, Orchard J, Parkinson R. The incidence of concussion in a professional Australian rugby league team, 1998–2012. J Sports Med 2013; online first.
42. Terwilliger VK, Pratson L, Vaughan CG, Gioia GA. Additional post-concussion impact exposure may affect recovery in adolescent athletes. J Neurotrauma. 2016;33:761–5.
43. Zuckerman SL, Yengo-Kahn AM, Buckley TA, Solomon GS, Sills AK, Kerr ZY. Predictors of postconcussion syndrome in collegiate student-athletes. Neurosurg Focus. 2016;40:E13.

Illicit Drug Use Among Gym-Goers: a Cross-sectional Study of Gym-Goers in Sweden

Yasmina Molero[1,2*], Ann-Sofie Bakshi[1] and Johanna Gripenberg[1]

Abstract

Background: The use of anabolic-androgenic steroids has increased among gym-goers, and it has been proposed that this may be part of a polysubstance use pattern that includes the use of illicit drugs. Still, epidemiological data on illicit drug use among gym-goers of both genders are meager. The aim of the present study was thus to examine the use of illicit drugs and its correlates in a large sample of men and women who engaged in weight training at gyms across Sweden.

Methods: In this cross-sectional study, a total of 1969 gym-goers who engaged in weight training in 54 gyms across Sweden were invited to fill in a questionnaire. The questionnaire included 25 items on background variables, weight training frequency, use of illicit drugs and doping substances, and non-medical use of benzodiazepines.

Results: Of the gym-goers, 19.6% reported having ever used illicit drugs, 6.5% reported use during the past 12 months, and 2.1% during the past 30 days. The most commonly used drug was cannabis, followed by cocaine, amphetamine, and ecstasy. Almost 40% of those who reported drug use had used more than one drug. Male participants and participants between 20 and 39 years of age made up the majority of users. Furthermore, 5.1% of the reported drug users had ever used a doping substance. There was an almost threefold higher odds (OR = 2.99, 95% CI = 1.16–7.66, $p < 0.023$) of doping use among people who had reported drug use as compared to non-users.

Conclusions: Training at gyms is typically considered a health-promoting behavior. However, our results revealed a slightly higher prevalence of illicit drug use among gym attendees as compared to the general population. Our findings may have captured an underrecognized group of young adult males who engage in weightlifting and use illicit drugs recreationally and/or as training aids. Developing knowledge is imperative in orientating preventive efforts among at-risk gym-goers.

Trial Registration: ISRCTN11655041

Keywords: Illicit drug use, Gym-goers, Anabolic-androgenic steroids, Cross-sectional study, Drug prevalence

Key Points

- Approximately one in five gym-goers report use of illicit drugs, most commonly cannabis and stimulants. The rates of drug use are higher among young adult males.
- Illicit drug use appears to be associated with the use of doping substances.
- Gyms could provide an innovative setting for intervention and prevention efforts targeting doping and illicit drug use, because such establishments already deal with health promotion.

* Correspondence: yasmina.molero.samuelson@ki.se
[1]STAD, Centre for Psychiatry Research, Department of Clinical Neuroscience, Karolinska Institutet, & Stockholm Health Care Services, Stockholm County Council, Norra Stationsgatan 69, SE-1113-64 Stockholm, Sweden
[2]Department of Medical Epidemiology and Biostatistics, Karolinska Institutet, Stockholm, Sweden

Background

Research shows that 65% of citizens in the European Union exercise at least once a week. Among this group, 30% exercise at sport clubs such as gyms and fitness centers [1]. In the USA, approximately 21% of adults reported exercising regularly [2], and more than 55 million memberships were purchased at health clubs and fitness centers in 2015 [3]. Exercise is a health-promoting activity associated with several benefits, including reduced risk of coronary heart disease, type 2 diabetes, breast and colon cancer, as well as premature mortality [4]. At the same time, there is growing evidence indicating that use of anabolic-androgenic steroids and non-medical use of prescription drugs have increased among gym-goers [5–7]. It has been proposed that this may be part of a polysubstance use pattern that involves other illicit drugs as well (e.g., cannabis and stimulants) [8]. Polysubstance use is associated with poorer mental health, sexual risk behavior, negative social consequences, and increased risk of infectious disease [9, 10]. Furthermore, concurrent use of substances may have synergistic negative effects on brain function [9]. It has been suggested that doping prevention efforts should target gym-goers [11]. Given the association between doping substances and illicit drugs [8, 12–14], prevention efforts could therefore also address the use of illicit drugs [6]. Still, the research base on illicit drug use among gym-goers is limited, and developing knowledge is imperative in orientating preventive efforts.

Several studies have examined the use of illicit drugs among sportspeople through questionnaires or toxicological testing [15–23]. Results from these studies indicate elevated rates of illicit drug use, with cannabis and stimulants being the most commonly used drugs. However, these samples have been restricted to elite athletes or adolescent populations. Epidemiological studies focusing on illicit drug use among adult gym-goers are few in number. One study on 311 gym-going gay men in New York showed that 6–35% (depending on the type of drug) reported having used a drug during the past 6 months [24]. Another study on 1592 gay men who attended gyms in London showed that 56% reported having used an illicit drug during the past year [25]. It was proposed that many of these men do not frequent gyms as a health-promoting activity, but rather to achieve an idealized muscular, physically strong body. This was suggested to be indicative of a gay subculture that focuses on physical prowess and risk behaviors, including illicit drug use [24]. However, results from these two studies may be difficult to generalize to other gym-attending populations and across gender.

The present study is part of a larger on-going project entitled 100% Pure Hard Training (100% PHT) [26]. In the 100% PHT project, the prevalence of doping substances (i.e., anabolic-androgenic steroids and growth hormones) and other illicit drugs is measured among gym-goers who engage in weight training (i.e., work with free weights or machines), and the effect of a doping prevention programme (i.e., 100% PHT) is examined. In the present study, the use of illicit drugs, benzodiazepines, and doping substances among gym-goers was assessed using a cross-sectional design. This assessment was carried out prior to implementation of the prevention programme.

The overall aim of the study is to examine the use of illicit drugs in a large sample of men and women who engage in weight training at gyms across Sweden. Specifically, we conducted a cross-sectional examination of the (a) frequency and type of illicit drugs used, (b) frequency of non-medical use of benzodiazepines, (c) age and sex differences in illicit drug use, (d) associations between use of illicit drugs and weight training frequency, and (e) associations between use of illicit drugs and use of doping substances.

Methods

Study Design

The present study has a cross-sectional study design.

Participants and Procedure

In the spring of 2015, a questionnaire was distributed to gym-goers at 54 gyms in Sweden. The gyms were recruited either through Prevention of Doping in Sweden (PRODIS; a national network comprising governmental agencies, universities, county administrative boards, municipal prevention coordinators, representatives from the police force and gyms, the Swedish Sports Confederation, and the Swedish Anti-Doping Hotline) or through the research centre STAD (Stockholm Prevents Alcohol and Drug Problems). The questionnaire was distributed prior to implementation of the doping prevention programme 100% PHT at the gyms. During data collection, research staff stood by the entrance of the gyms on a weekday afternoon or evening and asked arriving gym-goers above 16 years of age whether they were going to do weight training (i.e., work with free weights or machines). Those who replied in the affirmative were invited to participate in the study. Gym-goers who agreed to participate were asked to complete a questionnaire. To guarantee anonymity, participants completed the questionnaire anonymously and then placed it in an envelope and sealed it, before returning it to the research staff. For the study, 2631 gym-goers were asked to participate, and 1969 of them agreed (74.8% response rate). All gyms were located in urban areas; 39% of the gyms were located in a major city (i.e., more than 200,000 inhabitants), 37% in a large town (i.e., more than 50,000 inhabitants), and 13% in a small town (i.e., more than 15,000 inhabitants) [27]. For more details on the data collection, please see study protocol [26].

Measures

The questionnaire distributed to the participants was based on another questionnaire previously used in a Swedish study measuring anabolic-androgenic steroid use among gym-goers [28]. It included 25 items on background variables, weight training frequency, use of illicit drugs, doping substances, and nutritional supplements, as well as attitude items on doping prevention.

The questionnaire took 5 to 10 min to complete. The following measures were included in the current study:

Demographic Factors

Participants were asked to report their age, sex, employment, and highest educational attainment.

Weight Training Frequency

Participants were asked *"How often do you do weight training at the gym?"* Response alternatives were never, less than once a week, once or twice a week, three or four times a week, and five or more times a week.

Use of Illicit Drugs

Participants were asked *"Have you ever used any illicit drugs or prescription drugs without a doctor's order?"* Participants were then asked to specify the type of illicit drugs that they had used. Response alternatives were cannabis, amphetamines, cocaine, heroin, hallucinogens, ecstasy, benzodiazepines, or other. Furthermore, participants were asked *"Have you used any illicit drugs or prescription drugs without a doctor's order during the past 12 months?"* and *"Have you used any illicit drugs or prescription drugs without a doctor's order during the past 30 days?"*

Use of Doping Substances

To assess the use of doping substances, participants were asked *"Have you ever used any anabolic-androgenic substances, growth hormones or other doping substances without a doctor's order?"*

Statistical Analysis

First, frequencies and proportions of demographic factors and weight training intensity are presented for the whole sample (n = 1969). Illicit drug use and associated characteristics are also presented for the whole sample. In a subsequent step, drug characteristics are presented only for those who reported illicit drug use (n = 385). Logistic regression models were then calculated in the whole sample (n = 1969) to examine associations between illicit drug use and weight training frequency, as well as associations between illicit drug use and use of doping substances. Crude odds ratios (OR) and 95% confidence intervals (95% CI) are presented. Odds ratios were then adjusted; when examining associations between illicit drug use and weight training frequency, odds ratios were adjusted for age and sex. When examining associations between illicit drug use and the use of doping substances, odds ratios were adjusted for age, sex, weight training frequency, and number of illicit drugs used. IBM SPSS Statistics 24.0 was used in all analyses. The STrengthening the Reporting of OBservational studies in Epidemiology (STROBE) guidelines were followed (S1).

Power Analysis

Previous studies have shown that the effect of prevention programmes is rather low, typically about 15–20% [29, 30]. To measure the intervention effect, a power analysis was carried out a priori; a minimum of 40 gyms (20 intervention gyms and 20 control gyms) and a minimum of 1600 participants (800 individuals per condition) were required at each data collection point to achieve a power of 80% at an alpha level of .05 (two-tailed). In the current pre-intervention study, 27 intervention gyms and 27 control gyms have been enrolled, and a total of 1969 individuals completed the questionnaire.

Ethical approval

The present study adheres to the criteria of the World Medical Association Declaration of Helsinki, and has been approved by the regional ethical review board of Karolinska Institutet, Sweden (registration number: 2016/142-31/3).

Results

The present study included 1969 gym-goers from 54 gyms. The sample consisted of a large proportion of males (65.3%), and the majority of participants were below 40 years of age. Most gym-goers were employed, had completed secondary or tertiary education, and reported regular weight training. In the total sample of gym-goers, 2.0% (40) reported having ever used a doping substance (Table 1).

Among the participating gym-goers, 19.6% (385) reported having ever used an illicit drug or benzodiazepines without a prescription (Table 2). Furthermore, 6.5% reported that they had done so during the past 12 months and 2.1% during the past 30 days. Cannabis was the most commonly used illicit drug and had been used by 92.2% of participants reporting illicit drug use. Between 20 and 25.2% of the reported illicit drug users had used cocaine, amphetamine, and/or ecstasy. Heroin was the least common illicit drug. Among those who reported illicit drug use, 17.4% reported having used two drugs and 21.3% reported having used three or more drugs (Table 3). The prevalence of individuals who reported a lifetime use of doping substances was higher among those with prior illicit drug use (5.1%) than in the total sample. There were statistically significant gender differences in prevalence rates; males demonstrated higher rates of cannabis, amphetamine, cocaine, and ecstasy use. Males also demonstrated significantly higher rates of polysubstance use. Furthermore, there were statistically significant age differences; younger individuals (below age 40) demonstrated higher prevalence rates of

Table 1 Sample characteristics of gym-goers (n = 1969)

Sex[a]	
Male	63.5% (1251)
Female	35.8% (705)
Age[b]	
16–19 years	9.3% (184)
20–29 years	41.2% (811)
30–39 years	19.0% (375)
40–49 years	14.3% (281)
50–59 years	9.9% (194)
60 years and older	5.8% (114)
Occupation[c]	
Employed	71.4% (1406)
Unemployed	3.1% (62)
Studying	19.2% (378)
Retired	2.5% (49)
Sick leave	0.8% (16)
Other	2.1% (42)
Highest educational attainment[c]	
Primary education	8.2% (162)
Secondary education	42.7% (841)
Tertiary education	31.4% (619)
Weight training frequency[c]	
Never	1.1% (22)
Less than once a week	3.8% (75)
Once or twice a week	23.9% (470)
Three to four times a week	47.6% (937)
Five or more times a week	23.5% (463)
Lifetime use of doping substances	
Has ever used a doping substance	2.0% (40)

[a]Missing information for 13 individuals
[b]Missing information for 10 individuals
[c]Missing information for 16 individuals

Table 2 Lifetime drug use among gym-goers (n = 1969)

Lifetime drug use	
Has ever used drugs	19.6% (385)
Sex[a]	
Male	71.5% (274)
Female	28.2% (108)
Age[b]	
16–19 years	7.8% (30)
20–29 years	49.7% (191)
30–39 years	26.6% (102)
40–49 years	6.5% (25)
50–59 years	5.5% (21)
60 years and older	3.9% (15)
Recent illicit drug use	
Has used drugs during the past 12 months	6.5% (128)
Has used drugs during the past 30 days	2.1% (42)

[a]Missing information for three individuals
[b]Missing information for one individual

cannabis, amphetamine, cocaine, hallucinogen, and ecstasy use and also higher rates of polysubstance use (Table 3).

A logistic regression was performed to examine the relationship between weight training frequency and illicit drug use (Table 4). No statistically significant associations were found, neither in the crude analyses, nor when adjusting for sex and age. Another logistic regression was then performed to assess the relationship between illicit drug use and use of doping substances. The logistic regression model was statistically significant (χ^2 = 18.391, p < .001, df = 1), showing that individuals who reported illicit drug use were more than four times more likely to use doping substances compared to individuals without prior illicit drug use. When adjusting for age, sex, weight training frequency, and number of illicit drugs used, the model remained statistically significant (χ^2 = 38.514, p < .001, df = 5). Results showed that individuals who reported illicit drug use were almost three times more likely to use doping substances compared to individuals without prior illicit drug use.

Discussion

Discussion

In the present study, 1969 gym-goers at 54 gyms in Sweden completed a questionnaire covering the use of illicit drugs and prescription drugs. Results showed that 19.6% of gym-goers reported having ever used illicit drugs. Moreover, of this group, 6.5% reported use during the past 12 months and 2.1% during the past 30 days. Among those who reported illicit drug use, the most commonly used illicit drug was cannabis, followed by cocaine, amphetamine, and ecstasy. Furthermore, 5.1% of those reported a lifetime use of doping substances. Almost 40% of those reporting illicit drug use reported polysubstance use. Furthermore, male participants and participants between 16 and 39 years of age demonstrated significantly higher rates of illicit drug use and polysubstance use than female participants and participants above age 40, respectively.

Our findings are in line with two Swedish population-based surveys. In a survey from 2008/2009, 18% of respondents reported having used illicit drugs on at least one occasion in their lives [31]. In a survey from 2012, 3.1% of respondents had used an illicit drug during the past 12 months and 1.1% during the past 30 days [32].

Table 3 Drug characteristics among gym-goers who reported lifetime drug use (n = 385)

	All drug users	Males[a]	Females[a]	χ^2	p	Age 16–39[a]	Age 40 and over[a]	χ^2	p
Lifetime use of illicit drugs									
Cannabis	92.2% (355)	67.0% (258)	24.7% (95)	16.04	< 0.001	77.4% (298)	15.8% (56)	41.71	< 0.001
Cocaine	25.2% (97)	19.5% (75)	5.7% (22)	8.07	0.018	21.8% (84)	3.4% (13)	13.48	< 0.001
Amphetamine	21.8% (84)	16.1% (62)	5.5% (21)	10.47	0.005	17.7% (68)	4.2% (16)	5.07	0.024
Ecstasy	20.0% (77)	14.3% (55)	5.5% (21)	9.28	0.010	18.4% (71)	1.6% (6)	18.91	< 0.001
Hallucinogens	13.0% (50)	9.6% (37)	3.4% (13)	2.33	0.312	11.4% (44)	1.3% (5)	9.43	< 0.001
Benzodiazepines	8.6% (33)	6.8% (26)	1.8% (7)	3.26	0.196	7.0% (27)	1.6% (6)	2.25	0.133
Heroin	1.6% (6)	1.6% (6)	0.0% (0)	3.41	0.182	0.8% (3)	0.8% (3)	1.14	0.286
Other	3.1% (12)	2.9% (11)	0.3% (1)	4.05	0.132	2.6% (11)	0.3% (1)	2.71	0.100
Number of illicit drugs used (lifetime)									
One drug	59.7% (230)	41.3% (159)	18.2% (70)	15.55	0.001	48.3% (186)	11.4% (44)	41.73	< 0.001
Two drugs	17.4% (67)	13.5% (52)	3.9% (15)			14.8% (57)	2.3% (9)		
Three or more drugs	21.3% (82)	15.8% (61)	5.2% (20)			19.0% (73)	2.6% (10)		
Lifetime use of doping substances									
Doping substances	4.9% (19)	6.4% (17)	1.9% (2)	3.05	0.218	5.4% (17)	3.4% (2)	0.40	0.529

[a]Missing information for one individual

Training at gyms is typically a health-promoting behavior; hence, it could be hypothesized that the estimates in our sample would be lower than the rates found in the general population. However, our results pointed to a slightly higher prevalence of illicit drug use among gym-goers. The elevated rates in our study could be explained by age and sex differences in the samples; our study included more males and more individuals from younger age categories, where illicit drug use is generally more prevalent [31, 32].

Conversely, participants in the present study reported a lower lifetime prevalence of illicit drug use as compared to the European average. In the European Union, approximately 25% of 15- to 64-year-olds are estimated to have used an illicit drug [33]. Studies consistently indicate lower estimates of illicit drug use in Sweden compared to many countries [34–36], which also could be reflected among gym-goers [24, 25]. Further research is needed to specifically examine the use of illicit drugs and prescription drugs (beyond benzodiazepines) in gym settings and to assess between-country differences as well as associations with demographic factors. Prevalence rates in our study were higher than rates among elite athletes in Europe and Australia [17, 18, 21]. Higher estimates of illicit drug use among gym-goers might be expected, however, as elite athletes generally have a healthier lifestyle and are also subject to anti-doping tests, which may have a deterrent effect on illicit drug use [18].

Two studies have examined the use of illicit drugs among gay male gym-goers in New York and London, respectively. In these studies, prevalence rates were markedly higher than in our study; in the New York study, estimates ranged between 6% (for hallucinogen use) and 35% (for inhalant nitrite use) during the past 6 months [24]. Among the men recruited from London gyms, 56% reported having used an illicit drug during the past 12 months [25]. It was proposed that these studies largely reflected a specific subculture among gay and bisexual men who frequented clubs and engaged in risk behaviors (i.e., substance use and sexual risk behavior), which could explain the higher prevalence rates.

The most commonly used illicit drugs in our study were cannabis, cocaine, amphetamine, ecstasy, and hallucinogens—drugs that can be used both as training aids or "body image drugs," or recreationally as so-called club drugs [37–40]. Moreover, approximately 40% of the illicit

Table 4 Associations between illicit drug use and weight training frequency and use of doping substances, respectively (n = 1969)

	Crude			Adjusted		
	OR	95% CI	p	OR	95% CI	p
Weight training frequency	1.07	0.94–1.23	0.296	0.90[a]	0.78–1.04	0.143
Use of doping substances	4.40	2.28–8.46,	$p < 0.001$	2.99[b]	1.16–7.66	$p < 0.023$

OR odds ratio 95%, *CI* 95% confidence intervals
[a]Adjusted for sex and age
[b]Adjusted for sex, age, weight training frequency, and number of drugs used

drug users in our sample reported polysubstance use, and the rates were significantly higher among younger participants and males. Our results could also have captured a group of young adult males who focus on physical appearance and engage in partying and risk behaviors, comparable to the gay men in the gym studies discussed above. It has been suggested that drug use practices and weight training in a male "body subculture" can be understood as a way to construct a masculine identity and to achieve an idealized male body [41]. Our estimates were higher than the estimates in a study of anabolic substance use among 611 visitors to German fitness centers, where 15.9% reported using other illicit drugs [42]. Almost all participants in our study engaged in weight training, as opposed to 25% of the respondents in the German study. Again, the higher prevalence rates in our study could support the notion of a physical achievement-oriented group who engage in weight training and use illicit substances for ergogenic and/or recreational purposes.

In our study, however, we found no associations between weight training frequency and illicit drug use. Prior research on the association between physical activity and illicit drug use is mixed: Some studies suggest that the degree of sporting activity is negatively associated with substance use [43]. Others point to a curvilinear link between sporting activities and illicit drug use, i.e., that inactive and intensive levels are associated with greater use of illicit drugs than moderate levels are, particularly for strength sports (weightlifting and body-building) [19]. However, these studies have largely been based on adolescent populations, and it has been proposed that the relationship between physical activity and illicit drug use is affected by age [19], which could explain our differing results.

The overall prevalence of the lifetime use of doping substances (i.e., anabolic-androgenic substances and growth hormones) was lower in our total sample than in other gym samples [28, 42, 44–46]. Nonetheless, our results showed a threefold higher in odds of doping use among people who had reported illicit drug use as compared to non-users. Previous research has pointed to a strong relationship between use of doping substances and use of other illicit drugs [14, 47–49]. Illicit drugs may be used to increase or decrease the effects of anabolic-androgenic steroids (e.g., as pain relief to increase energy levels or to promote sleep) [6], and it has been proposed that doping prevention efforts should therefore address other illicit drugs as well [6]. The *European Commission Group of Experts on Anabolic Androgenic Steroid Use in Recreational Sports* has identified gyms as important target arenas for preventive efforts and has also suggested three key elements that should be included in research to inform policy, practice, and interventions: information on doping prevalence, use of other illicit drugs, and determinants and correlates [11].

Strengths and Limitations

The present study has both strengths and limitations that should be taken into account when interpreting the findings. One important strength is that we included a large sample of men and women and that participants were recruited from 54 gyms across the country. Limitations include a possible underestimation of illicit drug prevalence rates due to a higher degree of attrition among individuals who use illicit drugs or to recollection bias, social desirability, or fear that reported illicit drug use may attract unwanted attention to the gym [50]. Males and individuals under age 40 made up a large proportion of participants, which could limit the generalizability of the findings. Furthermore, the questionnaire was distributed on weekday afternoons and evenings, and only individuals who engaged in weight training were invited to participate, which could limit generalizability further. Although the questionnaire has been used in a prior study [28], its psychometric properties have not been validated. Another limitation was that the study was cross-sectional; thus, we could not establish causality in the association between illicit drug and doping use.

Conclusions

Our study examined illicit drug use in a large sample of male and female adult gym-goers. Illicit drug use estimates in our study were slightly elevated in comparison to estimates in population-based studies in Sweden [31, 32] and could simply reflect illicit drug use in the general population. This may seem contradictory, however, as training at gyms is typically considered a health-promoting behavior and prevalence rates could thus be expected to be lower among gym-goers. Our findings show that a substantial proportion of young adult males who lift weights have used several illicit drugs. This suggests that illicit drug use among sportspeople, possibly for ergogenic or analgesic purposes, is a public health problem not limited to elite athletes [17, 18, 21]. A proportion of younger recreational sportspeople may be at risk of developing substance abuse problems (including doping substances), yet there are few arenas on which young individuals can be reached other than nightlife settings and universities [50–52]. Previous research shows that young people who party frequent gyms to socialize, to offset the effects of substance use, or to purchase illicit drugs [53]. Gyms could thus provide an additional innovative setting for intervention and prevention efforts targeting doping and illicit drug use, because such establishments already deal with health promotion and do not allow on-site alcohol consumption.

Abbreviations

100% PHT: 100% Pure Hard Training; 95% CI: 95% confidence intervals; OR: Odds ratios; PRODIS: Prevention of Doping in Sweden; STAD: Stockholm Prevents Alcohol and Drug Problems; STROBE: STrengthening the Reporting of OBservational studies in Epidemiology guidance

Acknowledgements
The authors are grateful to Viveca Andersson, Kamilla Nylund, and Nicklas Kartengren for their help with the data collection and contributions to the manuscript, and to the PRODIS network and the participating gyms for their cooperation.

Funding
The study is funded by The Public Health Agency of Sweden (Grant Number 05522-2014-6.2). The funders play no role in the design of the study; the collection, analysis, and interpretation of the data; or in the writing of the manuscript.

Authors' contributions
JG conceived of the original idea and JG and ASB obtained the funding for the study. YM, JG, and ASB planned and designed the current study. YM carried out all the analyses, and YM, JG, and ASB interpreted the data. YM prepared the manuscript with the contribution of ASB and JG. All authors read and approved of the final manuscript.

Competing interests
Yasmina Molero, Ann-Sofie Bakshi, and Johanna Gripenberg declare that they have no conflict of interest.

References

1. Eurobarometer, Special. Eurobarometer 72.3. Sport and Physical Activity, Wave EB80 2. Brussels: Directorate General Education and Culture; 2010.
2. Facts about physical activity [Internet]. 2014. Available from: https://www.cdc.gov/physicalactivity/data/facts.htm. Accessed 28 Feb 2017.
3. Facts on Health & Fitness Clubs [Internet]. 2016. https://www.statista.com/topics/1141/health-and-fitness-clubs/. Accessed 28 Feb 2017.
4. Lee IM, Shiroma EJ, Lobelo F, Puska P, Blair SN, Katzmarzyk PT. Effect of physical inactivity on major non-communicable diseases worldwide: an analysis of burden of disease and life expectancy. Lancet (London, England). 2012;380(9838):219–29.
5. Baker JS, Graham MR, Davies B. Steroid and prescription medicine abuse in the health and fitness community: a regional study. European journal of internal medicine. 2006;17(7):479–84.
6. Sagoe D, McVeigh J, Bjornebekk A, Essilfie MS, Andreassen CS, Pallesen S. Polypharmacy among anabolic-androgenic steroid users: a descriptive metasynthesis. Subst Abuse Treat Prev Policy. 2015;10:12.
7. Sjoqvist F, Garle M, Rane A. Use of doping agents, particularly anabolic steroids, in sports and society. Lancet (London, England). 2008;371(9627):1872–82.
8. Dodge T, Hoagland MF. The use of anabolic androgenic steroids and polypharmacy: a review of the literature. Drug Alcohol Depend. 2011; 114(2–3):100–9.
9. Connor JP, Gullo MJ, White A, Kelly AB. Polysubstance use: diagnostic challenges, patterns of use and health. Current opinion in psychiatry. 2014; 27(4):269–75.
10. Midanik LT, Tam TW, Weisner C. Concurrent and simultaneous drug and alcohol use: results of the 2000 National Alcohol Survey. Drug Alcohol Depend. 2007;90(1):72–80.
11. Backhouse S, Collins C, Defoort Y, McNamee M, Parkinson A, Sauer M, et al. Study on doping prevention: a map of legal, regulatory and prevention practice provisions in EU 28. 2014.
12. Denham BE. Association between narcotic use and anabolic-androgenic steroid use among American adolescents. Subst Use Misuse. 2009;44(14): 2043–61.
13. Nyberg F, Hallberg M. Interactions between opioids and anabolic androgenic steroids: implications for the development of addictive behavior. Int Rev Neurobiol. 2012;102:189–206.
14. Kanayama G, Pope HG, Cohane G, Hudson JI. Risk factors for anabolic-androgenic steroid use among weightlifters: a case-control study. Drug Alcohol Depend. 2003;71(1):77–86.
15. Laure P, Lecerf T, Friser A, Binsinger C. Drugs, recreational drug use and attitudes towards doping of high school athletes. Int J Sports Med. 2004; 25(2):133–8.
16. Moore MJ, Werch CE. Sport and physical activity participation and substance use among adolescents. The Journal of adolescent health : official publication of the Society for Adolescent Medicine. 2005;36(6):486–93.
17. Thevis M, Sauer M, Geyer H, Sigmund G, Mareck U, Schanzer W. Determination of the prevalence of anabolic steroids, stimulants, and selected drugs subject to doping controls among elite sport students using analytical chemistry. J Sports Sci. 2008;26(10):1059–65.
18. Strano Rossi S, Botre F. Prevalence of illicit drug use among the Italian athlete population with special attention on drugs of abuse: a 10-year review. J Sports Sci. 2011;29(5):471–6.
19. Peretti-Watel P, Beck F, Legleye S. Beyond the U-curve: the relationship between sport and alcohol, cigarette and cannabis use in adolescents. Addiction. 2002;97(6):707–16.
20. Brisola-Santos MB, Gil F, Sampaio-Junior B, Marin MCD, de Andrade AG, Richter KP, et al. Prevalence and correlates of cannabis use among athletes—a systematic review. Am J Addict. 2016;(7):518-28.
21. Harcourt PR, Unglik H, Cook JL. A strategy to reduce illicit drug use is effective in elite Australian football. Br J Sports Med. 2012:bjsports-2012-091329.
22. Momaya A, Fawal M, Estes R. Performance-enhancing substances in sports: a review of the literature. Sports Med. 2015;45(4):517–31.
23. Reardon CL, Creado S. Drug abuse in athletes. Substance Abuse and Rehabilitation. 2014;5:95–105.
24. Halkitis PN, Moeller RW, Siconolfi DE, Jerome RC, Rogers M, Schillinger J. Methamphetamine and poly-substance use among gym-attending men who have sex with men in New York City. Annals of behavioral medicine : a publication of the Society of Behavioral Medicine. 2008;35(1):41–8.
25. Bolding G, Hart G, Sherr L, Elford J. Use of crystal methamphetamine among gay men in London. Addiction. 2006;101(11):1622–30.
26. Molero Y, Gripenberg J, Bakshi AS. Effectiveness and implementation of a community-based prevention programme targeting anabolic androgenic steroid use in gyms: study protocol of a quasi-experimental control group study. BMC sports science, medicine and rehabilitation. 2016;8:36.
27. Swedish Association of Local Authorities and Regions [Statens Kommuner och Landsting]. Division of municipalities 2017 [Kommungruppsindelning 2017]. Stockholm: Sveriges Kommuner och Landsting, ISBN: 978-91-7585-455-7; 2016.
28. Leifman H, Rehnman C, Sjoblom E, Holgersson S. Anabolic androgenic steroids—use and correlates among gym users—an assessment study using questionnaires and observations at gyms in the Stockholm region. Int J Environ Res Public Health. 2011;8(7):2656–74.
29. Skärstrand E. Prevention of alcohol and drug problems among adolescents: evaluating a Swedish version of the Strengthening Families Program: Inst för folkhälsovetenskap/Dept of Public Health Sciences. Solna: Karolinska Institutet; 2010.
30. Strandberg A. Evaluation of a Swedish parental prevention program: youth drunkenness, alcohol-specific parenting and gender differences: Inst för folkhälsovetenskap/Dept of Public Health Sciences. Solna: Karolinska Institutet; 2014.
31. The Public Health Agency of Sweden [Folhälsomyndigheten]. Drug use in Sweden [Narkotikabruket i Sverige]. Östersund: Folkhälsomyndigheten, ISBN: 978-91-7257-713-8; 2010.
32. Ramstedt M, Sundin E, Landberg J, Raninen J. Alcohol, narcotics, doping, and tobacco use and its negative consequences in the Swedish population—a study focused on misuse, abuse, and other problems related to alcohol, narcotics, doping, and tobacco [ANDT-bruket och dess negativa konsekvenser i den svenska befolkningen 2013—en studie med fokus på missbruk och beroende samt problem för andra än brukaren relaterat till alkohol, narkotika, doping och tobak]. Stockholm: STAD; 2014. ISBN: 978-91-85997-24-4.
33. European Monitoring Centre for Drugs and Drug Addiction. European drug report 2016: trends and developments. Luxembourg; 2016.
34. Degenhardt L, Bucello C, Calabria B, Nelson P, Roberts A, Hall W, et al. What data are available on the extent of illicit drug use and dependence globally? Results of four systematic reviews. Drug Alcohol Depend. 2011; 117(2–3):85–101.
35. Degenhardt L, Hall W. Extent of illicit drug use and dependence, and their contribution to the global burden of disease. Lancet (London, England). 2012;379(9810):55–70.

36. The Public Health Agency of Sweden (Folhälsomyndigheten). The 2013 national report (2012 data) to the EMCDDA by the Reitox National Focal Point Sweden. New development and trends. Östersund: STATENS FOLKHÄLSOINSTITUT A; 2013. p. 2.
37. Kanayama G, Hudson JI, Pope HG Jr. Illicit anabolic-androgenic steroid use. Horm Behav. 2010;58(1):111–21.
38. Clarkson PM, Thompson HS. Drugs and Sport. Sports Med. 1997;24(6):366–84.
39. Huestis MA, Mazzoni I, Rabin O. Cannabis in Sport. Sports Med. 2011;41(11): 949–66.
40. Kanayama G, Pope HG Jr, Hudson JI. "Body image" drugs: a growing psychosomatic problem. Psychother Psychosom. 2001;70(2):61–5.
41. Andreasson J. Reconceptualising the gender of fitness doping: performing and negotiating masculinity through drug-use practices. Soc Sci. 2015;4(3): 546–62.
42. Striegel H, Simon P, Frisch S, Roecker K, Dietz K, Dickhuth HH, et al. Anabolic ergogenic substance users in fitness-sports: a distinct group supported by the health care system. Drug Alcohol Depend. 2006;81(1):11–9.
43. Korhonen T, Kujala UM, Rose RJ, Kaprio J. Physical activity in adolescence as a predictor of alcohol and illicit drug use in early adulthood: a longitudinal population-based twin study. Twin research and human genetics : the official journal of the International Society for Twin Studies. 2009;12(3):261–8.
44. Sagoe D, Molde H, Andreassen CS, Torsheim T, Pallesen S. The global epidemiology of anabolic-androgenic steroid use: a meta-analysis and meta-regression analysis. Ann Epidemiol. 2014;24(5):383–98.
45. Nakhaee MR, Pakravan F, Nakhaee N. Prevalence of use of anabolic steroids by bodybuilders using three methods in a city of Iran. Addiction & health. 2013;5(3–4):77.
46. Alsaeed I, Alabkal JR. Usage and perceptions of anabolic-androgenic steroids among male fitness centre attendees in Kuwait—a cross-sectional study. Subst Abuse Treat Prev Policy. 2015;10:33.
47. Skarberg K, Nyberg F, Engstrom I. Multisubstance use as a feature of addiction to anabolic-androgenic steroids. Eur Addict Res. 2009;15(2):99–106.
48. Arvary D, Pope HG Jr. Anabolic-androgenic steroids as a gateway to opioid dependence. N Engl J Med. 2000;342(20):1532.
49. Kanayama G, Cohane GH, Weiss RD, Pope HG. Past anabolic-androgenic steroid use among men admitted for substance abuse treatment: an underrecognized problem? The Journal of clinical psychiatry. 2003;64(2): 156–60.
50. Gripenberg-Abdon J, Elgan TH, Wallin E, Shaafati M, Beck O, Andreasson S. Measuring substance use in the club setting: a feasibility study using biochemical markers. Subst Abuse Treat Prev Policy. 2012;7:7.
51. Nordfjaern T, Bretteville-Jensen AL, Edland-Gryt M, Gripenberg J. Risky substance use among young adults in the nightlife arena: an underused setting for risk-reducing interventions? Scandinavian journal of public health. 2016. [Epub ahead of print].
52. Bullock S. Alcohol, drugs and student lifestyle: a study of the attitudes, beliefs and use of alcohol and drugs among Swedish university students. Stockholm: SoRAD - Research Report nr 21 ISBN: 91-975134-7; 2004.
53. Lindsay J. 'Partying hard', 'partying sometimes' or 'shopping': young workers' socializing patterns and sexual, alcohol and illicit drug risk taking. Critical Public Health. 2003;13(1):1–14.

It's Time to Start Changing the Game: A 12-Week Workplace Team Sport Intervention Study

Andrew Brinkley*, Hilary McDermott, Rachel Grenfell-Essam and Fehmidah Munir

Abstract

Background: A 12-week multi-team sport programme was provided to employees of a large services organisation and conducted in workplaces. This programme was used to investigate the short-term effect of regular sports team participation on individual employee and organisational health.

Methods: A large services organisation participated in this study. Two regional worksites of office workers were assigned as the team sport (intervention) (n = 28 participants) or control (n = 20 participants) groups. The team sport sessions were underpinned by psychological behaviour change theory and consisted of weekly 1-h team sport sessions for 12 weeks. Measures of aerobic fitness, physical activity behaviour, group cohesion, interaction and communication, psychological wellbeing, health, anthropometrics and workplace experiences were recorded pre- and post-intervention. Data were analysed using a series of mixed ANOVAs.

Results: After 12 weeks significant improvements were observed in VO_2 max (+ 4.5 ± 5.8 ml/min kg, $P < .002$, $\eta_p^2 = .182$), interpersonal communication within teams (+ 3%, $P < .042$, $\eta_p^2 = .087$) and mean weekly physical activity duration (+ 154.74′, $P < .002$, $\eta_p^2 = .071$) in the intervention group. A significant ($P < .012$, $\eta_p^2 = .130$) effect on body composition was observed in the intervention group.

Conclusions: Participation in team sport may be an effective method to improve the aerobic fitness and physical activity behaviour of employees, and promote interpersonal communication between colleagues. Individual health outcomes and social interactions have the capacity to influence the health of the organisation. The extent of which these findings are replicable across a scope of organisations should be examined objectively over the long term.

Keywords: Communication, Fitness, Health, Quasi-experimental, Wellbeing, Workplace health, Workplace

Key Points

- This manuscript presents the first attempt to examine the efficacy of a workplace health promotion programme using a variety of team sports. This programme was the first of its kind implemented in a Financial Times and London Stock Exchange (FTSE 100) company and the first underpinned by self-determination theory.
- Past workplace team sport studies have examined markers of health without validated measures. This study tested the efficacy of workplace team sport across individual, social group and organisational health outcomes.
- This study provides support for the use of team sport to promote individual, social group and organisational health within a workplace setting.
- The findings of this study provide evidence for employers and occupational health teams considering implementing team sport into their workplaces.

* Correspondence: A.J.Brinkley@lboro.ac.uk
School of Sport, Exercise and Health Sciences, National Centre for Sport and Exercise Medicine, Loughborough University, Loughborough, Leicestershire LE11 3TU, UK

Background

Within Europe, almost half of working age adults are failing to meet physical activity (PA) guidelines [1]. Modifiable inactive behaviours are associated with non-communicable diseases (e.g. coronary heart disease and type-2 diabetes) and the prevalence of premature mortality [2]. An inactive workplace has been linked with diminished organisational health outcomes, increased sickness absence, reduced productivity and workplace engagement [3]. Workplace PA interventions can positively influence employee and organisational health [3]. Exercise/gym classes, walking, active-transport, educational training, active work stations and activity challenges have been utilised in the workplace with varying degrees of effectiveness [3]. However, research to date is yet to comprehensively examine the efficacy of sport and team sport on health outcomes [4]. Indeed, a further critique of workplace PA literature has been the failure to assess the efficacy of participation against social group and organisational health outcomes (e.g. communication, team performance, job satisfaction) [5].

Participation in workplace team sport has the capacity to improve individual, social group and organisational health outcomes [4]. Several randomised control trial (RCT) and quasi-experimental studies demonstrate that participation in competitive or non-competitive team sports can significantly improve cardiorespiratory fitness, musculoskeletal function [6–9] and psychological wellbeing [10]. These factors have the capacity to contribute to the reduced prevalence of non-communicable diseases associated with sickness absence, diminished productivity and all-cost mortality [2–5]. Qualitative studies suggest participation in team sports may also improve workplace relationships, communication and team cohesion [11–14].

Improvements in individual health and social group outcomes are known to contribute to the function of the organisation [3]. However, perhaps due to a limited level of funding and expertise, and the non-clinical community setting (i.e. the workplace), the research examining participation in team sport has been limited by the reliance on qualitative methods (e.g. focus groups and individual interviews) and interventions that lack strong theoretical underpinnings [4]. Researchers are yet to examine the impact of participation in workplace team sport on social group health outcomes (e.g. cohesion, communication, interpersonal relationships) with validated measures. Furthermore, the type of sport played is reported in most manuscripts but not the intensity it is played at, or the duration, volume and frequency of participation [11–14]. This challenges researchers in determining what 'dose' of team sport equals the benefits reported in the literature [4].

Participation in team sport is challenged by social comparisons with colleagues and superiors, the organisational culture and the facilities available within the workplace [15], and psychological barriers relating to autonomy, competence and relatedness [15, 16]. Self-determination theory (SDT) [17] suggests supporting people's innate needs for autonomy (i.e. feeling free and fully volitional to engage in team sport), competence (i.e. feeling capable to complete a skill in team sport) and relatedness (i.e. feeling supported, understood and valued by a social group) through the provision of an activity (e.g. team sport) may promote wellbeing and autonomous motivation [14–16]. Good evidence indicates supporting basic needs is an effective behaviour change strategy within a workplace, sports and exercise setting [15–17]. For these reasons, workplace team sport interventions should be underpinned by behaviour change theories with a focus on the social environment [15–17].

This study evaluated the impact of a workplace team sport intervention (i.e. 'Changing the Game'; CTG) underpinned by SDT. The primary intention of this study was to examine the impact of CTG on aerobic fitness (estimated VO_2 max). Secondary intentions were to investigate participation in CTG's impact on individual, social group and organisational health outcomes. These included subjective vitality, leisure-time PA, quality of life, occupational stress and fatigue, group cohesion, relationships with superiors and colleagues, communication, job satisfaction, individual and team job performance, and work engagement.

The intervention study was evaluated using a process evaluation underpinned by the RE-AIM approach [18]. This was conducted to evaluate the effectiveness of the intervention approach and its theoretical underpinning [18] and will be reported elsewhere (i.e. findings due for publication in late 2017[1]).

Methods

Design

The intervention was a 12-week non-randomised study (quasi-experimental design), which comprised two regional worksites from the same large service organisation (located an estimated 130 km apart). One worksite was assigned to the CTG (intervention group), while the other continued with normal working conditions (control group). Non-randomised intervention designs in health promotion are frequently adopted where feasibility and practicality issues challenge implementation [19]. In the current study, access to a local sport facility determined the intervention site. The participants were measured pre- (T^0) and post- (T^1) intervention at their respective workplaces. A schematic overview of the study's design, recruitment and attrition rate is provided in Fig. 1. Ethical approval was obtained from Loughborough University's Ethical Advisory Panel (Human Participants sub-committee). The study conforms to and was conducted in accordance with the Declaration of Helsinki.

Intervention

CTG consisted of 12 weekly 1-h lunchtime moderate-intensity team sport sessions in an indoor sports hall

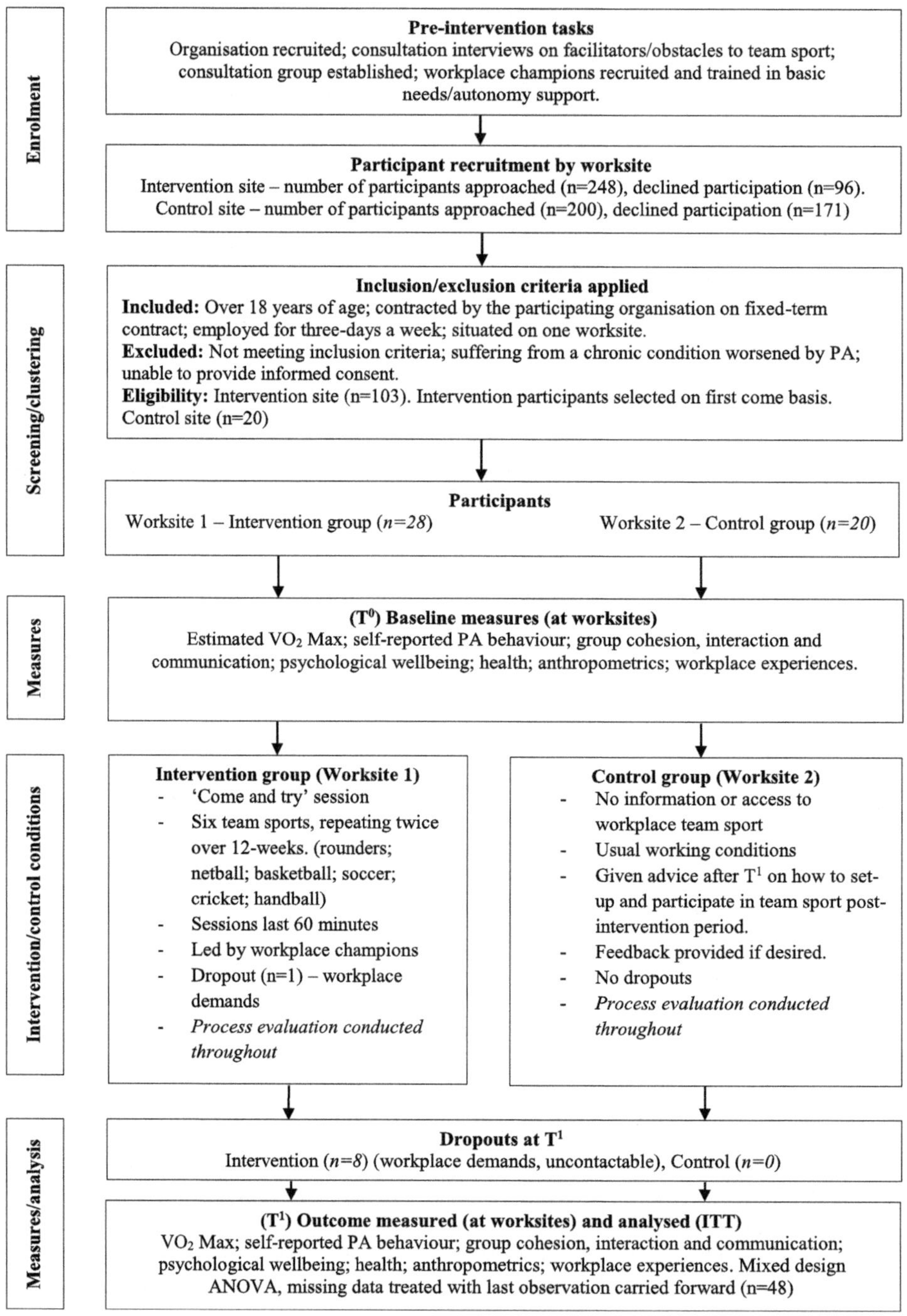

Fig. 1 Schematic overview of 'CTG'

(30 m × 18 m) located 400 m from the participating organisation. The sessions were funded by the researchers' university and consisted of rounders (weeks 1 and 7), netball (weeks 2 and 8), basketball (weeks 3 and 9), soccer (weeks 4 and 10), cricket (weeks 5 and 11) and handball (weeks 6 and 12). The sessions included a 10-min warm-up and familiarisation period, and a 40-min game (breaks given when requested by participants). The sports were chosen by the research team due to their moderate-intensity, transferability of skills and adaptability. Evidence suggests sports with transferable skills may support the needs for competence [15–17]. The sessions were delivered by two female workplace champions trained by the first author in the basic rules of each sport and in supporting basic needs for autonomy, competence and relatedness in their sports participation (training information available on request from the corresponding author). Prior to the intervention

participants were invited to take part in a taster session to help minimise perceptions of negative competence [15–17]. Throughout the CTG sessions, participants were encouraged to place an emphasis on having fun, to reflect on their individual and team skills development and social growth rather than competition and performance. Workplace champions discussed the potential benefits of participating in team sport with the participants who were able to opt out of any stage of the team sport sessions. Participants were given the opportunity to take ownership and alter any rule, skill or tradition associated with the sports as a team. This supportive leadership style can promote autonomous motivation and adherence to participation [15–17]. Adaptations made to the rules of each sport (e.g. removing double dribbles in basketball) has the capacity to support a participant's need for competence, provide self-efficacy and promote the adoption of more autonomous forms of motivation (i.e. identified, integrated and intrinsic regulation) [17]. Needs for relatedness refer to the development and maintenance of interpersonal relationships with individuals (e.g. colleagues) and within workplace teams or groups [16, 17]. Relatedness may have been fostered through the social support, group identity and cohesion of colleagues and superiors playing team sports [15–17].

Participants

A services organisation listed on the Financial Times and London Stock Exchange (FTSE) 100 located in the UK participated in this study. This organisation has a global workforce of 7048 employees (5080 operate in UK), across multiple worksites with employees in predominately office-based roles. This organisation was selected based on its size and structure and was recruited by email. A consultation group of employees, managers, workplace champions and employer representatives guided the intervention through a participatory approach [20]. The role of the consultation group was to advise on challenges specific to the participating organisation and discuss the implementation, delivery and evaluation of the programme within their organisation. Regular meetings were conducted with this working group throughout the intervention period.

Criterion-based sampling based on the inclusion and exclusion criteria was adopted.

Participants were recruited between May and June 2016, within the organisation through email, social media notifications and posters that outlined the purpose of the study. To ensure participants were motivated to participate, employees in both the intervention and control groups were recruited under the assumption they may be receiving team sport through their workplace. The intervention group was selected by access to a sports hall. More specifically, the intervention group was selected by its proximity to a sports hall, while the control group was selected from an isolated worksite. The control group did not have regular interactions with the intervention worksite. Employees interested in participating were sent an electronic or paper copy of the information sheet and informed consent form. Informed consent was obtained from all individual participants included in the study. Participants were screened and excluded from participation if they were under 18 years of age, were sub-contracted by another organisation, were contracted to work less than 3 days-a-week, had planned absences during the intervention period or were unable to provide informed consent. Following completion of the study, the control group was provided information on how to participate in workplace team sport.

Twenty eight participants (n = 8 females) in the intervention group were aged between 24 to 56 years (39.59 ± 9.11), and 20 participants (n = 12 females) in the control group age ranged between 24 to 64 years (40.75 ± 11.92). All participants worked within a team and represented a range of office-based job roles and levels of superiority (25% were in positions of superiority). The proportion of female participants (29%) reflects the proportion of females working within the organisation (i.e. 30% reported in 2016 annual report). Additional demographics are provided in Table 1.

Measures

Primary Outcome Measure

Estimated maximal oxygen consumption (i.e. VO_2 max) was recorded through a Chester step test (CST) [21]. The CST was conducted in accordance with a validated protocol [21]. Participants stepped on/off a 30-cm high exercise step until 80% MHR. Exercise heart rate was measured by a Polar™ T31 monitor and watch, and perceived exertion was indicated with the 15-point Borg scale [22]. The CST offers a feasible and ecologically valid means to examine maximal oxygen uptake with working age adults in community settings without discouraging participants prior to the intervention [23]. The CST was selected based on its re-test reliability [23]. A recent review [23] concluding the CST offers the most valid estimation of maximal oxygen uptake when compared to other step test protocols. The CST has correlated strongly (r = 0.92) with the output of VO_2 max gas analysis conducted on a maximal oxygen usage treadmill test [21].

Secondary Outcome Measures

To determine body mass index (BMI) (kg/m^2), height was measured to the nearest millimetre by a Leicester Height measure™, while weight in kilograms was measured by a Marsden™ M550 GP digital scale. The International PA Questionnaire 'Short Form' (IPAQ)

Table 1 Participant demographic and baseline data (T^0)

	Group				Sig
	Team sport		Control		
	M	SD	M	SD	
Age	39.59	9.11	40.75	11.92	.708
Gender (male = M, female = F)	M = 20, F = 8		M = 8, F = 12		.030*
Body mass index (BMI) (T^0)	27.71	4.49	26.28	5.09	.931
Tenure (months)	119.77	123.01	139.35	162.11	.640
Average working hours	38.74	7.15	34.65	4.96	.034*
Average number of teams	2	1.46	1.3	.73	.057
Average team size	9.29	6.68	11.45	9.11	.355
Number of superiors	18		10		.064
VO_2 max (ml/min/kg)	41.32	12.29	37.40	9.26	.236
Total MET per week	2474.08	2880.50	3444.40	2882.92	.256
Group cohesion	61.48▼	13.48	59.40	13.81	.604
Relationship superiors	47.92	16.33	57.07	11.12	.036*
Relationship colleagues	51.25	10.09	52.08	15.51	.850
Communication	74.42	10.74	79.40▼	11.71	.136
Subjective vitality	71.41	12.73	70.86	11.45	.878
Quality of life	68.57	16.51	74.42	16.69	.234
Stress	64.95	19.78	71.87	15.37	.198
Occupational fatigue	66.57	25.35	76.82▼	21.15	.147
Job satisfaction	75.51	9.41	75.71	10.46	.944
Job performance	82.75	9.38	83.57	10.44	.781
Team performance	63.27	14.70	68.29	15.11	.256
Work engagement	71.23	15.28	66.04	14.77	.246

Significant interactions indicated with $*P < .05$. Non-normally distributed data is indicated with ▼

estimated the total metabolic equivalent of task (MET) [24]. A self-report diary provided the day-to-day variation in frequency and duration of PA over the intervention period. PA diaries have strongly correlated with the output of objective measures of PA on indicators of duration (r = 0.82) [25]. Sub-scales from the Copenhagen Psychosocial Questionnaire-II were used to measure social cohesion and interpersonal relationships within the workplace [26]. Interpersonal communication within workplace teams was captured using five items reported in another study (Cronbach alpha = .95) [27]. Wellbeing was assessed using the Subjective Vitality Scale [28]; quality of life was measured with the Satisfaction with Life Scale [29]; the Perceived Stress Scale [30] measured self-reported stress; and occupational fatigue was assessed with the Need for Recovery Scale [31]. Job satisfaction was assessed with the Single-Item of Job Satisfaction [32]. Perceptions of individual job performance (four items) were measured on 5-point Likert scale [33]. Team performance was measured with the 'team effectiveness' sub-scale of the Aston Team Performance Inventory [34]. The Utrecht Work Engagement Scale (short form) captured work engagement [35]. All measures using scales were delivered in paper form and completed by hand.

Data Analysis

A meta-analysis found medium Cohen's effect sizes ranging from d = .47 to .57 for objectively estimated assessments of VO_2 max [5]. A power calculation using G*Power [36] indicated 36 participants were required to observe a medium effect in the primary outcome, where f = .25, power is .95 and the error of probability is set at .05. A 35% attrition rate was applied. Analysis was conducted using IBM SPSS Statistics version 23, and $P < .05$ was considered statistical significant. Outliers were winsorized to the nearest non-outlying value. Self-reported items are represented with 0–100 scores (i.e. 0 is unfavourable). Normality was assessed through a Shapiro-Wilk test. Typically, data were normally distributed; however, where this is not the case, this is indicated in tables with a ▼. The magnitude of change is represented by a 95% confidence interval. Differences at T^0 were assessed using a series of independent sample t

tests. The primary and secondary outcomes were assessed using mixed design ANOVAs under the intention-to-treat principle [37]. Missing data were treated with the last observation carried forward method. For clarity, data were also examined with a series of mixed design ANCOVAs controlling for T^0 data, gender, age, BMI and average working hours. These returned no contrasting findings. Significant findings were followed up with paired sample *t* tests. Data is represented by mean ± standard deviation.

Results

Observations at Baseline (T^0)

Participant demographic data at baseline is presented in Table 1. The number of participants differed on a week-by-week basis (between 12 and 27 participants). One participant dropped out without attending any sessions. A series of independent sample *t* test found that at T^0 the intervention and control groups did not significantly differ on the primary outcome of estimated VO_2 max, or on any of the secondary outcomes apart from relationships with superiors ($P < .036$). The groups did not significantly differ in age, tenure, average team size, number of workplace teams or superiority. However, the groups did significantly differ on gender ($P < .03$) and average hours worked ($P < .034$). More specifically, 29% of the intervention group were female, while 60% of the control group were female. The control group worked 4.0907 h less per week than the intervention group. These were controlled for in the subsequent analysis.

Main Analysis

Primary Outcome

Participation in workplace team sport significantly improved estimated VO_2 max ($P < .002$, $\eta_p^2 = .182$), when compared to the control group (see Table 2). A mixed design ANOVA captured a group × time interaction for mean estimated VO_2 max (see Fig. 2). Follow-up paired samples *t* test observed a significant ($P < .0001$, $d = .774$) increase in estimated VO_2 max of 4.5 ± 5.80 ml/min/kg (95% CI 2.248–6.752) in the intervention group. However, a non-significant reduction ($P < .568$, $d = .129$) of .65±5.00 ml/min/kg (95% CI – 2.299–1.694) was observed in the control group.

Secondary Outcomes

A mixed design ANOVA revealed a significant group × time interaction on PA duration (minutes) ($P < .002$,

Table 2 Individual health outcomes for the team sport (intervention) and control groups assessed at baseline (T^0) and at the end of the intervention (T^1)

	T^0		T^1		*F* statistic		
	M	SD	M	SD	Group × time	Time	Group
VO_2 max (ml/min/kg)	39.68	11.19	42.04	10.34	10.258**	5.733*	4.983*
Team sport	41.32	12.29	45.82	9.06			
Control	37.40	9.26	36.75	9.87			
Total MET per week	2878.38	2882.92	2830.58	2519.07	.472	.007	1.110
Team sport	2474.08	2880.50	2678.18	2282.26			
Control	3444.40	2882.92	3283.94	2840.80			
Subjective vitality	71.18	12.09	72.91	11.59	.437	.169	.919
Team sport	71.41	12.73	72.40	13.39			
Control	70.86	11.45	73.62	8.74			
Quality of life	71.01	16.67	70.41	17.05	.136	.493	.492
Team sport	68.57	16.51	69.69	16.91			
Control	74.42	16.69	71.24	17.63			
Stress	67.97	18.23	69.66	18.81	1.298	.358	.388
Team sport	64.95	19.78	68.97	19.72			
Control	71.87	15.37	70.62	17.92			
Occupational fatigue	70.84	24.00	74.06	25.36	.025	2.133	2.449
Team sport	66.57	25.35	69.49	27.90			
Control	76.82▼	21.15	80.45	20.27			
BMI (kg/m^2)	27.12	4.75	27.58	4.42	6.788*	13.091***	.608
Team sport	27.71	4.49	27.86	4.41			
Control	26.28	5.09	27.20	4.52			

Significant interactions indicated with *$P < .05$, **$P < .01$, ***$P < .001$. Non-normally distributed data is indicated with ▼

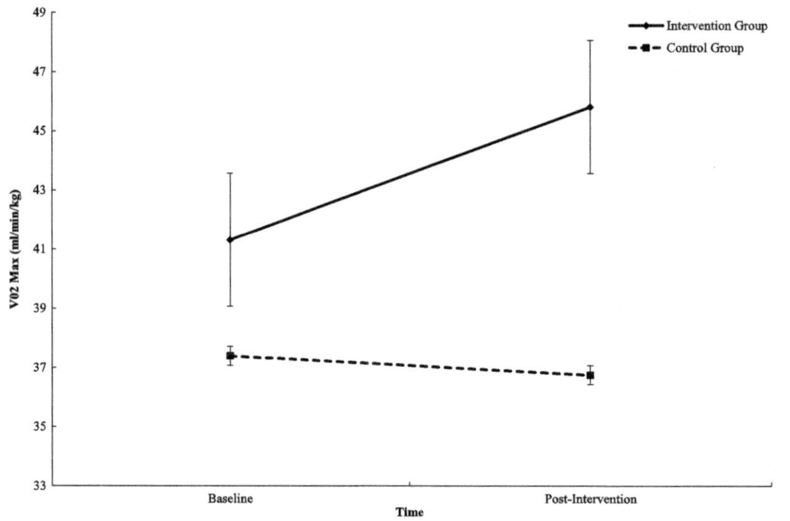

Fig. 2 Interaction effect between T^0 and T^1 for intervention and control group on estimated VO_2 max (ml/min/kg). Error bars represent standard error

η_p^2 = .071) (see Table 2). The intervention group participated in significantly ($P < .006$) more PA per week than the control group (154.74 min) (95% CI 47.36–261.85). A mixed design ANOVA detected a significant group × time interaction on communication ($P < .042$, $\eta_p^2 = .087$) (see Table 3). A follow-up paired samples *t* test observed a non-significant improvement ($P < .85$, $d = .337$) of 3.0 in interpersonal communication within workplace teams (95% CI − .446–6.446) in the intervention group and a non-significant ($P < .235$, $d = .274$) decrease of 2.6 (95% CI − 7.033–1.833) in the control group (see Fig. 3). A significant interaction was identified on relationships with colleagues over time only ($P < .045$, $\eta_p^2 = .085$) (see Table 3). Further, a mixed design ANOVA captured a group × time interaction for mean BMI ($P < .012$, $\eta_p^2 = .130$) (see Table 2). A follow-up paired samples *t* test observed a minor non-significant ($P < .203$, $d = .246$) increase in BMI of .146 ± .593 kg/m^2 (95% CI .0837–.3765) in the intervention group. However, a significant ($P < .008$, $d = .658$) increase in BMI of .920 kg/m^2 (95% CI .2659–1.574) was observed in the control group. All other secondary outcome variables were non-significant for group, time or group × time (see Tables 2, 3 and 4).

Discussion

Summary of Findings

This non-randomised intervention study examined the impact of participating in workplace team sport upon a primary outcome of estimated VO_2 max and secondary outcomes of individual, social group and organisational health. To our knowledge, this intervention study

Table 3 Social group outcomes for the team sport (intervention) and control groups at baseline (T^0) and at the end of the intervention (T^1)

	T^0		T^1		*F* statistic		
	M	SD	M	SD	Group × time	Time	Group
Group cohesion	60.61	13.51	62.81	12.43	.014	2.018	.417
Team sport	61.48	13.48	63.83	11.81			
Control	59.40	13.81	61.39	13.42			
Relationship superiors	51.73	14.97	51.02	14.19	3.067	.490	2.514
Team sport	47.92	16.33	49.80	15.44			
Control	57.07	11.12	52.73	12.40			
Relationship colleagues	51.60	12.49	48.10	13.95	1.220	5.006*	.091
Team sport	51.25	10.09	49.32	10.92			
Control	52.08	15.51	46.39	17.50			
Communication	76.50	11.33	77.16	11.66	4.386*	.022	.495
Team sport	74.42▼	10.74	77.42▼	12.03			
Control	79.40	11.71	76.80▼	11.43			

Significant interactions indicated with *$P < .05$. Non-normally distributed data is indicated with ▼

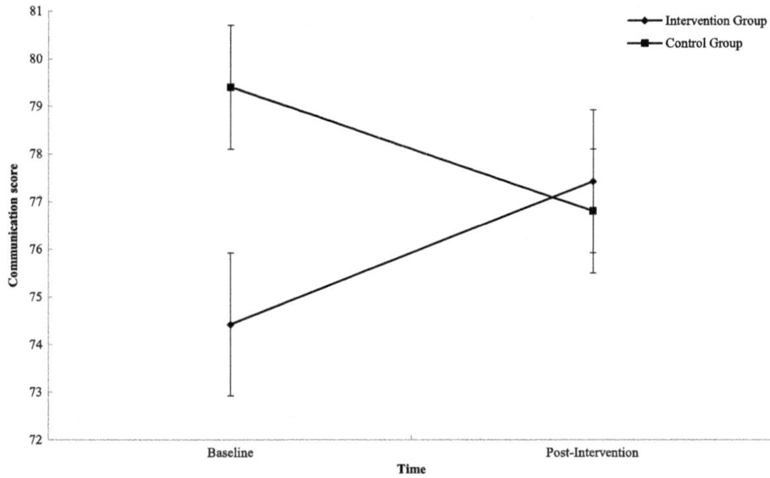

Fig. 3 Interaction effect between T^0 and T^1 for intervention and control group on interpersonal team communication. Error bars represent standard error

represents the first attempt to examine the impact of a multi-team sport programme within a workplace setting on multiple indicators of health.

A 10.32% increase in VO_2 max was observed in the intervention group. Other intervention studies examining the impact of workplace soccer on aerobic fitness have observed improvements of 5% [8, 9]. Improvements in VO_2 max are attributable to the prolonged exposure to high-intensity PA (HIPA) [9, 38]. HIPA improves cardiac output and skeletal muscle oxidation and capillarisation [8, 9, 38]. Decreased VO_2 max (– 1.75%) in the control group may be explained by the sedentary job roles performed by these employees [2]. A previous review of research with intervention designs suggests sedentary behaviour has a detrimental impact on cardiac output [2].

Team sport may have a protective effect on BMI. Increases in the control group's BMI (3.5%) may be attributable to the increased plasma glucose, triglycerides, lipoprotein and waist circumference associated with sedentary job roles [2]. Increases in energy expenditure in the intervention group may have caused participants to compensate by increasing nutritional intake and therefore BMI (.54%) [39]. This finding should be treated with caution given the absence of an RCT design, biomarkers, DEXA scans, skinfolds and nutritional intake. Adopting these measures may draw firmer conclusions.

Non-randomised (quasi-experimental) designs are however robust [18]. An RCT design may have been unethical, unfeasible or unrealistic to promote health within this workplace setting [18]. Likewise, quasi-experimental designs are effective at evaluating the

Table 4 Organisational health outcomes for the team sport (intervention) and control groups at baseline (T^0) and at the end of the intervention (T^1)

	T^0		T^1		*F* statistic		
	M	SD	M	SD	Group × time	Time	Group
Job satisfaction	75.59	9.75	77.08	8.19	1.906	.737	.556
Team sport	75.51	9.41	78.57	9.11			
Control	75.71	10.46	75.00	6.34			
Job performance	83.22	9.91	83.33	9.96	.687	.004	.597
Team sport	83.57	10.44	84.64	9.51			
Control	82.75	9.38	81.50	10.52			
Team performance	65.36	14.92	64.83	13.60	.181	.166	.267
Team sport	63.27	14.70	63.30	14.80			
Control	68.29	15.11	66.97	11.74			
Work engagement	69.06	15.13	67.30	15.99	.631	1.780	2.062
Team sport	71.23	15.28	70.53	15.77			
Control	66.04	14.77	63.30	15.72			

Non-normally distributed data is indicated with ▼

efficacy of interventions and may be preferred due to feasibility, and the practical challenges of conducting a controlled design [18].

CTG did improve interpersonal communication within teams over time (3% in intervention group). This finding provides the first empirical support for several qualitative studies exploring the benefits of participation in workplace team sport [10–13]. Improvements in communication may be explained by the time employees spent together participating in an activity of common interest with shared goals [10]. Qualitative evidence indicates employees learn more about their colleagues' communication style in a non-work environment with shared goals [10–13].

The employees in this study did not exclusively participate with their day-to-day colleagues, and therefore, the effect on working relationships, cohesion and team productivity may have been confounded. Future investigations examining workplace team sport may consider re-examining social group outcomes with a cluster RCT design whereby individual work teams are clustered into study arms. Although markers of individual health outcomes (e.g. psychological wellbeing) and organisational health outcomes (e.g. job satisfaction, productivity, work-engagement) did not significantly improve following participation, it would be unwise to suggest that team sport does not influence individual and organisational health. Rather, post hoc power analysis using G*Power [36] revealed most secondary outcome measures were unpowered (apart from quality of life) and unable to detect a significant interaction. Quality of life has shown to be a subjective state, and therefore, our findings may have been confounded by factors internal (e.g. salary, working practises) and external (e.g. personal relationships, lifestyle choices) [40] to the intervention. It may be of interest to researchers to re-examine markers of individual and organisational health with adequately powered outcome measures through day level (i.e. directly pre-post team sport) and over the long term (e.g. 6 months, 12 months).

Limitations

The participants in this study represent a one large private services organisation. To prevent contamination, care was taken to select two isolated regional worksites. The groups did however differ in gender and average working hours at T^0. Therefore, the study groups may not have been counterfactual. Given the absence of a RCT design and these differences between the groups, the results may have been confounded and caution should be applied when interpreting these findings. Although CTG was successful at recruiting female participants, only 29% of the intervention group were female. While this figure is proportionate to the number of females who work in the organisation (30% reported in 2016 annual report), researchers still may wish to understand why less female employees participate in team sport with their colleagues. Likewise, 89% of intervention group and 85% of control group participants reported meeting PA guidelines [1]. This figure is higher than the national average for working-age adults (67% of males, 55% of females). This may suggest workplace team sport attracts primarily active employees, rather inactive employees at risk of non-communicable illnesses and diseases. Future research may consider investigating the impact of workplace team sport with inactive employees.

A further limitation is the low number of employees initially recruited into a fully funded study from a large organisation. The current study's process evaluation indicates recruitment over a 1-month period and ineffective communication strategy reduced the reach of the programme (process evaluation due for publication in 2017[1]). Intrapersonal, interpersonal, organisational and environmental factors may have facilitated participation or created obstacles for attendance [15]. Consistent with previous qualitative research, workplace demands, culture and practises challenged the consistent participation of employees [15]. Future research should continue to account for these factors using a participatory approach to implementation [20].

PA behaviour may be influenced by team sport participation over time. While the IPAQ and self-reported diary provide adequate psychometric properties, future research measuring PA would benefit from the addition of objective measures [41]. To maintain self-efficacy and competence, the current study avoided examination of sport intensity with heart rate monitors. While logical, this is a limitation of the study. Further, research may consider measuring intensity with heart rate monitors or perceived exertion (RPE) (e.g. the Borg Scale). Finally, data representing communication and occupational fatigue was not normally distributed and should be treated with caution. Future research may consider readdressing team sports impact on these outcomes.

Conclusions

The current study examined the impact of a 12-week workplace team sport intervention on individual, social group and organisational health outcomes. Results indicate workplace team sport can improve aerobic fitness, PA behaviour and interpersonal communication within teams. These results suggest team sport may be an effective and viable form of health promotion within a workplace setting. Promoting forms of PA such as team sport within workplace settings is required to meet UK public health guidelines and reduce the financial and societal burden faced as attributable to an inactive population [42]. Therefore, it remains important to continue to understand why employees choose to participate in team sport and promote programmes which encourage participation. The current study suggests this may be achieved by promoting team sports which are supportive of autonomy, competence and relatedness. Researchers should consider testing the efficacy of a multi-team sport programme within a workplace setting over the long term with cluster RCT designs (i.e. randomise on work-place team level) and further objective measures of health (e.g. objective measures of physical activity, skin-fold, DEXA scans, sickness absence).

Endnotes

[1]The process evaluation referenced in this article is due for publication in 2017. More specifically, this study is under-review at the time of acceptance of the current study. The process-evaluation provides further detail and information regarding the CTG's reach, efficacy, adoption (e.g. participant adherence), implementation (e.g. theoretical underpinnings) and potential maintenance.

Acknowledgements

The authors of this study would like to thank the participants who took part in this study.

This activity was conducted under the auspices of the National Centre for Sport and Exercise Medicine (NCSEM) England. The NCSEM is a collaboration between several universities, NHS trusts and sporting and public bodies. The research was supported by the National Institute for Health Research (NIHR) Leicester Biomedical Research Centre, which is a partnership between University Hospitals of Leicester NHS Trust, Loughborough University and the University of Leicester. The views expressed are those of the authors and not necessarily those of the NCSEM, NHS, the NIHR or the Department of Health.

Funding

The project of which the intervention is a part of was a fully funded studentship by the authors' university.

Authors' Contributions

AB, HM and FM designed the study. AB recruited, collected measures and managed the intervention. AB and RGE conducted the analysis. All authors contributed to the manuscript and interpretation of the results.

Competing Interests

Andrew Brinkley, Hilary McDermott, Rachel Grenfell-Essam and Fehmidah Munir declare that they have no conflicts of interest relevant to this intervention study.

References

1. Townsend N, Wickramasighe K, Williams J, Bhatnager P, Rayner M. Physical activity statistics 2015. London: British Heart Foundation; 2015.
2. Hamilton MT, Healy GN, Dunstan DW, Zderic TW, Owen N. Too little exercise and too much sitting: inactivity physiology and the need for new recommendations on sedentary behaviour. Curr Cardiovasc Risk Reps. 2012; 2(4):292–8. doi: 10.1007/s12170-008-0054-8
3. Batt ME. Physical activity interventions in the workplace: the rationale and future direction for workplace wellness. Br J of Spor Medi. 2009;43(1):47–8. doi: 10.1136/bjsm.2008.053488
4. Brinkley A, McDermott H, Munir F. What benefits does team sport hold for the workplace? A systematic review. J Spor Sci. 2017;35(2):136–48. doi: 10.1080/02640414.2016.1158852
5. Conn VS, Hafdahl AR, Cooper PS, Brown LM, Lusk SL. Meta-analysis of workplace physical activity interventions. Am J Prev Med. 2009;37(4):330–9. doi: 10.1016/j.amepre.2009.06.008
6. Barene S, Holtermann A, Oseland H, Brekke OL, Krustrup P. Effects on muscle strength, maximal jump height, flexibility and postural sway after soccer and zumba exercise among female hospital employees: a 9-month randomised control trial. J Spor Sci. 2016; doi: 10.1080/026404414.2016.1140906
7. Barene S, Krustrup P, Holtermann A. Effects of the workplace health promotion activities soccer and zumba on muscle pain, work ability and perceived physical exertion among female hospital employees. PLoS One. 2014;9(12) doi: 10.1371/journal.pone.0115059
8. Barene S, Krustrup P, Brekke OL, Holtermann A. Soccer and Zumba as health-promoting activities among female hospital employees: a 40-weeks cluster randomized intervention study. J Spor Sci. 2014;32(16):1539–49. doi: 10.1080/02640414.2014.906043
9. Barene S, Krustrup P, Jackman SR, Brekke OL, Holtermann A. Do soccer and Zumba exercise improve fitness and indicators of health among female hospital employees? A 12-week RCT. Scand J Med Sci Spor. 2013;24(6):990–9. doi: 10.1111/sms.12138
10. Scherrer P, Sheridan L, Sibson R, Ryan MM, Henley N. Employee engagement with a corporate physical activity program: the global corporate challenge. Inter J Bus Stud. 2010;18(1):125–39.
11. Joubert YT. Sports contribution to open communication in a workplace: a qualitative study. J Psych Afr. 2014;24(2):203–6. doi: 10.1080/14330237.2014.903072
12. Joubert YT, De Beer H. Experiences of employees who participate in organisational team sport activities. J Emerg Trends Econo Manag Sci. 2010; 1(1):51–9.
13. Joubert YT, De Beer JJ. Benefits of team sport for organisations. S Afr J Res Spor Phys Educ Recreat. 2011;33(3):59–72.
14. Lee AL. Sports in the workplace do they pay? In: Diamant L, editor. Psychology of sports, exercise, and fitness: social and personal issues. New York: Hemisphere Publishing Corporation; 1991. p. 167–86.
15. Brinkley A, Freeman J, McDermott H, Munir F. What are the facilitators and obstacles to participation in workplace team sport? A qualitative study. AIMS Pub Heal. 2017;4(1):94–126. doi: 10.3934/publichealth.2017.1.94
16. Gucciardi DF, Jackson B. Understanding sport continuation: an integration of the theories of planned behaviour and basic needs theory. J Sci Med Spor. 2015;18(1):31–6. doi: 10.1016/j.jsams.2013.11.011
17. Deci EL, Ryan RM. The "what" and "why" of goal pursuits: human needs and the self-determination of behavior. Psycho Inqu. 2000;11(4):227–68. doi: 10.1207/S15327965PLI1104_01
18. Dzewaltowski DA, Glasgow RE, Klesges LM, Estabrooks PA, Brock E. RE-AIM: evidence-based standards and a web resource to improve translation of research into practice. Ann Behav Med. 2004;28(2):75–80. doi: 10.1207/s15324796abm2802_1
19. Schelvis RMC, Oude Hengel KM, Burdorf A, Blatter A, Strijk JE, van der Beek AJ. Evaluation of occupational health interventions using a randomized controlled trial: challenges and alternatives research designs. Scand J Work Environ Heal. 2015;41(5):491–503.
20. Nielsen K, Randall R, Holten AL, González ER. Conducting organisational-level occupational health interventions: what works? Work Stress. 2010;24(3): 234–59. doi: 10.1080/02678373.2010.515393
21. Sykes K, Roberts A. The Chester step test—a simple yet effective tool for the prediction of aerobic capacity. Physiother. 2004;90(4):183–8.
22. Borg G. Psychophysical scaling with applications in physical work and the perception of exertion. Scand J Work Environ Heal. 1990;16(1):55–8.
23. Bennett H, Parfitt G, Davidson K, Eston R. Validity of submaximal step tests to estimate maximal oxygen uptake in healthy adults. Spor Med. 2015; doi: 10.1007/s40279-015-0445-1
24. Craig CL, Marshall AL, Sjöström M, Bauman AM, Booth ML, Ainsworth BE, et al. International physical activity questionnaire: 12 country reliability and validity. Med Sci Spor Exerc. 2003;195(9131/03):3508–1381. doi: 10.1249/01.MSS.0000078924.61453.FB
25. Connor SO, McCafferey N, Whyte E, Moran K. The novel use of a SenseCam and accelerometer to validate training load and training information in self-recall training diary. J Spor Sci. 2016;34(3):303–10. doi: 10.1080/02640414.2015.1050600
26. Kristensen TS. A new tool for assessing psychosocial work environment factors: the Copenhagen psychosocial questionnaire. In M Hagberg, B

Knave, L Lillienberg, H Westberg (Ed's). x2001—expo and assess in Epidem and Pract. 2001; 210-213.
27. González-Romá V, Hernández A. Climate uniformity: its influence on team communication quality, task conflict, and team performance. J Appl Psych. 2014;99(6):1042–58. doi: 10.1037/a0037868
28. Frederick CM, Ryan RM. Differences in motivation for sport and exercise and their relations with participation and mental health. J Spor Behav. 1993;16(3):124.
29. Diener E, Emmons RA, Larsen RJ, Griffin S. The satisfaction with life scale. J Pers Assess. 1985;49(1):71–5. doi: 10.1207/s15327752jpa4901_13
30. Cohen S, Kamarck T, Mermelstein R. A global measure of perceived stress. J Heal Soci Behav. 1983;24(4):385–96. doi: 10.2307/2136404
31. Veldhoven VM, Broersen S. Measurement quality and validity of the "need for recovery scale". Occup Environ Med. 2003;60(1):3–9. doi: 10.1136/oem.60.suppl.1.i3
32. Dolbier CL, Webster JA, McCalister KT, Mallon MW, Steinhardt MA. Reliability and validity of a single-item measure of job satisfaction. Am J Heal Promot. 2005;19(3):194–8. doi: 10.4278/0890–1171-19.3.194
33. Munir F, Houdmont J, Clemes S, Wilson K, Kerr R, Addley K. Work engagement and its association with occupational sitting time: results from the Stormont study. BMC Publ Heal. 2015;15(1):30. doi:10.1186/s12889-015-1427-9
34. West MA, Markiewicz L, Dawson JF. Aston team performance inventory: management set. London: ASE; 2006.
35. Schaufeli WB, Bakker AB, Salanova M. The measurement of work engagement with a short questionnaire a cross-national study. Educ Psych Meas. 2006;66(4):701–16. doi: 10.1177/0013164405282471
36. Faul F, Erdfelder E, Lang AG, Buchner A. G*Power 3: a flexible statistical power analysis program for the social, behavioural, and biomedical sciences. Behav Res Meth. 2007;39(2):175–91. doi: 10.3758/BF03193146
37. Elkins MR, Moseley AM. Intention-to-treat analysis. J Phys 2015; 61(3): 165-167. doi: 10.1016/j.jphys.2015.013.
38. Krustrup P, Christensen JF, Randers MB, Pedersen H, Sundstrup E, Jakobsen MD, et al. Muscle adaptations and performance enhancements of soccer training for untrained men. Eur J Appl Physiol. 2010;108(6):1247–58. doi: 10.1007/s00421-009-1319-8
39. King NA, Horner K, Hills AP, Byrne NM, Wood RE, Bryant E, et al. Exercise, appetite and weight management: understanding the compensatory responses in eating behaviour and how they contribute to variability in exercise-induced weight loss. Br J Spor Med. 2012;46(5):315–22. doi: 10.1136/bjsm.2010.082495
40. Gill DL, Hammond CC, Reifsteck EJ, Jehu CM, Williams RA, Adams MM, et al. Physical activity and quality of life. J Prev Medi Publ Heal. 2013;46(1):28–34. doi: 10.3961/jpmph.2013.46.S.S28
41. Kelly P, Fitzsimons C, Baker. Should we reframe how we think about physical activity and sedentary behaviour measurement? Validity and reliability reconsidered. Int J Behav Nutr Phys Act. 2016; doi: 10.1186/s12966-016-0351-4
42. Department of Health. Start active, stay active: a report on physical activity for health from the four home countries' chief medical officers. London: UK Government; 2011.

11

The Reproducibility of 4-km Time Trial (TT) Performance Following Individualised Sodium Bicarbonate Supplementation: a Randomised Controlled Trial in Trained Cyclists

Lewis Anthony Gough*, Sanjoy Kumar Deb, Andy Sparks and Lars Robert McNaughton

Abstract

Background: Individual time to peak blood bicarbonate (HCO_3^-) has demonstrated good to excellent reproducibility following ingestion of both 0.2 g kg^{-1} body mass (BM) and 0.3 g kg^{-1} BM sodium bicarbonate ($NaHCO_3$), but the consistency of the time trial (TT) performance response using such an individualised $NaHCO_3$ ingestion strategy remains unknown. This study therefore evaluated the reproducibility of 4-km TT performance following $NaHCO_3$ ingestion individualised to time to peak blood bicarbonate.

Methods: Eleven trained male cyclists completed five randomised treatments with prior ingestion of 0.2 g kg^{-1} (SBC2) or 0.3 g kg^{-1} BM (SBC3) $NaHCO_3$, on two separate occasions each, or a control trial entailing no supplementation. Participants completed a 4-km cycling TT on a Velotron ergometer where time to complete, power and speed were measured, whilst acid-base blood parameters were also recorded (pH and blood bicarbonate concentration HCO_3^-) and lactate [La^-].

Results: Alkalosis was achieved prior to exercise in both SBC2 and SBC3, as pH and HCO_3^- were greater compared to baseline ($p < 0.001$), with no differences between treatments ($p > 0.05$). The reproducibility of the mean absolute change from baseline to peak in HCO_3^- was good in SBC2 ($r = 0.68$) and excellent in SBC3 ($r = 0.78$). The performance responses following both SBC2 and SBC3 displayed excellent reproducibility (r range = 0.97 to 0.99).

Conclusions: Results demonstrate excellent reproducibility of exercise performance following individualised $NaHCO_3$ ingestion, which is due to the high reproducibility of blood acid-base variables with repeat administration of $NaHCO_3$. Using a time to peak HCO_3^- strategy seems to cause no dose-dependent effects on performance for exercise of this duration and intensity; therefore, athletes may consider smaller doses of $NaHCO_3$ to mitigate gastrointestinal (GI) discomfort.

Keywords: Buffering, Alkalosis, Performance, Acid-base balance, Ergogenic aids, Reliability

* Correspondence: goughl@edgehill.ac.uk
Sports Nutrition and Performance Group, Department of Sport and Physical Activity, Edge Hill University, Ormskirk, Lancashire L39 4QP, UK

Key Points

- Time to peak blood bicarbonate (HCO_3^-) induced via ingestion of sodium bicarbonate ($NaHCO_3$) produces consistent physiological responses prior to, during and post-exercise.
- Four-kilometre TT performance displays excellent reliability following repeat administration of 0.2 and 0.3 g kg body mass (BM) $NaHCO_3$ individualised to time to peak HCO_3^-.
- Athletes need to be aware that the gastrointestinal (GI) discomfort response is varied even with repeated administration; therefore, this needs to be monitored.

Background

Personalised nutrition has gathered recent attention as individual characteristics (i.e. genetics, training status and nutrition) can potentially improve or reduce the physiological adaptation from the same intervention [21]. Through personalising nutrition strategies, both the individual bioavailability and bioefficacy can be quantified to maximise the effects of an intervention within individuals [23]. This concept can also be applied to the use of nutritional ergogenic aids aimed to enhance human physiology and exercise performance; however, common practice of ergogenic aid research determines the effectiveness of a single treatment by evaluating the mean differences between groups or trials [15]. As a result, the inter- and intra-individual responses are seldom considered. To account for this, repeat administration of the experimental treatment is plausible, thereby allowing assessment of the reproducibility of nutritional ergogenic aids [18, 19]. This method permits athletes to appropriately evaluate the effectiveness of ergogenic aids and to assess if they can provide consistent benefits to exercise performance upon repeated use during training and/or competition [4].

The use of over-the-counter sodium bicarbonate ($NaHCO_3$) is one example of a supplement that allows for repeated administration by representing a low cost and easy digestion. Primarily, $NaHCO_3$ is used as an ergogenic aid to mitigate the effects of metabolic acidosis (i.e. decline in pH) by increasing bicarbonate (HCO_3^-) buffering capacity during short distance/duration high-intensity exercise of between 1 and 10 min [27]. Traditionally, $NaHCO_3$ is administered in a single 0.3 g kg^{-1} body mass (BM) dose at a standardised time prior to exercise ranging between 1 and 4 h [26, 32, 34]. It was originally suggested that the point of peak alkalosis (measured by either peak pH and/or HCO_3^-) occurred between 60 and 90 min post $NaHCO_3$ ingestion [29, 32, 34]. This same peak has also been suggested to occur up to 180 min in other studies however [6, 22, 35], whilst more recently, it has been shown to range between 40 and 140 min following both 0.2 and 0.3 g kg^{-1} BM $NaHCO_3$ [14]. These data therefore suggest that there is a large individual variation in time to peak alkalosis. Consequently, some athletes may not be ingesting this supplement at a time that corresponds to their peak buffering capacity, which might limit the resulting ergogenic effect.

To account for such inter-individual variation an individualised $NaHCO_3$ strategy has recently been recommended, which entails administering $NaHCO_3$ at a time point to ensure peak pH and/or HCO_3^- concentrations at the beginning of exercise [10, 14, 22, 28, 33]. By identifying peak alkalosis, it ensures that the HCO_3^- buffering capacity is maximised, compared to a standardised ingestion strategy where some participants may not begin exercise at peak alkalosis. This methodological alteration may therefore account for some of the equivocal performance data which has been observed using $NaHCO_3$ [5, 13, 16, 32]. Gough et al. [14] have displayed using an individualised $NaHCO_3$ time to peak strategy that time to peak blood HCO_3^- was highly repeatable using intraclass correlation coefficient (ICC) analysis (r = 0.77 to 0.94). The authors also reported the mean HCO_3^- change from baseline to peak was + 5.7 mmol l^{-1} following 0.2 g kg^{-1} BM $NaHCO_3$, which is greater than the + 3.9 ± 0.9 mmol l^{-1} mean change reported in a meta-analysis from a 0.3 g kg^{-1} BM dose [5]. This suggests that using an individualised $NaHCO_3$ ingestion strategy may elicit more reproducible biological acid-base balance changes, whilst a smaller 0.2 g kg^{-1} BM $NaHCO_3$ dose induces a change in HCO_3^- greater than the mean change observed using a standardised 0.3 g kg^{-1} BM $NaHCO_3$ dose. This smaller dose therefore represents a viable option for the athlete, and the performance responses following this dose are worthwhile to determine.

A factor that may hamper the use of $NaHCO_3$ in a practical sense is the onset of gastrointestinal (GI) discomfort. Common symptoms include nausea, belching, diarrhoea and vomiting, which can have both practical and perceived impacts on the efficacy of this supplement for performance enhancements [32]. Therefore, whilst it is important to initially heighten the level of peak alkalosis, it is of equal importance to mitigate GI discomfort. One strategy to reduce the severity of GI discomfort is a lower dose (0.2 g·kg^{-1} BM), which has been shown to reduce the severity of the symptom suffered compared to 0.3 g kg^{-1} BM [13, 26]. This dose might not have been used as widely in previous research due to the previous standardised times of ingestion, and the early findings of McNaughton [26] reporting 0.3 g kg^{-1} BM produced greater ergogenic benefits compared to 0.2 g kg^{-1} BM $NaHCO_3$. Nonetheless, with an individualised ingestion strategy, an increase in HCO_3^- (~ 5 mmol l^{-1}) should be reached with a lower amount of $NaHCO_3$ (i.e. 0.2 g kg^{-1} BM $NaHCO_3$), whilst also reducing the severity of GI discomfort [14, 22].

In studies utilising standardised $NaHCO_3$ ingestion strategies, equivocal performance responses have been reported across consecutive repeated trials [6, 12]. Dias et al. [12] reported when four seperate cycling bouts at 110% peak power output until time to exhaustion (TTE) were performed with ingestion of 0.3 g kg^{-1} BM $NaHCO_3$, ten participants improved performance in at least one trial, whilst only one participant improved in all trials. Although blood pH and HCO_3^- were generally repeatable in this study, a factor contributing to this variation may have been the exercise test employed. A high variation in responses has been displayed in TTE tests [17], particularly in untrained individuals which feature in the Dias et al. [12] study, and compared to time trial (TT) tests [7, 9, 16, 24]. The lack of consistent improvements in response to $NaHCO_3$ may therefore be due to the exercise protocol adopted, not the failure of $NaHCO_3$'s buffering mechanism to enhance performance. In a further study, Carr et al. [6] reported that performance responses were repeatable for mean power during a 2000-m rowing TT performance displaying a typical error (TE) of 2.1%. The authors, however, reported the change in HCO_3^- from baseline to pre-exercise displayed a very large TE (2.5%) and coefficient of variation (CV) (7%), which may explain why no performance effect was observed. This evidence suggests the blood responses following $NaHCO_3$ may not be consistent following 0.3 g kg^{-1} BM $NaHCO_3$. Furthermore, both Dias et al. [12] and Carr et al. [6] utilised a standardised $NaHCO_3$ ingestion strategy and only reported mean blood responses, which may have adversely affected the blood and performance responses and thus, the interpretation of the data. Only two studies have evaluated the repeatability of the performance responses following acute ingestion of $NaHCO_3$ and reported equivocal findings, meaning further enquiry is required. The aim of this study was therefore to investigate the reproducibility of blood acid-base, performance and GI discomfort responses following two individualised $NaHCO_3$ doses.

Methods

Participants

Eleven trained male cyclists volunteered for a randomised, double-blind, crossover design study (height 182 ± 8 cm, body mass 86.4 ± 12.9 kg, age 32 ± 9 years, maximal oxygen consumption (VO_{2max}) 58.0 ± 3.8 ml kg min^{-1}, peak power 4.5 ± 0.5 W kg^{-1}). The participant inclusion required individuals to meet the criteria of 'trained cyclist' as outlined by De Pauw et al. [11], be between 18 and 50 years of age, training for a minimum of 4 h $week^{-1}$ and have 2 years continuous cycling experience. Participants were also excluded if they had ingested any intra/extracellular buffer in the prior 6 months before data collection. Ethical approval was obtained from the Departmental Research Ethics Committee, and each participant provided written informed consent prior to any data collection, with the research conducted in accordance with the Declaration of Helsinki.

Participants visited the laboratory in a 4-h postprandial state to limit confounding nutritional effects on exercise performance and at the same time of day to control for circadian rhythms [30]. Participation in any strenuous/unaccustomed exercise and alcohol intake was prohibited for the 24 h prior to each treatment arm. Caffeine was also to be avoided for the 12 h prior. Compliance with the above procedures was checked via written logs of nutritional intake, and participants were asked to replicate nutritional practices for subsequent trials (adherence = 100%).

Determination of Maximal Oxygen Consumption and Time to Peak Blood Bicarbonate

Participants initially completed an incremental exercise test on an electromagnetically braked cycle ergometer (Excalibur Sport, Lode, Netherlands) to determine VO_{2max} and peak power output (PPO). After a self-selected warm-up, the cycling protocol began at 75 W for 1 min and then increased by 1 W every 2 s (30 W min^{-1}) until the point of volitional exhaustion. This was determined by the inability for the participant to sustain their self-selected cadence for longer than 5 s, whereby they were given an initial warning, and the test was then terminated on the subsequent occurrence.

Two trials were conducted in a randomised order to identify time to peak blood HCO_3^- following ingestion of either 0.2 g kg^{-1} $NaHCO_3$ (SBC2) or 0.3 g kg^{-1} BM $NaHCO_3$ (SBC3). This was ingested as a drink and mixed with 400 ml of water and 50 ml double strength blackcurrant sugar-free squash. The use of time to peak HCO_3^- was utilised as this has displayed greater reproducibility compared to time to peak pH [14]. Finger prick capillary blood samples were taken prior to $NaHCO_3$ ingestion in a seated position and collected within a 100-µl heparin-coated glass clinitube for analysis of blood pH and HCO_3^- (ABL800 BASIC, Radiometer Medical Ltd., Denmark). Subsequent blood samples were drawn every 10 min over a 180-min period to identify time to peak HCO_3^-. The double-blind nature of the study was maintained by a volunteer outside of the research team, who identified the time to peak HCO_3^-.

Familiarisation and Experimental Treatment Arms

The participants then performed a 4-km TT familiarisation trial, followed by a further five separate visits requiring completion of the same exercise following ingestion of either 0.2 g kg^{-1} BM $NaHCO_3$ twice (SBC2a and SBC2b), 0.3 g kg^{-1} BM $NaHCO_3$ twice (SBC3a and SBC3b) or a control treatment entailing no supplementation in a randomised order. A control trial was conducted to obtain a reference point measure of performance. Blood samples were taken at rest, at time to peak HCO_3^- and post-exercise to analyse blood pH and HCO_3^-, with the addition of a 5-μl sample for blood lactate [La^-] (Lactate Pro 2, Arkray, Japan). Ingestion of either SBC2 or SBC3 was completed within 10 min, and participants remained seated and rested until their respective time to peak. A questionnaire to assess the severity gastrointestinal (GI) discomfort was used every 10 min until individual time to peak HCO_3^- [14, 28].

Each TT was completed on a Velotron Racermate™ cycle ergometer interfaced with Velotron 3D coaching software (Racermate, USA). Frame geometry (handlebars, seat position) and gear ratios were selected by the participant to match their preferred riding style to be replicated for each subsequent trial. Strong and consistent verbal encouragement was provided throughout the TT. Participants were blinded from the clock, but were provided with feedback on distance covered, watts (W) and cadence (rev min^{-1}) via the display [38]. This feedback was provided as cyclists used in this study were not habitually completing 4-km TT distances in competition.

Statistical Analysis

Shapiro-Wilk test and standard graphical methods (Q-Q plots) were used to assess normality of the data, and the Mauchly test was used for homogeneity and variance. Both the severity and time to peak GI discomfort were considered non-normally distributed by the respective normality tests. Therefore, a Friedman rank test was used as an alternative and is reported with z score (significance) and effect size (d) calculated by $Z/\sqrt{n}$. Interpretation was then considered as small (0.10), medium (0.24) and large (> 0.37) [20]. Mean speed, power and time to complete were compared between treatment arms using a repeated measures analysis of variance (ANOVA). Haematological data such as pH, HCO_3^- and [La^-] were analysed using a two-way (treatment × time) repeated measures ANOVA. Post hoc comparisons were determined by Bonferroni correction. Effect size is reported as partial η^2 value and considered trivial (< 0.20), small (0.20–0.49), moderate (0.50–0.79) and large (≥ 0.80) in accordance with the conventional Cohen's d interpretations [8].

Limits of agreement (LOA) with 95% percent limits and Bland-Altman plots were initially used to determine if data was heteroscedastic [3]. The repeatability of both blood acid-base balance and performance responses to SBC2 and SBC3 was determined using intraclass correlation coefficients (ICC) with r value and significance level (i.e. p value) as per previous recommendations [2, 39]. Interpretation of reproducibility was categorised by the respective r value with categories of poor ($r \leq 0.40$), fair ($r = 0.40$–0.59), good ($r = 0.60$–0.74) and excellent ($r \geq 0.74$). Typical error (TE) is reported and calculated using the method of Hopkins [19], with categories of small (≤ 0.2–0.6), moderate (0.6–1.2), large (1.2–2.0), very large (2.0–4.0) and extremely large (≥ 4.0%) used to interpret the data. Coefficient of variation (CV) was reported using SD/mean × 100. Statistical procedures were completed using SPSS version 22 (IBM, Chicago, USA), and calculations were carried out using Microsoft Excel 2013 (Microsoft Inc., USA). All data are presented as mean ± SD unless otherwise stated. Statistical significance was set at $p > 0.05$.

Results

Reliability of Treatments

The blood responses following SBC treatments were largely reproducible (Tables 1 and 2). Individual blood responses displaying absolute changes from baseline to peak pH and HCO_3^- are depicted in Table 3. The only inconsistency observed was the absolute change in pH from baseline to peak in SBC3, revealing a poor ICC. Excluding that case, blood responses pre-, during and post-exercise ranged from good to excellent for all SBC treatments (ICC range $r = 0.68$ to 0.95).

Excellent reproducibility of time to complete the 4-km TT was observed in both SBC2 ($r = 0.97$, $p < 0.001$) and SBC3 ($r = 0.99$, $p < 0.001$) with a low TE (range = 0.3 to 0.5%; Table 4). Mean power displayed excellent reproducibility in both SBC2 ($r = 0.96$, $p < 0.001$; TE = 0.6%) and SBC3 ($r = 0.98$, $p < 0.001$; TE = 0.4%). Mean speed also displayed excellent reproducibility in SBC2 ($r = 0.97$, $p < 0.001$; TE = 0.6%) and SBC3 ($r = 0.98$, $p < 0.001$; TE = 0.4%). Eight participants reported symptoms of GI discomfort (Table 5). The severity of GI discomfort displayed good reproducibility in SBC2 ($r = 0.72$, $p = 0.023$; TE = 1.3%) in comparison to excellent in SBC3 ($r = 0.76$, $p = 0.017$; TE = 1.3%). The time to peak GI discomfort displayed excellent reproducibility in both SBC2 ($r = 0.99$, $p < 0.001$; TE = 0.2%) and SBC3 ($r = 0.84$, $p = 0.005$; TE = 1.1%).

Effect of Treatment

In the initial treatments to identify time to peak alkalosis, peak HCO_3^- was achieved between 40 and 110 min (median 50 min) following SBC2 and between 40 and 100 min (median 70 min) following SBC3. There was a large inter-individual variation as the CV range was between 27 and 33% for SBC treatments. A + 5.5 ± 0.7 mmol l^{-1} change in HCO_3^- from baseline to peak was observed following SBC2, compared to + 6.5 ± 1.3 mmol l^{-1} in SBC3, respectively (Table 2). Both

Table 1 Overview of intraclass correlation coefficients (ICC) and typical error (TE) statistical analysis following sodium bicarbonate ($NaHCO_3$) treatments (SBC2 and SBC3) on pre-, during and post-exercise blood pH, bicarbonate (HCO_3^-) and lactate

Absolute change from baseline to peak (including initial TTP trial)								
HCO_3^-	SBC2	SBC3	pH	SBC2	SBC3			
ICC			ICC					
r value	0.79	0.69	*r* value	0.79	0.17			
p value	< 0.001	0.006	*p* value	< 0.001	0.326			
Typical error %	1.2	1.4	Typical error %	1.4	1.7			
Interpretation	Excellent	Good	Interpretation	Excellent	Poor			
During exercise								
Decline in HCO_3^-	SBC2	SBC3						
ICC								
r value	0.69	0.95						
p value	0.026	< 0.001						
Typical error %	1.3	0.6						
Interpretation	Good	Excellent						
Post-exercise								
Blood lactate	SBC2	SBC3	HCO_3^-	SBC2	SBC3	pH	SBC2	SBC3
ICC			ICC			ICC		
r value	0.91	0.92	*r* value	0.89	0.95	*r* value	0.92	0.95
p value	< 0.001	< 0.001	*p* value	< 0.001	< 0.001	*p* value	< 0.001	< 0.001
Typical error %	0.7	0.8	Typical error %	0.8	0.6	Typical error %	0.6	0.6
Interpretation	Excellent	Excellent	Interpretation	Excellent	Excellent	Interpretation	Excellent	Excellent

SBC treatments displayed a large CV ranging from 14 to 19%. In comparison, peak pH from baseline was achieved between 50 and 80 min (median 60 min) following SBC2 and between 50 and 90 min (median 70 min) following SBC3. Similarly, a large CV range was also observed (18 to 22%). The change from baseline to peak was + 0.07 ± 0.02 in SBC2 and + 0.09 ± 0.03 in SBC3, again with a large CV from 29 to 34% (Table 2).

Following $NaHCO_3$ ingestion, HCO_3^- was greater compared to baseline in both SBC2 and SBC3, revealing a main effect for time ($p < 0.001$, $\eta^2 = 0.932$); however, no difference between treatments was observed ($p = 0.184$, $\eta^2 = 0.010$; Table 2). This trend was similar for pH with a main effect for time ($p \leq 0.001$, $\eta^2 = 0.983$) and no difference between SBC treatments ($p = 0.512$, $\eta^2 = 0.003$). During exercise, there was no difference in the decline of HCO_3^- following both SBC2 and SBC3 ($p = 0.251$, $\eta^2 = 0.129$). Post-exercise [La^-] also displayed no difference between SBC treatments ($p = 0.494$, $\eta^2 = 0.076$; Table 2).

The time to complete the 4 km distance was similar for both SBC2 (combined mean = 373.6 ± 13.3 s) and SBC3 (373.5 ± 13.1 s) (mean diff = 0.01 s; $p = 0.929$, $\eta^2 = 0.015$; Table 3). Compared to the control treatment arm, both SBC2 and SBC3 produced faster completion times (mean difference SBC2 = − 8.0, $p \leq 0.001$ and 8.8 s, $p = 0.006$; SBC3 = − 8.2, $p = 0.005$ and 8.6 s, $p = 0.006$). There was no difference between SBC2 and SBC3 for either mean power ($p = 0.966$, $\eta^2 = 0.009$) or mean speed ($p = 0.746$, $\eta^2 = 0.040$). Severity of GI discomfort in SBC3 was marginally greater (3.4 ± 3.0 and 4.6 ± 3.6) compared to SBC2 (2.8 ± 3.4 and

Table 2 Mean (± SD) blood pH, bicarbonate (HCO_3^-) and lactate responses following sodium bicarbonate ($NaHCO_3$)

Baseline to pre-exercise	Ind. time to peak SBC2	SBC2	SBC2	Ind. time to peak SBC3	SBC3	SBC3
pH	0.07 ± 0.02	0.06 ± 0.01	0.07 ± 0.02	0.09 ± 0.03	0.06 ± 0.02	0.07 ± 0.02
HCO_3^- (mmol l^{-1})	5.5 ± 0.7	4.9 ± 0.8	5.2 ± 1.1	6.5 ± 1.3	5.6 ± 1.0	5.7 ± 1.1
During exercise						
HCO_3^- usage (mmol l^{-1})		12.7 ± 2.6	13.9 ± 1.7		13.8 ± 2.7	13.2 ± 2.5
Post-exercise						
Blood lactate (mmol l^{-1})		16.1 ± 3.4	17.2 ± 3.7		16.1 ± 3.4	16.3 ± 3.8

Table 3 Individual blood responses for both blood pH and bicarbonate (HCO_3^-) following sodium bicarbonate ($NaHCO_3$)

Blood HCO_3^-	Absolute change in mmol l^{-1}							Blood pH	Absolute change					
Participant number	Ind. dose	SBC2	SBC2	Ind. dose	SBC3	SBC3	CON	Ind. dose	SBC2	SBC2	Ind. dose	SBC3	SBC3	CON
1	5.5	5.4	5.7	4.9	4.1	4.8	0.0	0.06	0.07	0.04	0.09	0.09	0.08	0.00
2	6.8	5.6	5.1	5.6	4.1	4.9	0.1	0.08	0.08	0.07	0.05	0.04	0.05	0.00
3	5.6	4.7	7.2	5.0	6.2	6.9	− 0.5	0.07	0.05	0.06	0.07	0.05	0.08	0.00
4	6.2	4.5	5.0	8.1	7.2	7.2	0.0	0.05	0.03	0.08	0.10	0.02	0.03	0.01
5	5.8	5.5	6.3	8.1	5.8	4.9	0.0	0.09	0.05	0.06	0.06	0.08	0.07	0.00
6	5.3	5.4	5.0	6.5	5.4	6.9	0.0	0.09	0.08	0.11	0.16	0.05	0.04	0.00
7	4.7	3.3	2.9	7.6	6.5	4.2	0.1	0.07	0.06	0.06	0.10	0.07	0.08	0.00
8	3.8	3.8	4.3	7.8	6.4	6.1	− 0.1	0.06	0.05	0.05	0.09	0.06	0.06	0.00
9	5.3	5.6	5.2	4.6	4.8	4.8	0.3	0.05	0.06	0.06	0.06	0.09	0.09	0.00
10	5.4	5.8	6.0	7.0	6.0	6.9	0.0	0.05	0.04	0.04	0.09	0.05	0.04	0.00
11	5.9	4.9	5.2	6.4	5.6	5.7	0.0	0.11	0.07	0.12	0.09	0.10	0.11	0.01
Mean	5.5	5.0	5.3	6.5	5.6	5.8	0.0	0.07	0.06	0.07	0.09	0.06	0.07	0.00
SD	0.7	0.8	1.1	1.3	0.9	1.0	0.2	0.02	0.02	0.02	0.03	0.02	0.02	0.00

1.4 ± 1.5), however not significantly (z = 0.268, d = 0.08) (Table 5). Likewise, time to peak GI discomfort was around 20 min later in SBC3 (41 ± 27 and 43 ± 31 min) compared to SBC2 (23 ± 25 and 20 ± 24 min), although again not significantly (z = 0.197, d = 0.06; Table 5).

Discussion

The aim of this study was to investigate the reproducibility of both blood acid-base analytes and performance responses following repeated ingestion of $NaHCO_3$. The present study is the first to demonstrate that both the physiological and performance responses are reproducible when the ingestion time for $NaHCO_3$ is determined by individual time to peak HCO_3^-. This provides a legitimate and workable strategy to elicit consistent performance responses on exercise of this duration and intensity. The primary findings are in contrast to those of the previous research which has reported large inter- and intra-individual variability in both performance responses [12] and blood acid-base responses [6] following a standardised $NaHCO_3$ ingestion strategy. It would therefore appear that an individual time to peak HCO_3^- ingestion strategy is more efficacious in eliciting consistent responses.

Table 4 Individual 4-km TT performance differences between sodium bicarbonate ($NaHCO_3$) treatments (SBC2 and SBC3)

Participant number	Difference in seconds between treatments		% difference between treatments	
	SBC2 vs. SBC2	SBC3 vs. SBC3	SBC2 vs. SBC2	SBC3 vs. SBC3
1	1.4	2.3	0.4	0.6
2	2.5	1.1	0.7	0.3
3	0.5	3.0	0.1	0.9
4	11.2	4.3	2.9	1.1
5	0.2	0.4	0.1	0.1
6	4.6	0.4	1.2	0.1
7	5.6	1.9	1.5	0.5
8	7.8	2.5	2.1	0.7
9	3.0	5.2	0.8	1.3
10	1.6	2.4	0.4	0.7
11	2.7	1.7	0.7	0.4
Mean	3.7	2.3	1.0	0.6
SD	3.2	1.4	0.8	0.4
TE %	0.5		0.3	

Table 5 Individual severity and time to peak gastrointestinal (GI) responses in participants who reported symptoms only (n = 8)

	SBC2			SBC2			SBC3			SBC3		
Participant number	Severity	Peak GI (min)	Symptom	Severity	Peak GI (min)	Symptom	Severity	Peak GI (min)	Symptom	Severity	Peak GI (min)	Symptom
1	6	30	Diarrhoea/bowel urgency	2	30	Belching	4	50	Belching	3	60	Belching
2	3	30	Belching	3.5	20	Belching	0	0	None	0	0	None
3	10	50	Diarrhoea/bowel urgency	3	40	Belching	5	60	Belching	0	0	None
4	3	70	Stomach bloating	3	70	Stomach bloating	10	60	Diarrhoea/bowel urgency	10	90	Diarrhoea/bowel urgency
5	0	0	None	0	0	None	3	80	Stomach cramp	10	80	Diarrhoea/bowel urgency
6	0	0	None	0	0	None	3	40	Nausea/bloating	4	40	Diarrhoea/bowel urgency
7	0	0	None	0	0	None	2	40	Bloating	5.5	30	Bloating/belching
8	0	0	None	0	0	None	0	0	None	4	40	Stomach cramp
Mean	2.8	23		1.4	20		3.4	41		4.6	43	
SD	3.4	25		1.5	24		3.0	27		3.6	31	

Performance following $NaHCO_3$ displayed excellent reproducibility within the trained cyclist cohort used in this study. The TE values for the time to complete the 4-km cycling TT in the present study are consistent with a previous investigation of the reliability of TT cycling of the same distance without $NaHCO_3$ ingestion. Stone et al. [36] reported a TE of 0.9% which is similar to both the SBC conditions in the present study (TE ≤ 0.5%), whilst mean speed also displayed similar TEs (< 1%). These consistent values may be evident due to the high training status of the cyclists used in each respective study and the well-reported reliability of 4 km TT cycling performance under laboratory conditions [1, 23, 38]. The present study data suggests the inclusion of $NaHCO_3$ did not compromise the reliability of the performance responses, and therefore, it can be recommended to elicit consistent performance responses during this type of exercise. The present study also displays the intra-individual variation between conditions (i.e. SBC2 vs. SBC2). The intra-individual variation was larger in SBC2 than in SBC3, although this was largely due to participant 4 who displayed an 11-s difference between the two SBC2 treatments. With participant 4 removed from the analysis, a 3-s change would have occurred which is more akin to SBC3. In contrast, four of the sample reported a difference < 1 s between SBC conditions. Athletes should therefore be aware of this variation and monitor accordingly if they consider using $NaHCO_3$ on a consistent basis.

The primary findings agree with Carr et al. [6] who reported a low TE (2.1%) for 2000 m rowing ergometry following $NaHCO_3$. In contrast, a lack of repeatability was observed in a later study [12] reporting a mean CV of 7.4 ± 3.2% (range = 2.5 to 14.8%) and large intra-individual variation following $NaHCO_3$. This is considerably higher than the CV of Carr et al. [6] (1.6%) and the present study (3.5%), which is likely due to the lower training status of the participants used by Dias et al. [12]. Equally, both the study of Carr et al. [6] and the present study used TT simulation compared to a cycling TTE protocol at 110% peak power output [12]. It is suggested the 'open-ended' nature, the lack of control over power output and motivational differences during a TTE test explain the greater variation compared to TT simulation [24]. In a study by Saunders et al. [31], however, an identical protocol as used by Dias et al. [12] displayed excellent test-retest reliability in ICC analysis (r = 0.88), suggesting the exercise protocol did not negate the reliability of responses following $NaHCO_3$. It is more likely, therefore, that the training status of participants may have caused the greater variation in responses compared to that of Carr et al.'s [6] and the present study, as a trained athlete is likely to be able to produce a similar effort compared to a recreationally active participant.

The present study reports similar reproducibility of blood acid-base balance variables following $NaHCO_3$ in previous studies [6, 12]. Carr et al. [6] reported a high variation in HCO_3^- post-supplementation (TE = 2.4%), whilst Dias et al. [12] highlighted a discrepancy of 0.02 pH units between two $NaHCO_3$ treatment arms. Likewise, the present study reported similar inconsistencies such as a 0.03 pH unit discrepancy between the SBC3 individual TTP experiment and SBC3, and a 0.9 mmol l^{-1} HCO_3^- discrepancy in the same SBC3 treatment. Whether such small discrepencies are practically meaningful however, is abtruse. Nontetheless, individual analysis revealed a small number of inconsistencies in blood acid-base balance, as participant 4's absolute HCO_3^- change from baseline to peak was + 4.7 mmol l^{-1} in SBC2a, compared to a + 7.2 mmol l^{-1} change in SBC2b. Likewise, the change from baseline to peak for participant 8 was + 2.3 mmol l^{-1} different in SBC3 (+ 6.5 vs. + 4.2 mmol l^{-1}). Some degree of inconsistency was subsequently evident in performance times, particularly with participant 4, who was around 11 s slower in SBC2a than in SBC2b, whereas participant 8 was slower in SBC3a by around 3 s, despite the greater change in HCO_3^-, compared to SBC3b. These inconsistencies add to previous findings that have reported whilst the majority of blood responses were reproducible, some individuals display large variability following $NaHCO_3$ [14]. Given these inconsistencies, individuals should monitor the performance effects following $NaHCO_3$ ingestion across multiple trials to ensure similar responses are elicited.

The physiological responses pre, during and post the TTs displayed good to excellent reproducibility following both $NaHCO_3$ doses used in this study. During exercise, the change in HCO_3^- was highly repeatable for all SBC conditions and the values were reflective of a recent study following $NaHCO_3$ during a 3-min 'all-out' cycling test compared to a placebo [10]. Of particular interest is the lack of a difference in blood responses during experimental trials between the $NaHCO_3$ doses in the present study. The absolute HCO_3^- change from baseline was similar for both SBC conditions, as only a 0.5 mmol l^{-1} greater increase was observed in SBC3 compared to SBC2. Likewise, the increases in pH following $NaHCO_3$ ingestion were similar between the SBC conditions. This may explain why no dose-dependent performance effects were observed in this study, as buffering capacity would have been increased to a similar extent and therefore lead to equal amounts of H^+ buffering by circulating HCO_3^-. Moreover, in respect of blood lactate, a low TE range of 0.7 to 0.8% was displayed along with excellent ICC values (r = 0.91 to 0.92). This is in contrast to previous research displaying a TE of ~ 7% [6]. Nonetheless, some small inconsistencies were apparent as participants

6, 8 and 10 reported values with at least 2 mmol l^{-1} difference in SBC2, whilst participants 3 and 9 displayed this effect in SBC3. The reasons for this are unclear, although it may be due to the technical error associated with the lactate analyser used in this study [37]. Nonetheless, the present study displays that the physiological responses are consistent with repeated use of $NaHCO_3$ meaning the primary acting mechanisms for performance enhancement should be in place if the athlete is seeking a performance enhancement.

A unique finding of the present study is that the performance responses following $NaHCO_3$ were not dose dependent, akin to previous research [25]. The fastest 4-km TT completion time was observed in SBC2b although the other SBC treatments were not significantly slower (range + 0.2 to 0.9 s; % diff < 0.5%), suggesting a smaller dose of $NaHCO_3$ may be plausible to prompt similar physiological and performance responses. A consideration of this study however is that no placebo treatment was utilised to identify if these responses were ergogenic. The central aim of the study was to quantify the reproducibility of performance following repeated $NaHCO_3$ ingestion; therefore, this comparison was not included. Nonetheless, a control trial was conducted and our SBC conditions were significantly faster by 2.1 and 2.3% for SBC2 and 2.2 and 2.3% faster for SBC3. This suggests an ergogenic effect was apparent, in agreement with other studies using a time to peak alkalosis $NaHCO_3$ ingestion strategy [10, 28]. Yet, further research should address this by comparing such performance responses to a placebo.

A practical benefit of utilising smaller doses of $NaHCO_3$ is to minimise GI discomfort, as smaller doses have been shown to reduce the severity of symptoms [14, 26]. McNaughton [26] reported anecdotally as the amount of $NaHCO_3$ ingested increased from 0.1 to 0.5 g kg^{-1} BM the severity of GI discomfort increased, however since this study, comparisons between doses have been sparse. Indeed, the severity and time to peak GI discomfort was reproducible in the present study using ICC analysis (ICC range r = 0.72 to 0.99); however, in some cases, the symptom suffered varied despite a similar rating of severity and time to peak. Participant 8 for instance suffered from nausea and bloating in SBC3a but then suffered diarrhoea and bowel urgency in SBC3b. The reasons for the discrepancies in symptoms remain inconclusive, as previous research seemed to suggest it was not linked to pre-exercise nutrition (carbohydrate, protein, fat and sodium intake) or the change in sodium (Na^+) following $NaHCO_3$ [14, 22], although further research is warranted. Nonetheless, this provides a challenge to the individual considering routine use of $NaHCO_3$ as the symptom suffered may change with no clear pattern, which subsequently could impact the ability or desire to perform exercise, although the time to peak GI discomfort does seem to occur at the same time point. This influence of GI discomfort should therefore be monitored during training prior to use in competition.

Conclusions

This study is the first to display consistent performance responses from $NaHCO_3$ ingestion when exercise begins at the individual time of peak HCO_3^-. These datum support the use of individualised $NaHCO_3$ supplementation strategies prior to performance to elicit reproducible physiological and performance responses. The use of personalised nutrition to maximise the bioavailability of HCO_3^- and produce reliable responses in exercise that is competitive in nature is therefore recommended. Accompanying this finding, both 0.2 and 0.3 g kg^{-1} BM $NaHCO_3$ produced similar blood acid-base balance and performance reliability, with no difference between doses, suggesting both amounts can be used as an ergogenic strategy. Lastly, the use of $NaHCO_3$, irrespective of dose and repeated ingestion, appears to have a varied response on GI discomfort. Athletes should therefore monitor these responses, in an attempt to mitigate the impact of GI discomfort on exercise performance.

Acknowledgements

The first author would like to thank Dr. Craig Bridge for his input into the study design and kind words of advice.

Funding

No funding was received for this study.

Disclosures and Grants

Lewis Gough, Sanjoy Deb, Andy Sparks and Lars McNaughton can confirm that there are no conflicts of interest, and no grants or funding were received for this work.

Authors' Contributions

LG designed the study initially, with contributions from LM, AS and SD. The data collection was completed by LG and SD. The manuscript was written by LG, with feedback provided by LM, AS and SD. All authors read and approved the final manuscript.

Competing Interests

Lewis Gough, Sanjoy Deb, Andy Sparks and Lars McNaughton can confirm that there are no conflicts of interest.

References

1. Altareki N, Drust B, Atkinson G, Cable T, Gregson W. Effects of environmental heat stress (35° C) with simulated air movement on the thermoregulatory responses during a 4-km cycling time trial. Int J Sports Med. 2009;30(01):9–15.
2. Atkinson G, Nevill AM. Statistical methods for assessing measurement error (reliability) in variables relevant to sports medicine. Sports Med. 1998;26:217–38.
3. Bland JM, Altman GD. Statistical methods for assessing agreement between two methods of clinical measurement. Lancet. 1986;1(8476):307–10.

4. Burke LM. Practical issues in evidence-based use of performance supplements: supplement interactions, repeated use and individual responses. Sports Med. 2017;47:1–22.
5. Carr AJ, Hopkins WG, Gore CJ. Effects of acute alkalosis and acidosis on performance: a meta-analysis. Sports Med. 2011;41:801–14.
6. Carr AJ, Slater GJ, Gore CJ, Dawson B, Burke LM. Reliability and effect of sodium bicarbonate: buffering and 2000-m rowing performance. Int J Sports Physiol Perform. 2012;7:152–60.
7. Castell LM, Stear SJ, Burke LM. Nutritional supplements in sport, exercise and health. London: Routledge; 2015.
8. Cohen J. Statistical power analysis for the behavioural science. New York: Routledge.
9. Costa VP, Matos DG, Pertence LC, Martins JAN, Lima JRP. Reproducibility of cycling time to exhaustion at VO_{2Max} in competitive cyclists. JEP Online. 2011;14(1):28–34.
10. Deb SK, Gough LA, Sparks SA, McNaughton LR. Determinants of curvature constant (W') of the power duration relationship under normoxia and hypoxia: the effect of pre-exercise alkalosis. Eur J Appl Physiol. 2017;117:901–12.
11. De Pauw K, Roelands B, Cheung SS, De Geus B, Rietjens G, Meeusen R. Guidelines to classify subject groups in sport-science research. Intern J Sport Physiol Perf. 2013;8(2):111–22.
12. Dias GF, Silva V, de Salles Painelli V, Sale C, Artioli GG, Gualano B, Saunders B. (In) consistencies in responses to sodium bicarbonate supplementation: a randomised, repeated measures, counterbalanced and double-blind study. PLoS One. 2015;10(11):e0143086.
13. Flinn S, Herbert K, Graham K, Siegler JC. Differential effect of metabolic alkalosis and hypoxia on high-intensity cycling performance. J Strength Cond Res. 2014;28(10):2852–8.
14. Gough LA, Deb SK, Sparks SA, McNaughton LR. The reproducibility of blood acid base responses in male collegiate athletes following individualised doses of sodium bicarbonate: a randomised controlled crossover study. Sports Med. 2017; https://doi.org/10.1007/s40279-017-0699-x. [Epub ahead of print]
15. Hecksteden A, Kraushaar J, Scharhag-Rosenberger F, Theisen D, Senn S, Meyer T. Individual response to exercise training—a statistical perspective. J Appl Physiol. 2015;118:1450–9.
16. Higgins MF, James RS, Price MJ. The effects of sodium bicarbonate ($NaHCO_3$) ingestion on high intensity cycling capacity. J Sports Sci. 2013;31:972–81.
17. Higgins MF, James RS, Price MJ. Familiarisation to and reproducibility of cycling at 110% peak power output. J Sports Med Phys Fitness. 2014;54(2):139–46.
18. Hopkins WG. Measures of reliability in sports medicine and science. Sports Med. 2000;30:1–15.
19. Hopkins WG. Individual responses made easy. J Appl Physiol. 2015;118: 1444–6.
20. Ivarsson A, Andersen MB, Johnson U, Lindwall M. To adjust or not adjust: nonparametric effect sizes, confidence intervals, and real-world meaning. Psych Sport Exc. 2013;14:97–102.
21. Jeukendrup AE. Periodized nutrition for athletes. Sports Med. 2017:1–13.
22. Jones RL, Stellingwerff T, Artioli GG, Saunders B, Cooper S, Sale C. Dose-response of sodium bicarbonate ingestion highlights individuality in time course of blood analyte responses. Int J Sport Nutr Exerc Metab. 2016;26(5):445–53.
23. Kussmann M, Fay LB. Nutrigenomics and personalized nutrition: science and concept. Personalized Med. 2008;5:447–55.
24. Laursen PB, Francis GT, Abbiss CR, Newton MJ, Nosaka K. Reliability of time-to-exhaustion versus time-trial running tests in runners. Med Sci Sports Exerc. 2007;39(8):1374–9.
25. McKenzie DC, Coutts KD, Stirling DR, Hoeben HH, Kuzara G. Maximal work production following two levels of artificially induced metabolic alkalosis. J Sports Sci. 1986;4(1):35–8.
26. McNaughton LR. Bicarbonate ingestion: effects of dosage on 60 s cycle ergometry. J Sports Sci. 1992;10:415–23.
27. McNaughton LR, Gough L, Deb S, Bentley D, Sparks SA. Recent developments in the use of sodium bicarbonate as an ergogenic aid. Curr Sports Med Rep. 2016;15(4):233–44.
28. Miller P, Robinson AL, Sparks SA, Bridge CA, Bentley DJ, McNaughton LR. The effects of novel ingestion of sodium bicarbonate on repeated sprint ability. J Strength Cond Res. 2016;30:561–8.
29. Price MJ, Singh M. Time course of blood bicarbonate and pH three hours after sodium bicarbonate ingestion. Int J Sports Physiol Perform. 2008;3:240–2.
30. Reilly T. Human circadian rhythms and exercise. Crit Rev Biomed Eng. 1990;18:165–80.
31. Saunders B, Sale C, Harris RC, Morris JG, Sunderland C. Reliability of a high-intensity cycling capacity test. J Sci Med Sport. 2013;16:286–9.
32. Saunders B, Sale C, Harris RC, Sunderland C. Sodium bicarbonate and high-intensity-cycling capacity: variability in responses. Int J Sports Physiol Perform. 2014;9:627–32.
33. Sparks SA, Williams EL, Bentley D, Bridge CA, McNaughton LR. Sodium bicarbonate ingestion and individual variability in time to peak pH. Res Sports Med. 2017;25(1):58–66.
34. Siegler JC, Midgley AW, Polman RC, Lever R. Effects of various sodium bicarbonate loading protocols on the time-dependent extracellular buffering profile. J Strength Cond Res. 2010;24:2551–7.
35. Siegler JC, Marshall PW, Bray J, Towlson C. Sodium bicarbonate supplementation and ingestion timing: does it matter? J Strength Cond Res. 2012;26(7):1953–8.
36. Stone MR, Thomas K, Wilkinson M, Gibson ASC, Thompson KG. Consistency of perceptual and metabolic responses to a laboratory-based simulated 4,000-m cycling time trial. Eur J Appl Physiol. 2011;111(8):1807–13.
37. Tanner RK, Fuller KL, Ross ML. Evaluation of three portable blood lactate analysers: lactate pro, lactate scout and lactate plus. Eur J Appl Physiol. 2010;109(3):551–9.
38. Thomas K, Goodall S, Stone M, Howatson G, Gibson ASC, Ansley L. Central and peripheral fatigue in male cyclists after 4-, 20-, and 40-km time trials. Med Sci Sports Exerc. 2015;47:537–46.
39. Vincent W, Weir J. Statistics in kinesiology. 4th ed. Human Kinetics: Champaign; 2012.

12

Observational study of potential risk factors of immersion pulmonary edema in healthy divers: exercise intensity is the main contributor

A. Boussuges[1*], K. Ayme[1], G. Chaumet[2], E. Albier[3], M. Borgnetta[3] and O. Gavarry[4]

Abstract

Background: The risk factors of pulmonary edema induced by diving in healthy subjects are not well known. The aim of the present study was to assess the parameters contributing to the increase in extravascular lung water after diving.

Methods: This study was carried out in a professional diving institute. All divers participating in the teaching program from June 2012 to June 2014 were included in the study. Extravascular lung water was assessed using the detection of ultrasound lung comets (ULC) by chest ultrasonography. Clinical parameters and dive profiles were recorded using a questionnaire and a dive computer.

Results: One-hundred six divers were investigated after 263 dives. They used an open-circuit umbilical supplying compressed gas diving apparatus in 202 cases and a self-contained underwater breathing apparatus in 61 cases. A generalized linear mixed model analysis was performed which demonstrated that the dive induced a significant increase in ULC score (incidence rate ratio: 3.16). It also identified that the predictive variable of increased extravascular lung water after the dive was the exercise intensity at depth ($z = 3.99$, $p < 0.0001$). The other parameters studied such as the water temperature, dive profile, hyperoxic exposure, or anthropometric data were not associated with the increase in extravascular lung water after the dive.

Conclusions: In this study, the exercise intensity was the main contributor to the increase in extravascular lung water in healthy divers. To improve the prevention of immersion pulmonary edema, the exercise intensity experienced during the dive should thus be adapted to the aerobic fitness level of the divers.

Keywords: Diving medicine, Pulmonary edema, Ultrasound, Chest ultrasonography

Key points

- This is the first prospective study investigating the factors implicated in the increase in extravascular lung water after diving.
- An important increase in extravascular lung water rarely occurs after a well-controlled dive.
- The main contributor to the increase in extravascular lung water in a healthy diver is the exercise intensity.

* Correspondence: alain.boussuges@univ-amu.fr; alain.boussuges@gmail.com
[1]UMR MD2, Dysoxie-Suractivité, Aix-Marseille Université et Institut de Recherche Biomédicale des Armées (IRBA), Faculté de Médecine Nord, Marseille, France
Full list of author information is available at the end of the article

Background

Pulmonary edema (PE) induced by SCUBA diving has been described in 1981 by Wilmshurst et al. [1]. Since this initial report, several cases of PE induced by various aquatic activities such as swimming, aquagym, breath-hold diving, and SCUBA diving have been reported [2–5]. The injuries may be under-reported, as the intensity of the clinical disorders may vary from minimal symptoms (transitory cough) to acute respiratory distress. Consequently, some divers may not apply for medical attention. However, diagnosis remains important because when recurrent injuries have been reported, the second episode of PE can be fatal [6]. In some cases, PE occurred in divers with cardiac disease [7–9]. Most frequently, the injury affected divers with an apparently normal heart [10]. A deeper understanding of the pathophysiology of the SCUBA diving-induced PE is important to better prevent the injury. Risk factors probably included environmental stressors and individual factors of susceptibility. Environmental stressors experienced during SCUBA diving such as water immersion, cold exposure, exercise intensity, hyperoxia, and decompression have been implicated in the pathogenesis [11]. Furthermore, the injury occurred more frequently in one sole diver among a group of divers performing the same dive profile, suggesting that some individual risk factors existed. In a recent review, Peacher et al. [12] reported that among recreational divers, risk factors of cardio-respiratory disorders are more frequent than initially estimated (from 44 to 72%). Other risk factors such as female gender [13, 14], advanced age [4], consumption of fish oil [14] or anti-platelet agent [2], hypertension [15], and obesity [12] have also been suggested.

For a better understanding of the pathogenesis of this injury, a prospective study is needed. Nevertheless, immersion pulmonary edema (IPE) is a rare event. The frequency of the disease has been assessed in an epidemiologic study performed on 1250 divers and swimmers. From this group, 1.1% presented symptoms related to IPE [4]. To undertake a prospective study, a procedure that can detect clinically silent PE would be advantageous. Chest ultrasonography is recognized as an interesting tool to visualize alveolo-interstitial syndrome using specific images called ULC (Ultrasound lung comets, Fig. 1) [16]. It has been used to quantify extravascular lung water (EVLW) in detecting minor PE in both climbing victims of mountain sickness [17] and athletes performing heavy exercise at sea level [18]. Chest ultrasonography has also been performed after apnea competitions demonstrating that breath-hold diving could increase the ULC score (ULCs) particularly in divers with clinical troubles [19, 20].

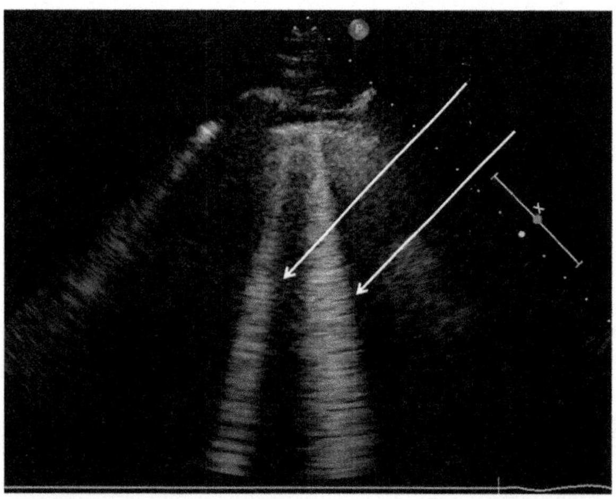

Fig. 1 Two ultrasound lung comets (arrows) arising from the pleural line

The present study was therefore designed to assess the environmental and individual factors promoting an increase in EVLW in a large population of professional divers with no medical history of cardio-respiratory disease. We hypothesized that risk factors suggested in previous studies such as cold temperature, heavy exertion, and stressors induced by the dive profile are implicated in the increase in EVLW after diving.

Methods

This prospective study consisted in an assessment of EVLW using ultrasonographic chest examinations in healthy volunteers who performed dives in the Mediterranean Sea.

Population studied

Our study was an observational study performed during the daily activity of the French National Institute of Professional Diving. All divers participating in the teaching program (8 weeks) were included in the study from June 2012 to June 2014. While the frequency of the injury is rather low (around 1%), the increase in EVLW, suggesting minor pulmonary edema, is more frequent. For example, in the study of Castagna et al. [21], an EVLW accumulation was reported in 73% of divers. Consequently, the investigation of a population larger than 100 individuals was considered to be appropriate for the aim of our study.

Each subject passed a screening examination, which included a physical examination and a review of their medical history. The baseline investigations, including chest ultrasonography, were performed between the third and the eighth day after entering the diving center, in a period without diving activity. During the study, the subjects were investigated directly in the boat, inside a cabin with a controlled ambient temperature (25 °C), before and after the dives. The number of dives per subject varied according to the availability of the investigators and the weather conditions. In the case of several examinations for the same diver, the recordings were performed before and after each dive. The post-dive investigations, which included chest ultrasonography, were recorded between 5 and 60 min after the end of the dive. This delay was considered appropriate because Ljubkovic et al. [22] have reported that ULC disappeared within 2 or 3 h after surfacing. The diving parameters were also recorded (depth, duration at the bottom, duration of immersion, breathing apparatus, decompression stop duration, gas at depth and during decompression stops, diving suit type, and water temperature). The dive profile was recorded using a dive computer (Galileo Sol, Scubapro-Uwatec, Antibes, France). Furthermore, the occurrence of respiratory symptoms such as coughing, shortness of breath, expectorations or hemoptysis, during or after the dive was systematically researched. Lastly, the exercise intensity (using the Borg Rating of Perceived Exertion Scale—RPE) and cold perception (using a visual analog scale—VAS cold) experienced during the dive were quantified. The training program and the dive profiles were decided by the diving instructors. Consequently, the investigators were blinded to the dive profiles as well as to the stressors experienced by the divers during exercise at depth.

Chest ultrasonography

The ultrasonographic examinations were carried out by experienced investigators using a commercially available Doppler echocardiograph (Esaote Mylab 30CV, Genoa, Italy) connected to a 2.5–3.5 MHz transducer array. The researchers were blinded to the clinical status as well as to the results of the questionnaire. Detection of ULC was performed using a recognized method [16, 19, 23] previously used for breath-hold divers [20]. A small number of ULC can be found in healthy subjects. In our work, according to past studies [24–26], an increase in ULC number of more than four artifacts when compared with the examination performed before the corresponding dive and a score greater than 5 was considered as a sign of increase in EVLW. The investigations were recorded on computers and were subsequently read by two independent observers.

Statistical analysis

Continuous variables were expressed as mean ± standard deviation. All the statistical analyses were performed with R statistical software [27]. Each subject served as his own control. Two series of measurements were obtained: the first as a control before each dive and the second after the dive. We then searched for the factors associated to the increase in ULC number. First, linear relationship between our variables was described by using Spearman's correlation.

Ultrasound examinations of the chest were performed between 2 and 12 times per subject, before and after diving. Number of diving instances per subject varied between one and six. Thus, we needed to take this source of randomness into account and assess the implied unbalance of our protocol. Because Ancova based on linear model with imbalanced data produced numerous difficulties [28], we used the most appropriate statistical tool, i.e., a mixed model with the following fixed effects: protocol factor, diving, individual factors such as age, weight, etc. and characteristics of the dive profile (e.g., duration of the dive, water temperature, etc.) and random effect: subjects.

Wald statistic was calculated and reported (z value) for each fixed effect. The z value is the Wald statistic for testing the hypothesis that the corresponding parameter (regression coefficient) is zero. Under the null hypothesis, it has an approximately N(0,1) distribution. $P(>|z|)$ is the tail area in a two-tail test, i.e., the test within a two-sided outer hypothesis. Our dependent variable, a sign of increase in EVLW, is considered a rare event in a healthy population. Thus, we used a negative binomial model that takes into account overdispersion in the distribution of events.

We compared two models by Akaike information criterion (AIC) [29]: the first was composed by all the predictive variables with no interaction and a second with all the variables plus age crossed with the physical activity intensity level (Borg scale). Model with the lowest AIC was kept. The lme4 package [30] was used for these analyses. The incidence rate ratio was calculated with the exponent of the estimate when appropriate. To assess the stability of our results, we produced power calculation through simulation process: 100 new dependant variables were generated and 100 new mixed model calculations were computed thus proportion of success (p value equal or inferior to 0.05) defines as power.

Results

Population studied

One-hundred six divers (104 men, 2 women) were included in the study. Their mean age was 31 ± 7 years (from 19 to 58) with most divers (75%) between 27 (first quartile) and 35 years old (third quartile). The mean weight was 80 ± 12 kg, and the mean height was 178 ± 6 cm. At baseline (at admission into the diving institute), all divers had a number of ULC lower than 5: 76 divers had no ULC, 22 divers had 1 ULC, 4 divers had 2 ULC, 3 divers had 3 ULC, and 1 diver had 4 ULC. These ULC were mainly recorded on the lower intercostal spaces on the antero-lateral chest (parasternal, mid-clavicular, anterior axillary, and mid-axillary lines) on the right side (41% of cases) and on the left side (31%). ULC were more rarely recorded on the posterior chest (posterior axillary, scapular and paravertebral lines) on the right (16%) or on the left side (13%).

Dives studied

In total, 263 dives (Table 1) were investigated (from one to six dives per subject). The water temperature was 16 ± 3 °C (range 10–23 °C). The divers breathed air at the bottom. They were submitted to a maximal partial pressure of oxygen (O_2) from 0.38 to 1.22 ATA. The ascent rate was 9 to 15 msw.min^{-1}, with a decompression

Table 1 Characteristics of the dives studied

	HOOKAH	SCUBA
	Mean ± SD (min–max)	Mean ± SD (min–max)
Number of dives	202	61
Diving suit	Dry	Wet
Depth (msw)	30 ± 12 (8–48)	33 ± 11 (10–48)
Duration at the bottom (min)	43 ± 15 (9–77)	20 ± 7 (9–30)
Total duration of immersion (min)	64 ± 13 (18–113)	29 ± 7 (15–45)

HOOKAH dives performed with an open-circuit umbilical supplying compressed gas diving apparatus
SCUBA dives performed with a self-contained underwater breathing apparatus

stop at 3 and/or 6 msw and sometimes 9 msw, according to the recommendations of the decompression tables developed by the French Ministry of Labor in 1992 (MT92 table) [31]. During the decompression period at 3 and 6 msw, the divers breathed 100% O_2; they breathed air at 9 msw. Forty-three successive dives were investigated.

Examinations after the dives

Two divers reported one episode of breathlessness during the decompression stops. In the two cases, these troubles disappeared before the end of the water immersion stay and no respiratory trouble was recorded during the ultrasonographic examinations performed after the dive. In one diver, a significant increase in ULC number was recorded by chest ultrasonography, while in the other diver, no ULC was observed.

Linear relationship between the variables

To assess relationship between the studied variables, a correlation matrix was performed (Spearman's rho). The correlation plot is reported in Fig. 2. High linear relationships were observed between diving duration (scaled) and material (SCUBA = 1, HOOKAH = 0), gas during decompression stops (O_2 = 1, Air = 0) and material, gas during decompression stops and diving duration (scaled), height (scaled) and weight (scaled) VAS cold, and material. ULC number has linear relationship with only two variables: diving and RPE (Borg scale).

Association and potential predictors

When comparing model with all variables plus interaction between age × Borg scale (RPE) and model with all variables without interaction, AIC was lower (923.89 vs. 925.64) for the model with no interaction. The simpler model (without interaction) was kept for the following analysis.

Results of the generalized linear mixed-effects model for the negative binomial family are reported in Table 2. Diving increased ULC number by 3.16 (IRR confidence interval, 2.01–4.57, $z = 6.42$, $p = 1.37 \times 10^{-10}$). The only other predictive variable of an increasing number of ULC was the exercise intensity (RPE) at depth ($z = 3.99$, $p = 0.0000659$). As seen in 3.4, diving has no significant linear relationship with other variables than ULCs, and RPE has weak linear relationship with material, gas during decompression stops, weight (scaled) VAS cold, and ULCs restraining confounding of a third variable.

Discussion

The present study provides several interesting findings on the risk of increase in EVLW after diving in healthy subjects.

Increase in extravascular lung water after diving

First, the occurrence of respiratory troubles in the context of well-controlled dives is rare. In the population studied, only 2 divers out of 106 reported one episode of breathlessness at the end of the dive during the decompression stop. These respiratory symptoms quickly disappeared, and the divers were asymptomatic when they were submitted to the investigations on board. In our work, chest ultrasonography was used to detect an increase in EVLW. One diver with breathlessness during the decompression stop had an elevated ULCs whereas the other had no ULC. Consequently, the respiratory troubles could not be related to minor pulmonary edema.

In the whole population, although a significant increase in ULC number was recorded after the dives, ULC number remained low. At the baseline examination, ULC number was lower than 5 in all volunteers. After the dives, few divers presented a ULC number greater than 5. According to the criteria chosen to define a significant increase in ULC number, only 8 divers out of 106 had ultrasonographic signs of increase in EVLW. This increase was recorded in 12 dives out of 263 investigated. Consequently, it can be concluded that an increase in EVLW rarely occurs after a well-controlled dive in healthy subjects. Given the infrequent occurrence of the increase in EVLW reported in our population of divers (104 men and only 2 women), our results should be interpreted with cautions.

The contribution of exercise in the increase in extravascular lung water

The statistical analysis demonstrated that the intensity of exercise was the main contributor to the increase in EVLW. This result, recorded in our population of healthy subjects, agreed with physiological knowledge and previous case series of IPE. It is well recognized that strenuous exercise on land can induce PE in healthy subjects [32, 33]. During exercise on land, hemodynamic changes include an increase in both the cardiac output

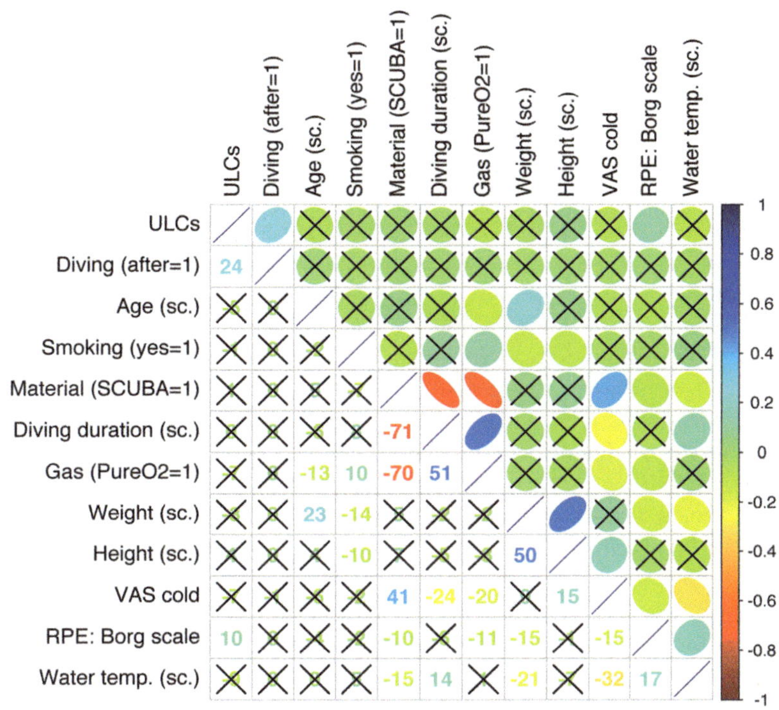

Fig. 2 Correlogram reporting the relationship between the variables. Positive relationship is in color blue and negative relationship in red color. Absence of relation is in white. Non-significant correlations are crossed ($p > .05$). In the upper part, an ellipse represents the orientation and the strength of the relation, the narrower the ellipse is, the higher the strength is. In the lower part, the rounded Spearman rho is indicated. Order of the variables is determined by hierarchical clustering with the "complete" agglomeration method. "sc." is an abbreviation for scaled (centered and scaled). *ULC* ultrasound lung comet, *SCUBA* self-contained underwater breathing apparatus, *Gas* gas during decompression stop, O_2 oxygen, *VAS* visual analog scale, *RPE* rating of perceived exertion, *Temp.* temperature

Table 2 Estimate, standard error of estimate, confidence intervals of estimate obtained by bootstrap, *z* value, *p* value, and post hoc power are represented for fixed effects of generalized linear mixed-effects model for the negative binomial family

	Estimate	Std. error	2.5%	97.5%	*z* value	Pr(> |z|)	1-β
(Intercept)	−3.14	0.84	−4.11	−2.21	−3.74	0.000186*	1
Diving (after)	1.15	0.179	0.696	1.53	6.42	1.37×10^{-10}*	1
Age (scaled)	−0.141	0.139	−0.414	0.126	−1.01	0.312	0.72
Smoking (yes)	−0.000678	0.279	−0.63	0.507	−0.0024	0.998	0.56
Material (SCUBA)	−0.0576	0.516	−0.898	0.602	−0.112	0.911	0.56
Total duration (scaled)	0.133	0.155	−0.167	0.397	0.857	0.392	0.69
Decompression Gas (O_2)	−0.511	0.499	−1.3	0.171	−1.02	0.306	0.76
Weight (scaled)	−0.0603	0.143	−0.408	0.271	−0.421	0.674	0.55
Height (scaled)	0.175	0.151	−0.122	0.488	1.16	0.248	0.78
Coldness (VAS)	−0.0244	0.0617	−0.208	0.0899	−0.396	0.692	0.61
Water temperature (scaled)	−0.169	0.116	−0.376	0.0491	−1.46	0.145	0.8
RPE (Borg scale)	0.172	0.0431	0.106	0.229	3.99	6.59×10^{-05}*	1

Diving (after) is the impact of the dive on the ULCs—examinations before and after the dive
O_2 oxygen, *SCUBA* self-contained underwater breathing apparatus, *VAS* visual analog scale, *RPE* rating of perceived exertion
*Significant difference

and pressure in pulmonary and systemic circulation. The increase in the pulmonary arterial pressure, leading to pulmonary capillary leakage and pulmonary capillary stress failure, is likely to be implicated in the pathophysiology of exercise pulmonary edema. In some individuals, such as subjects with left diastolic function impairment, an increase in both left atrial pressure and pulmonary capillary pressure can contribute to the pulmonary edema [34].

In water, supplementary cardio-respiratory strains are experienced. The high density of water in comparison to the air density, leads to an increase in ambient pressure. In SCUBA diving, it has been reported that the wet suit contributes to the increase in hydrostatic pressure [35]. This external hydrostatic pressure is transmitted to the smooth wall peripheral vessels reducing their compliance and leading to a blood mass transfer towards the central circulation [36–38]. In addition, the hydrostatic pressure also triggers a capillary shift of interstitial fluid into the blood compartment, which after some delay significantly increases the plasma volume [39–41]. The hemodynamic changes have been investigated at depth using underwater Doppler-echocardiography. A restrictive transmitral filling pattern, in favor of an impairment in left ventricular diastolic function leading to an increase in both left atrial pressure and pulmonary arterial wedge pressure, has been reported [42].

Furthermore, the myocardial wall stretch, due to the blood mass transfer, leads to the release of natriuretic peptides in the plasma, and is reported both after water immersion or SCUBA diving [22, 41, 43, 44]. Natriuretic peptides are recognized to increase endothelial permeability [45]. Lastly, the specific stressors induced by SCUBA breathing during exercise at depth might contribute to the development of PE through the increased workload of breathing, thus leading to great pleural pressure variations and subsequently to great variations in cardiac preload and after load [11]. Consequently, the cardiac, respiratory, and humoral alterations induced by water immersion could explain that exercising in water was the main contributor to the increase in EVLW in our study.

The role of other environmental stressors

The other environmental stressors investigated in our work were not related to the increase in ULCs.

Cold exposure has been implicated in the pathogenesis of IPE [15]. Nevertheless, PE have also been described after diving in warm water [3, 20, 46]. In our study, the statistical analysis did not demonstrate a correlation between ULCs and water temperature or coldness. Consequently, cold exposure did not seem to be a major contributor to the increase in EVLW. Nevertheless, our study was carried out in the Mediterranean Sea and the water temperature ranged from 10 to 23 °C. One could object that the cold stressor was not sufficient enough. Further studies in fresh water would be interesting to better assess the contribution of cold in the pathogenesis of IPE.

No correlation between the increase in ULCs and the parameters of the dive profile was recorded in our work. The magnitude of the decompression stressor induced by the dive seemed unrelated to the increase in EVLW. This result agreed with the previous studies. In a study performed in 12 divers, Dujic et al. [47] did not observe any significant increase in ULCs after a no-decompression dive performed at 33 msw. In this work, a high bubble grade was recorded in the divers. In the study of Dujic et al. [47] and the present study, the profiles were controlled and the decompressions were performed according to the recommendations of the Norwegian and French diving tables, respectively. These results did not disagree with the fact that pulmonary edema can be induced by a major decompression stress such as pulmonary decompression sickness, i.e., “chokes” [48].

Lastly, hyperoxia might be implicated in the pathogenesis of IPE through an increase in the production of oxygen-free radicals. Indeed, it has been demonstrated that a long duration exposure to an increase in oxygen partial pressure was associated to endothelial damages in the pulmonary capillaries and alveoli, resulting in interstitial and alveolar edema [49]. In our work, for short duration dives (37 ± 16 min at the bottom) performed by healthy subjects, hyperoxia did not contribute to the increase in ULCs. This result could be related to the fact that the risk of IPE in military divers using oxygen-enriched gas mixtures through rebreathers did not seem to be higher than in swimmers or recreational divers [50, 51]. On the other hand, a protective effect of hyperoxia has been recently evoked. When compared with normoxia, hyperoxia counteracted the increase in both central venous pressure and mean arterial pulmonary pressure recorded at depth (4.7 ATA) during exercise [52]. In our work, no difference in ULCs was found after the dives between subjects breathing oxygen and subjects breathing air at the decompression stop. Nevertheless, our study was performed in a diving school of professional divers leading to the use of specific procedures and materials such as a HOOKAH. The decompression stops were most frequently performed using oxygen breathing (88% of cases). A few SCUBA dives, breathing air for the whole duration of the dive, were investigated (31 dives). Although these SCUBA divers did not develop more numerous ULC after diving than others (232 dives), the small sample studied led to an impairment of the power of the statistical analysis. Furthermore, if the protective effect of hyperoxia is real, the procedure used in our diving center could explain the scarcity of the increase in EVLW recorded after the dives, when compared with the recent study of Castagna et al. [21]. Consequently, it seems important to perform further studies on the potential protector effect of hyperoxia against IPE, in particular among SCUBA divers.

Conclusions

According to the results of our prospective study, the main contributor to the increase in EVLW in healthy divers is exercise intensity. The other environmental stressors investigated such as the temperature of the water, the dive profile, and the hyperoxic exposure were not significantly related to the increase in ULC number assessed by chest ultrasonography. These findings are important to improve the prevention of IPE in divers. Indeed, before dive training, it is important to assess the aerobic fitness of the divers and subsequently adapt the exercise intensity experienced during the dive to the aerobic fitness level of the individual diver.

Abbreviations

AIC: Akaike information criterion; ATA: Atmosphere absolute; EVLW: Extra vascular lung water; HOOKAH: Open-circuit umbilical supplying compressed gas; IPE: Immersion pulmonary edema; msw: meters of sea water; O_2: Oxygen; PE: Pulmonary edema; SCUBA: Self-contained underwater breathing apparatus; ULC: ultrasound lung comets; ULCs: ULC score

Acknowledgements

The authors gratefully acknowledge the volunteers. This work was made possible through the support of the French National Institute of Professional Diving and its director, Commandant Paul Gavarry.

Funding

This study was supported by a French Ministry of Defense research grant (Direction Générale de l'Armement, PDH-1-SMO-2-0701). The funds were used to pay the rent of the ultrasound machine.

Authors' contributions

AB and OG conceived and designed the study. AK, EA, and MB assisted with the technical aspects of the protocol, recruited all the participants, and were involved in the acquisition of the data. AB and KA analyzed the data and GC performed the statistical analysis. AB, GC, and OG have drafted the article while MB and EA revised it critically for important intellectual content. All the authors have given final approval of the version to be published.

Competing interests

Alain Boussuges, Karine Ayme, Guillaume Chaumet, Eric Albier, Marc Borgnetta, and Olivier Gavarry declare that they have no conflict of interest.

Author details

[1]UMR MD2, Dysoxie-Suractivité, Aix-Marseille Université et Institut de Recherche Biomédicale des Armées (IRBA), Faculté de Médecine Nord, Marseille, France. [2]Altrabio, Lyon, SA, France. [3]Institut National de Plongée Professionnelle, Port de la Pointe Rouge, Marseille, France. [4]Laboratoire HandiBio EA 4322, Université de Toulon, La Garde, France.

References

1. Wilmshurst PT, Nuri M, Crowther A, et al. Forearm vascular responses in subjects who develop recurrent pulmonary edema when SCUBA diving : a new syndrome. Br Heart J. 1981;45:349.
2. Boussuges A, Pinet C, Thomas P, et al. Haemoptysis after breath-hold diving. Eur Respir J. 1999;13:697–9.
3. Hampson NB, Dunford RG. Pulmonary oedema of SCUBA divers. Undersea Hyperb Med. 1997;24:29–33.
4. Koehle MS, Lepawsky M, McKenzie DC. Pulmonary oedema of immersion. Sports Med. 2005;35:183–90.
5. Pons M, Blickenstorfer D, Oechslin E, et al. Pulmonary oedema in healthy persons during scuba-diving and swimming. Eur Respir J. 1995;8:762–7.
6. Cochard G, Arvieux J, Lacour JM, et al. Pulmonary edema in scuba divers: recurrence and fatal outcome. Undersea Hyperb Med. 2005;32:39–44.
7. Dwyer N, Smart D, Reid DW. SCUBA diving, swimming and pulmonary oedema. Intern Med J. 2007;37:345–7.
8. Gempp E, Boussuges A, Poyet R, et al. Acute coronary event revealed by diving-related pulmonary edema. Ann Cardiol Angeiol. 2009;58:240–3.
9. Kenealy H, Whyte K. Diving-related pulmonary oedema as an unusual presentation of alcoholic cardiomyopathy. Diving Hyperb Med. 2008;38:152–4.
10. Ludwig BB, Mahon RT, Schwartzman EL. Cardiopulmonary function after recovery from swimming-induced pulmonary edema. Clin J Sports Med. 2006;16:348–51.
11. Slade JB Jr, Hattori T, Ray CS, et al. Pulmonary edema associated with scuba diving: case reports and review. Chest. 2001;120:1686–94.
12. Peacher DF, Martina SD, Otteni CE, et al. Immersion pulmonary edema and comorbidities: case series and updated review. Med Sci Sports Exerc. 2015;47:1128–34.
13. Coulange M, Rossi P, Gargne O, et al. Pulmonary oedema in healthy SCUBA divers: new physiopathological pathways. Clin Physiol Funct Imaging. 2010;30:181–6.
14. Miller CC III, Calder-Becker K, Modave F. Swimming-induced pulmonary edema in triathlete. Am J Emerg Med. 2010;28:941–6.
15. Wilmshurst PT, Nuri M, Crowther A, et al. Cold-induced pulmonary edema in scuba divers and swimmers and subsequent development of hypertension. Lancet. 1989;1(8629):62–5.
16. Lichtenstein D, Mézière G, Biderman P, et al. The comet-tail artifact. An ultrasound sign of alveolar-interstitial syndrome. Am J Respir Crit Care Med. 1997;156:1640–6.
17. Pratali L, Cavana M, Sicari R, et al. Frequent subclinical high-altitude pulmonary edema detected by chest sonography as ultrasound lung comets in recreational climbers. Crit Care Med. 2010;38:1818–23.
18. Pingitore A, Garbella E, Piaggi P, et al. Early subclinical increase in pulmonary water content in athletes performing sustained heavy exercise at sea level: ultrasound lung comet-tail evidence. Am J Physiol Heart Circ Physiol. 2011;301:H2161–7.
19. Frassi F, Pingitore A, Cialoni D, et al. Chest sonography detects lung water accumulation in healthy elite apnea divers. J Am Soc Echocardiogr. 2008;21:1150–5.
20. Boussuges A, Coulange M, Bessereau J, et al. Ultrasound lung comets induced by repeated breath-hold diving: a study in underwater fishermen. Scand J Med Sci Sports. 2011;21:e384–92.
21. Castagna O, Gempp E, Poyet R, et al. Cardiovascular mechanisms of extravascular lung water accumulation in divers. Am J Cardiol. 2017;119:929–32.
22. Ljubkovic M, Gaustad SE, Marinovic J, et al. Ultrasonic evidence of acute interstitial lung edema after SCUBA diving is resolved within 2-3h. Respir Physiol Neurobiol. 2010;171:165–70.
23. Agricola E, Bove T, Oppizzi M, et al. Ultrasound comet-tail images: a marker of pulmonary edema. Chest. 2005;127:1690–5.
24. Picano E, Frassi F, Agricola E, et al. Ultrasound lung comets: a clinically useful sign of extravascular lung water. J Am Soc Echocardiogr. 2006;19:356–63.
25. Gargani L. Lung ultrasound: a new tool for the cardiologist. Cardiovasc Ultrasound. 2011;9:6.
26. Lambrechts K, Germonpré P, Charbel B, et al. Ultrasound lung "comets" increase after breath-hold diving. Eur J Appl Physiol. 2011;111(4):707–13.
27. R Core Team. R: A language and environment for statistical computing. Vienna, Austria; 2015. URL https://www.r-project.org/. 2015-03-09.

28. Shaw RG, Mitchell-Olds T. ANOVA for unbalanced data: an overview. Ecology. 1993;74:1638–45.
29. Akaike H. A new look at the statistical model identification. IEEE Trans Autom Control. 1974;19:716–23.
30. Bates D, Maechler M, Bolker B, et al. Fitting linear mixed-effects models using lme4. J Stat Softw. 2015;67:1–48.
31. Imbert JP. Calcul des tables du Ministère du travail MT92. In: Broussolle B, Méliet JL, editors. Physiologie et Médecine de la Plongée. Paris: Ellipses; 2006. p. 530–40.
32. Hopkins SR, Schoene RB, Henderson WR, et al. Intense exercise impairs the integrity of the pulmonary blood-gas barrier in elite athletes. Am J Respir Crit Care Med. 1997;155:1090–4.
33. Zavorsky GS. Evidence of pulmonary edema triggered by exercise in healthy humans and detected with various imaging techniques. Acta Physiol (Oxf). 2007;189:305–17.
34. Agricola E, Picano E, Oppizzi M, et al. Assessment of stress-induced pulmonary edema by chest ultrasound during exercise echocardiography and its correlation with left ventricular function. J Am Soc Echocardiogr. 2006;19:457–63.
35. Castagna O, Blatteau JE, Vallee N, et al. The underestimated compression effect of neoprene wetsuit on divers hydromineral homeostasis. Int J Sports Med. 2013;34:1043–50.
36. Arborelius M Jr, Balldin UI, Lilja B, et al. Hemodynamic changes in man during immersion with the head above water. Aerosp Med. 1972;43:592–8.
37. Gabrielsen A, Johansen LB, Norsk P. Central cardiovascular pressures during graded water immersion in humans. J Appl Physiol. 1993;75:581–5.
38. Risch WD, Koubenec HJ, Beckmann U, et al. The effect of graded immersion on heart volume, central venous pressure, pulmonary blood distribution, and heart rate in man. Pfluggers Arch. 1978;374:115–8.
39. Khosla SS, DuBois AB. Osmoregulation and interstitial fluid pressure changes in humans during water immersion. J Appl Physiol Respir Environ Exerc Physiol. 1981;51:686–92.
40. Miki K, Hajduczok G, Hong SK, et al. Plasma volume changes during head-out water immersion in conscious dogs. Am J Phys. 1986;251:R582–90.
41. Ayme K, Rossi P, Gavarry O, et al. Cardiorespiratory alterations induced by low-intensity exercise performed in water or on land. Appl Physiol Nutr Metab. 2015;40:309–15.
42. Marabotti C, Cialoni D, Pingitore A. Environment-induced pulmonary oedema in healthy individuals. Lancet Respir Med. 2017;5:374–6.
43. Norsk P, Bonde-Petersen F, Christensen NJ. Catecholamines, circulation, and the kidney during water immersion in humans. J Appl Physiol. 1990;69:479–84.
44. Passino C, Franzino E, Giannoni A, et al. B-type natriuretic peptide secretion following scuba diving. Biomark Med. 2011;5:205–9.
45. Curry FR. Atrial natriuretic peptide: an essential physiological regulator of transvascular fluid, protein transport, and plasma volume. J Clin Invest. 2005;115:1458–61.
46. Gnadinger CA, Colwell CB, Knaut AL. Scuba diving-induced pulmonary edema in a swimming pool. J Emerg Med. 2001;21:419–21.
47. Dujic Z, Marinovic J, Obad A, et al. A no-decompression air dive and ultrasound lung comets. Aviat Space Environ Med. 2011;82:40–3.
48. Kondo Y, Shiohira S, Kamizato K, et al. Vascular hyperpermeability in pulmonary decompression illness: 'the chokes. Emerg Med Australas. 2012;24:460–2.
49. Crapo JD. Morphologic changes in pulmonary oxygen toxicity. Annu Rev Physiol. 1986;48:721–31.
50. Arieli R, Shochat T, Adir Y. CNS toxicity in closed-circuit oxygen diving: symptoms reported from 2527 dives. Aviat Space Environ Med. 2006;77:526–32.
51. Gempp E, Louge P, Blatteau JE, et al. Descriptive epidemiology of 153 diving injuries with rebreathers among French military divers from 1979 to 2009. Mil Med. 2011;176:446–50.
52. Peacher DF, Pecorella SR, Freiberger JJ, et al. Effects of hyperoxia on ventilation and pulmonary hemodynamics during immersed prone exercise at 4.7 ATA: possible implications for immersion pulmonary edema. J Appl Physiol. 2010;109:68–78.

13

Vision and Visual History in Elite/Near-Elite-Level Cricketers and Rugby-League Players

Brendan T. Barrett[1*], Jonathan C. Flavell[1,2], Simon J. Bennett[3], Alice G. Cruickshank[1], Alex Mankowska[1], Julie M. Harris[4] and John G. Buckley[5]

Abstract

Background: The importance of optimal and/or superior vision for participation in high-level sports remains the subject of considerable clinical research interest. Here, we examine the vision and visual history of elite/near-elite cricketers and rugby-league players.

Methods: Stereoacuity (TNO), colour vision, and distance (with/without pinhole) and near visual acuity (VA) were measured in two cricket squads (elite/international-level, female, $n = 16$; near-elite, male, $n = 23$) and one professional rugby-league squad (male, $n = 20$). Refractive error was determined, and details of any correction worn and visual history were recorded.

Results: Overall, 63% had their last eye examination within 2 years. However, some had not had an eye examination for 5 years or had never had one (near-elite cricketers 30%; rugby-league players 15%; elite cricketers 6%). Comparing our results for all participants to published data for young, optimally corrected, non-sporting adults, distance VA was ~1 line of letters worse than expected. Adopting $\alpha = 0.01$, the deficit in distance VA was significant, but only for elite cricketers ($p < 0.001$) (near-elite cricketers, $p = 0.02$; rugby-league players, $p = 0.03$). Near VA did not differ between subgroups or relative to published norms for young adults ($p > 0.02$ for all comparisons). On average, near stereoacuity was *better* than in young adults, but only in elite cricketers ($p < 0.001$; $p = 0.03$, near-elite cricketers; $p = 0.47$, rugby-league players). On-field visual issues were present in 27% of participants and mostly (in 75% of cases) comprised uncorrected ametropia. Some cricketers (near-elite 17.4%; elite 38%) wore refractive correction during play, but no rugby-league player did. Some individuals with prescribed correction choose not to wear it when playing.

Conclusions: Aside from near stereoacuity in elite cricketers, the basic visual abilities we measured were not better than equivalent, published data for optimally corrected adults; 20–25% exhibited sub-optimal vision, suggesting that the clearest possible vision might not be critical for participation at the highest levels in the sports of cricket or rugby league. Although vision could be improved in a sizeable proportion of our sample, the impact of correcting these, mostly subtle, refractive anomalies on playing performance is unknown.

Keywords: Vision, Eye, Eyesight, Elite sports, Ametropia, Refractive error, Cricket, Rugby league

* Correspondence: b.t.barrett@bradford.ac.uk
[1]School of Optometry and Vision Science, University of Bradford, Bradford, UK
Full list of author information is available at the end of the article

Key Points

- Around two thirds of elite- and near-elite-level rugby-league players and cricketers had their eyes examined in the past 2 years, but 20–25% had either never had an eye examination or had had their last examination ≥ 5 years ago.
- Twenty to twenty-five per cent had an anomaly of vision in their habitual playing state, which, in ~ 75% of cases, was due to uncorrected refractive error; such errors are easily treatable using contact lenses.
- Findings suggest that the basic, clinically measured vision of high-level cricket and rugby-league players is frequently sub-optimal. However, the extent to which correction of these, mostly subtle, anomalies of refraction would lead to improved, on-field performance is not known.

Background

Vision plays a key role in interceptive tasks that are ubiquitous features of human action and interaction in our world, for example when shaking hands or crossing the street. Interceptive tasks are also a key component of many sports, such as when catching and/or striking a ball.

While some minimum level of vision is obviously important for participation in most sports, the requirement to optimise retinal image clarity in order to maximise sporting performance is contested. There are claims that vision is superior in elite athletes compared to the general population [1–6] or in elites compared to sub-elite athletes or novices [7–9]. Most of these claims have been made for sports which feature a small, fast moving target such as in baseball [5]. Also, vision measures and oculomotor behaviour (e.g. where and/or when the eyes are looking) may differ between elite individuals from different sports [10, 11] or between players in different positions in the same sports (e.g. fielders and pitchers in baseball [12], hitters and pitchers in baseball [13]; but see [14]). One interpretation of these findings is that excellent vision has contributed to the potential for 'eliteness'. This is supported by studies suggesting (i) that vision can be trained (e.g. in terms of where and/or when to look) or possibly even improved (i.e. made more acute) [2, 14–17], (ii) that better vision is associated with better on-field performance [18, 19], and (iii) that vision training can enhance performance in the field [16, 20].

However, counter evidence suggests that optimal and/or superior vision is not required to fulfil the potential for eliteness. Firstly, there are examples of elite-sporting individuals whose vision was sub-optimal. Mansoor Ali Khan (1941–2011) became the captain of the Indian cricket team at the age of 21 having lost sight in one eye when aged 16 [21], and there are also questions about the vision of the legendary Babe Ruth [22]. Secondly, low to moderate levels of retinal-image blur, simulating uncorrected myopia, may not necessarily impact negatively on performance in sporting tasks [23, 24], even in tasks where the visual demands are high [25–27]. Also, the uptake of eye care amongst elite-level athletes may be low; hence, suboptimal vision (e.g. due to uncorrected refractive error) may well exist amongst some elite sportspeople [28–32]. Finally, a number of studies have concluded that claims that vision can be trained or improved remain unproven [18, 33–35].

As outlined above, the evidence that high-level sports players need to have superior vision is equivocal. The importance of 'vision' depends not only on the sport, and in some cases, on the position played in that sport (e.g. bowling or batting or fielding in cricket), but also on precisely which aspect of *vision* is being considered (e.g. which of the many different tests of vision are used to evaluate vision). While visual acuity (the ability to resolve static, black letters of decreasing size on a white background) is the most well-known measure of acuteness of vision, there are many measures that reflect different visual abilities; these include stereoacuity, visual acuity for dynamic targets ('dynamic VA') [4, 12, 36], contrast sensitivity [37], and positional acuity [38], to name but a few. Different measures of vision may reflect, to a greater or lesser extent, the demands associated with particular tasks on the field of play. Further, if they exist at all, differences in vision between elites and sub-elites or novices may not emerge as differences in raw visual performance measures, but they might instead arise from differences in *how* vision is used. That is, elites, either through experience or through training, may adopt a better strategy than sub-elites for knowing where and when to look in order to access the most useful information at the most appropriate time [39]. For example, in a study of anticipation and visual search behaviour by Savelsbergh et al. [40] in which expert soccer goalkeepers were classified as successful or unsuccessful based on performance on a film-based test of anticipation, the 'successful' experts appeared to spend longer periods of time fixating on the non-kicking leg compared with non-successful experts. In putting, Vickers [41] found that better golfers exhibited longer fixation durations on the ball and target and fewer fixations on the club and surface. In cricket, Land and McLeod's study [42] led them to conclude that a cricket player's eye movement strategy contributes to skill in the game (see also [43]).The distinction between visual ability measures and the use of different visual strategies has been compared to the hardware versus software (respectively) distinction in computing [44]. Adopting this analogy, many believe that while changes to the hardware (improvements in visual ability, e.g. visual acuity and stereoacuity) are not achievable (but see [20]), changes to the software (e.g. improvements in visual strategies) may be both possible and effective [18]. It is possible that either 'hardware' or 'software' differences in vision contribute to the potential for sporting eliteness or that neither do. It is also possible that the two might interact so that for example, reduced vision (e.g. due to significant uncorrected refractive error) may limit a player's ability to employ a particular visual strategy.

Based upon the computing analogy outlined above, investigations into whether differences exist in vision between elites and sub-elite or novices, it is possible to divide such studies into comparisons between players and non-players in terms of vision abilities or of visual strategy. The current study is concerned with the former. Surprisingly, there have been no studies of eye care and basic (i.e. standard) visual abilities amongst UK-based high-level sportspeople. Here, we examine vision and visual history in UK-based elite/sub-elite players from two sports with very different visual demands, cricket and rugby league. The impact of sub-optimal vision may be greater in cricketers due to the demands of the game which features a small, often very fast moving object (the cricket ball). We gathered information about the visual history of our sports players to examine basic visual abilities in high-level cricketers and rugby-league players and to compare these visual measures with published normative values from young adults. Our aim was to understand the importance of optimally corrected vision for high-level participation in these sports and to look for evidence for better-than-normal vision. To our knowledge, this is the first study to measure the basic vision abilities and visual history of athletes who play the popular UK sports of cricket and rugby league.

Methods

Participants

Between September 2014 and October 2015, we conducted clinical visual assessments in 59 high-level sports players. Our rugby-league player sample consisted of 20 males from a 'Super-League' (professional) team. There were two cricketing samples. The first consisted of 23 male, near-elite-level players who represent the best players from universities in the north of England and who formed the Leeds/Bradford Marylebone Cricket Club. Several of these cricketers had played for periods with English county teams and together this group had played as a team against first-class, English county cricket teams. The second sample of cricketers was female and consisted of 16 members of England's international women's cricket team. Age details are provided in Table 1.

Protocols and Clinical Data Gathered

We gathered data from the participant groups described above. The results from our participants were compared with published data from young non-sporting individuals (see the 'Statistical Analysis' section below).

We measured the monocular (each eye) and binocular visual acuities (VA) at distance (6 m) and near (40 cm). Vision was measured in the habitual 'sports participation' state, i.e. with optical correction if worn when playing sports. Distance vison measures were taken using a logMAR chart [45, 46], and near vision was measured using an MNRead chart [47], which has a similar scoring system to logMAR distance VA measurement. We also determined whether distance VA in each

Table 1 Details of clinical visual measures

Group	Age (years, mean ± SD, range)	Distance visual acuity (habitual[a]) (LogMAR) (average ± SD) [range]	Number (%) showing improvement of ≥ 1 line with pinhole disc in at least 1 eye	Near visual acuity (habitual[a]) (LogMAR) (average ± SD) [range]	Stereoacuity (", seconds of arc)	Number (%) with red/green colour vision deficit
Elite cricketers ($n = 16$)	25.6 ± 2.9 [range 22–30]	− 0.07 ± 0.08 [+ 0.10 to − 0.18] (*p < 0.001*)[b]	1 (6%)	− 0.19 ± 0.05 [− 0.09 to − 0.26] ($p = 0.02$)[b]	Average 34.2" Median 30" Range 15–60" IQR 22.5"–45" (*p < 0.001*)[c]	0 (0%)
Near-Elite cricketers ($n = 23$)	20.7 ± 1.5 [range 17–23]	− 0.04 ± 0.21 [+ 0.20 to − 0.18] ($p = 0.02$)[b]	2 (8.7%)	− 0.18 ± 0.22 [+ 0.77 to − 0.30] ($p = 0.64$)[b]	Average 36" Median 22.5" Range 15–120" IQR 15"-52.5" ($p = 0.03$)[c]	2 (8.7%)
Rugby players ($n = 20$)	22.8 ± 3.5 [range 17–28]	− 0.09 ± 0.13 [+ 0.24 to − 0.20] ($p = 0.03$)[b]	2 (10%)	− 0.19 ± 0.08 [0 to − 0.30] ($p = 0.07$)[b]	Average 61" Median 30" Range 15–240" IQR 30"–60" ($p = 0.47$)[c]	0 (0%)

P values in italics met the criterion for statistical significance ($p < 0.01$)

[a]Habitual means with both eyes open, wearing any correction, that is normally worn when playing or without correction if not

[b]Results of statistical comparison using *t* tests of distance and near (VA) visual acuity for our three samples to the average value (− 0.16 logMAR) expected in young adults with normal or correct-to-normal vision [49, 50]

[c]Results of statistical comparison using *z* testing of TNO stereoacuity for our three samples against an average value for stereoacuity measured in young adults with the TNO test (50")[51–55]

eye improved when participants viewed through a pinhole (1 mm) because any improvement would suggest that the existing habitual refractive status was non-optimal [48]. We assessed stereoacuity using the TNO stereotest (version no. 14, 2014 TNO Stereotest. Boca Raton, FL: Richmond Products). When only one of the two plates at the next level was correctly identified, stereoacuity (in seconds of arc, ″) was taken as the average of the two levels. Colour vision was assessed using the Ishihara test (24-plate edition, Kanehara & Co. Ltd., Tokyo, Japan), and we determined the type and extent of any refractive error using an auto-refractor (Shin-Nippon, NVision-K 5001, Shin-Nippon Corporation, Japan).

We recorded the frequency of eye examinations, whether glasses or contact lenses are worn while playing, and whether there was any history of eye injury or eye disease. Using a questionnaire, participants were asked about the use of an eye patch as a child and any previous participation in eye/vision-training programmes. The complete list of questions is given in Table 2. Our aim was to gather detailed information about the clinically measured visual function, the perceived level of vision, and the visual history of each participant. All but two questionnaires (both from the rugby-league sample) were completed, though not all questions were answered by every participant (Table 2).

Statistical Analyses

For each sub-group, we used z tests to compare near and distance VA, and stereoacuity against published values from young adults. We also compared performance on each of these tests between the participant sub-groups using t tests. For both z and t tests, we adopted an α-criterion of 0.01.

Ethics, Consent, and Permissions

The study was approved by the ethics committee at the University of Bradford, and the tenets of the Declaration of Helsinki were followed. Written, informed consent was obtained from all participants included in the study.

Results

Clinically Measured Level of Visual Function

Stereoacuity and VA data are presented in Table 1 and Fig. 1. There were no statistically significant differences in VA (distance or near) between the three subgroups ($p > 0.01$ for all comparisons). In all sub-groups, the average distance VA was ~ 1 line of letters worse than the level which the published literature indicates can be expected in young, optimally corrected, non-sporting adults [49], i.e. those who have undergone an eye examination and are wearing the optical prescription that maximises their visual acuity. However, the deficit we identified in distance VA was only statistically significant for the elite cricketers (Table 1). The modest levels of distance VA mainly reflect the fact that a number of individuals had under- or uncorrected refractive error (see below). This is consistent with the finding that pinhole viewing improved VA by ≥ 1 line in 8.5% of participants (Table 1). Levels of near VA were consistent with those expected in young adults [50] (Table 1, Fig. 1).

Overall, the median near stereoacuity was 30″. Stereoacuity did not differ significantly between the three sub-groups (Table 1, Fig. 1). Stereoacuity in elite cricketers was significantly better ($p < 0.001$) than 50″, which is a consistently reported average value for TNO stereoacuity in young adults [51–55]. However, stereoacuity in the near-elite cricketers ($p = 0.03$) and rugby-league players ($p = 0.47$) was not better than the 50″ criterion. While median stereoacuity was good in all sub-groups (Table 1), three rugby-league players (15%) and two near-elite cricketers (~ 9%) had stereoacuity worse than 60″. These two cricketers were 'lower-order' batters, meaning that they are less-able at batting than some of their teammates and that their primary contribution to the team is in the form of bowling and fielding. None of the elite cricketers had stereoacuity worse than 60″.

Colour vision testing suggested normal performance in all participants except two near-elite cricketers. Thus, overall, 4.7% of our males had red/green colour deficiency compared to an expected 8% in European Caucasian males [56], who comprised the overwhelming majority of our males. This discrepancy may be due to our modest sample size, but it is consistent with findings that colour vision deficits are under-represented in high-level cricketers in England [57] and with another study [58] in which fewer first-grade cricketers than expected were found to be colour-vision deficient. None of the female cricketers were found to be colour deficient, and this is consistent with the much lower prevalence of red/green deficiency expected in females compared to males [56].

Residual Visual Issues

Residual visual issues (i.e. uncorrected, possibly unknown, anomalies of vision/visual system that could impact upon play) were found in 27.1% (16/59) of participants. Amongst the sub-groups, this varied from 18.8 to 35% (Table 2). Of the 16 individuals, most ($n = 12$, 75%) had uncorrected (92%) or under-corrected (8%) refractive error, and the pinhole test revealed improved VA in 5 of these 12 cases. In 6 of the 12 cases, the last eye examination had taken place > 5 years previously or no examination had ever taken place. In 4 of the 12 cases, correction for mild refractive error (up to 1 dioptre of myopia or astigmatism) was worn but not during play.

No cases of undetected ocular pathology existed, but one player (near-elite bowler) had significant, known ocular pathology that impacted on vision during play (Table 3). Three cases of binocular vision anomalies existed (Table 3).

Table 2 Eye examination history, refractive correction worn (including when playing), and refractive/other visual conditions identified

Group	Last eye examination			Wears specs or CLs?	Wears specs or CLs while playing?	Refractive error corrected by specs or CLs	Number (%) where residual visual issues were identified	Details of residual issues identified
	Within 2 years	2–5 years	5+ years or never					
Elite cricketers (*n* = 16)	11 (69%)	4 (25%)	1 (6%)	Neither: 8 (50%) Spectacles only: 3 (19%) CLs only: 2 (12%) Both: 3 (19%)	6 (38%) [5 of the 6 wear CL during play]	Of the 8 (50%) with refractive correction, 5 are primarily wearing correction for myopia, 2 for astigmatism, and 1 for hypermetropia	3 (18.8%)	2 of those who have spectacles (for mild myopia and astigmatism correction) do not wear these during play and do not wear contact lenses. In 1 other individual, vision was reduced due to myopia for which no correction was worn (spectacles or contact lenses). Aside from these uncorrected refractive error cases, there were no other residual visual issues that could affect play.
Rugby-league players (*n* = 20)	14 (70%)	3 (15%)	3 (15%)	Neither: 18 (90%) Spectacles only: 2 (10%) CLs only: 0 (0%) Both: 0 (0%)	0 (0%)	Of the 2 players (10%) with refractive correction (spectacles), both are primarily worn for the correction for myopia.	5 (25%)	Neither of the 2 spectacle wearers have contact lenses; hence, no refractive correction is worn by them during play. In 1 other individual, vision was reduced due to myopia for which no correction was worn (spectacles or contact lenses). The remaining 2 visual issues are binocular vision issues. Neither of these were previously diagnosed [i.e. participant unaware]; 1 (convergence insufficiency) is potentially treatable, while the other (ocular motility disorder) is not. The extent to which they would affect vision during play is uncertain.
Near-elite cricketers (*n* = 23)	12 (52.2%)	4 (17.4%)	7 (30.4%)	Neither: 19/23 (82.6%) Spectacles only: 0/23 (0%) CLs only: 0/23 (0%) Both: 4/23 (17.4%)	4 (17.4%) [all 4 wear CL during play]	Of the 4 (17.4%) with refractive correction, 2 are primarily wearing correction for myopia and 2 for hypermetropia.	8 (35%)	6 of the eight cases are refractive in origin (5 where no refractive correction is worn, 1 where only a partial correction is worn). The remaining 2 cases had (a) an ocular disease (macular dystrophy, diagnosed, not treatable, likely to have substantial impact on vision on the field) and (b) a binocular vision issue (convergence insufficiency, potentially treatable, not previously diagnosed, uncertain impact on vision on the field).

CL contact lenses

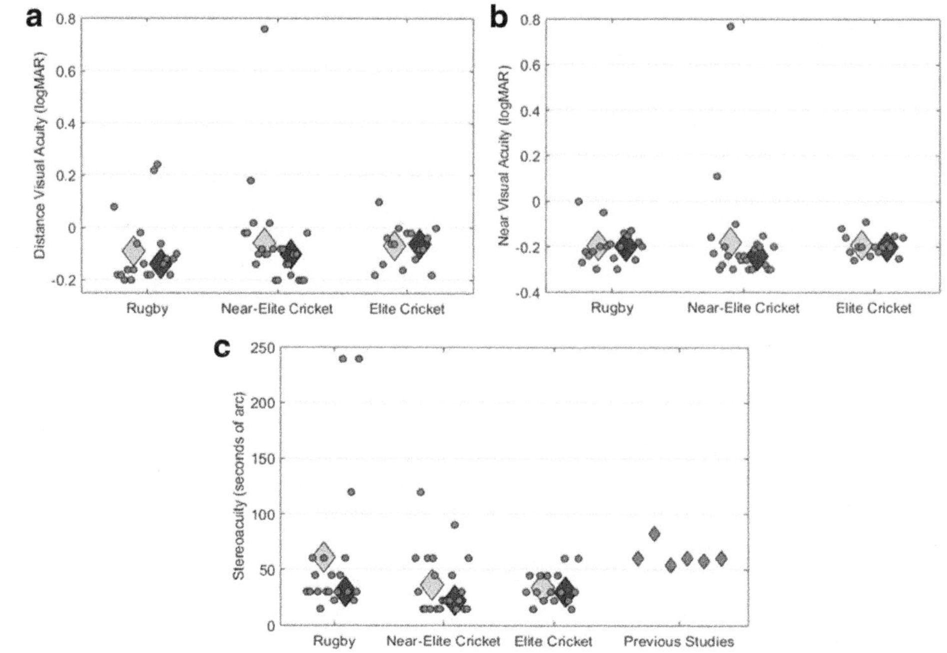

Fig. 1 **a** Distance visual acuity (VA) with habitual prescription worn for sports, if any. Circles represent data for individual subjects. These data are jittered on the *x*-axis to enhance legibility. Pale and darker diamond symbols represent the average and median values, respectively (see Table 1). **b** Same as for **a**, except for near VA. **c** Same as **a** except for TNO stereoacuity. Results from previous studies of near stereoacuity in young adults are also shown. From left to right, these data are from [52](median), [52] (average), [51] (average), [53] (average), [54] (average), and [53] (median). There were no differences in distance VA (**a**), near VA (**b**), or stereoacuity (**c**) between the three samples that participated in this study (all $p > 0.10$)

Uptake of Eye Care

Sixty-three per cent of all participants had their last eye examination within the past 2 years. However, there were substantial differences between the groups (Table 2); ~ 30% of near-elite cricketers had their last eye examination > 5 years before or had never had one, compared to 15% of rugby-league players and 6% of elite cricketers. Across the full sample, the figure was 18.6% (Table 2). In the questionnaire, only ~ 50% of the cricketers (elite and near-elite) and ~ 40% of the rugby-league players indicated that they regularly undergo eye examinations at least every 2 years (Table 3). Overall, 24.6% (Table 3) said they have eye examinations at ≥ 5 yearly intervals.

Refractive Correction Worn During Play

17.4% of near-elite cricketers and 38% of elite cricketers reported using refractive correction during play, but none of the rugby-league players did (Table 3). In all except one case, this consisted of contact lenses. 62.2% of cricketers wore (non-corrective) sunglasses in bright playing conditions (Table 3). No participant had refractive surgery.

Perceived Level of Visual Function

Overall, 84.2% of players rated their vison as 'good' or 'excellent' (Table 3). Around 20% of the near-elite cricketers rated their vision as only 'moderate' or 'poor', compared to 11 and 6% of the rugby-league players and elite cricketers, respectively (Table 3). The majority of players (5/8, 62.5%) who rated their vision as 'moderate' or 'poor' had uncorrected/under-corrected refractive error.

Although over 90% of elite cricketers rated their vision as 'good' or 'excellent', ~ 30% reported visual difficulties during play, compared with only 16.7% of rugby-league players and 8.7% of near-elite cricketers (Table 3). The discrepancy between the proportion of players with residual visual issues (see above) and the proportion who report visual problems during play for the elite cricketers (18.8 versus 30%, respectively), near-elite-level cricketers (35 versus 8.7%), and rugby-league players (25 versus 16.7%) suggests that perceived level of vision may not be a reliable guide to clinically measured vision and vice-versa (Tables 2 and 3).

History of Eye Disease, Eye Accidents, and Vision Training

Table 3 contains details of sports-related eye injuries (one rugby-league player), ocular disease (one near-elite cricketer), and vision training (two near-elite cricketers) to improve sports performance.

Discussion

To our knowledge, there have been no previous studies of eye care and basic (i.e. standard) visual abilities

Table 3 Questionnaire responses

	Elite cricketers (*n* = 16)	Near-elite cricketers (*n* = 23)	Rugby-league players (*n* = 18)
How would you describe your eyesight?	Excellent: 18.8% Good: 75.0% Moderate: 6.3% Poor: 0%	Excellent: 60.9% Good: 13.0% Moderate: 13.0% Poor: 8.7% No response: 4.3%	Excellent: 38.9% Good: [50.0% Moderate: 5.6% Poor: 5.6%
Do you ever notice problems with your vision when playing?	Y: 31.3% N: 68.7%	Y: 8.7% N: 91.3%	Y: 16.7% N: 83.3%
Do you ever wear sunglasses when playing?	Y: 56.3% N: 31.3% No response: 12.5%	Y: 60.9% N: 30.4% No response: 8.7%	N/A
How frequently do you have your eyes examined?	Every year: 31.3% 1–2 years: 18.8% 2–5 years: 31.3% 5+ years/never: 12.5% No response: 6.3%	Every year: 30.4% 1–2 years: 17.4% 2–5 years: 13.0% 5+ years/never: 34.9% No response: 4.3%	Every year: 27.8% 1–2 years: 11.1% 2–5 years: 5.6% 5+ years/never: 22.2% No response: 33.3%
Did you wear an eye patch as a child?	Y: 0% N: 100%	Y: 0% N: 100%	Y: 5.6% N: 94.4%
Have you have any kind of eye surgery?	Y: 0% N: 100%	Y: 0% N: 95.7% No response: 4.3%	Y: 5.6% (1 case; for detached retina) N: 94.4%
Any injury to your eyes or eye condition that caused you to visit Doctor/Hospital?	Y: 0% N: 100%	Y: 35.3% [not sports-related: 3 × corneal scratch, 1 × conjunctivitis, 1 × macular dystrophy; sports related: 1 × sub-conjunctival haemorrhage caused by ball to face (no lasting damage)]. N: 95.7%	Y: 5.6% (1 case: for detached retina) N: 94.4%
Any difficulty seeing colours?	Y: 0% N: 100%	Y: 4.3% N: 91.4% No response: 4.3%	Y: 0% N: 83.3% No response: 16.7%
Have you ever taken part in an eye/vision training programme designed to improve your sports performance?	Y: 0% N: 100%	Y: 12.9% [in all cases, this was suggested by coach, was 'cricket specific' visual training; for 0.5 to 1 h per day over 2–5 months. Deemed 'useful' by the player in 2 of 3 cases; 'not useful' in other case] N: 87.1%	Y: 0/18 [0%] N: 100%

amongst UK-based high-level sports players in the games of cricket or rugby league. This work represents a preliminary attempt to understand whether having optimal and/or superior vision is important for elite-level participation in these sports. Our sample size is modest which reduces the power of our statistical analyses. Having said this, groups of elites are by their very nature small because they represent the best of their sports, e.g. our cricketing elites were, at the time, more or less the entire England's ladies cricket squad. We did not gather equivalent data in a control group of non-sporting, age-matched individuals. Instead, we compared the results in our sports players with published results from young, optimally corrected, non-sporting adults. Thus, while these comparisons are between samples of broadly similar age, they are not specifically age-matched nor of the same sample size. We believe this was a better approach because published data on young adults are generally of studies involving larger sample sizes, which we believed there was no need to try to replicate.

Is 'Excellent' Vision a Prerequisite for Participation in Elite Cricket/Rugby League?

Our results show that our samples of elite and near-elite sports players do not have basic visual characteristics which could be considered excellent/superior. Aside from the possible exception of near stereoacuity, we did not find superior visual function relative to published values for young, optimally corrected adults [48–55]. The latter finding is at odds with studies of sports people in which the average level of vision (e.g. distance VA) was found to be excellent [5, 59, 60], but it is supported by studies which, like the present study, found that the average level of vision was no better than would be expected compared to the levels found in young adults (e.g. [61, 62]). On a similar note, we are not the first to find a significant proportion of high-performance athletes with either sub-optimal VA or other visual issues [28, 30]. For example, one study [63] reported that 28% of their sample of elite sportspersons had distance VA poorer than +0.10logMAR using the refractive correction habitually worn for sports.

Since uncorrected/under-corrected refractive error in young adults is more likely to impact on distance vision than on near vision [64], it follows that there might not be an adverse effect on stereoacuity taken at near (40 cm). Indeed, this is what we found, with very good median near stereoacuity in all sub-groups. Previous studies have found better-than-average stereoacuity in elite ball-sports athletes (i.e. baseball) [5, 8, 59], though whether this applies to both distance and near stereoacuity remains unclear [5, 65]. The possible importance of stereoacuity for sports is strengthened by the fact that individuals with naturally occurring, poor stereopsis exhibit poorer catching ability [66] and much reduced learning on a catching task by comparison with those with good stereopsis [67]. Interestingly, with some notable exceptions [21, 22], there are few reports of individuals with poor stereopsis reaching elite levels in sports, though of course this could be the result of children with a binocular disorder not being encouraged to participate in sports. If good or excellent stereoacuity is associated with elite-level sports, it is not clear what the nature of this association is, since disparity processing is temporally slow compared with that of luminance [68]. It is also not clear whether the better stereopsis that we and others [5, 8, 59] have reported in elite sportspeople leads to faster motion-in-depth perception. There appear to be two mechanisms for motion-in-depth perception, one based on sensitivity to retinal disparity and the other based on a comparison of motion signals in the two eyes. The relative importance of these two mechanisms for judging motion-in-depth is still debated [69, 70], but the mechanism comparing motion signals is thought to be independent of the one that uses binocular disparity. Thus, good motion in depth perception is not necessarily dependent on good stereopsis.

Uptake of Eye Examinations and Prevalence of Visual Disorders

Twenty to twenty-five per cent of our participants reported either never having an eye examination or that their examination interval was ≥ 5 years. This is consistent with a study [63] conducted in the USA between 1992 and 1995 on junior Olympic competitors and in other elites in which 25% had never had an eye examination. Given that we also found that 20–25% of the players had a vision/visual system anomaly in the habitual sports visual status, it is tempting to conclude that simply uncovering and addressing these anomalies through more frequent eye examinations would have a significant impact on the on-field vision of a sizeable proportion of players. This is partly supported by our finding that most residual visual anomalies consisted of uncorrected refractive error in individuals who had not had an eye examination within the past 5 years. However, while some players only became aware of the fact that their vision could be improved as a result of the examination we conducted, this was not the case for all of the players. Notably, four players (25% of those with residual visual anomalies) were aware they required refractive correction, but they chose not to wear it while playing. Also, another four players had anomalies that were non-refractive and which may not be treatable or their impact on vision during play was uncertain. Thus, while greater uptake of eye examinations will improve on-field VA in a selection of players, the proportion likely to benefit is probably considerably smaller than the overall 20–25% in whom we, and others [63], found anomalies.

Beckermann and Hitzeman [63] found that 29% of their sample had visual symptoms. We found that overall 17.5% reported vision difficulties when playing, with the highest proportion of these coming from the elite cricketers. Curiously, this group had the lowest proportion of residual visual anomalies found during clinical examination (Table 2). Discrepancies between perceived and clinically measured deficits in vision may arise because clinical measures do not reflect the visual demands on-the-field or because some reduction in clinically measured visual function can exist without impacting on perceived vision on the field (or both).

Other ways to Study the Nature of the Relationship between Vision and Elite Sports

The current study has been concerned with understanding whether superior vision is important for elite sports participation, and as such, we examined the basic visual attributes and the visual history of elite/near-elite cricketers and rugby-league players. Other ways to examine the relationship between vision and high-level sports participation/performance include artificially generating a visual problem in visual normals. Mann and colleagues [25, 26] found that low-to-moderate levels of simulated myopia did not affect cricket batting and there are other examples of resistance to defocus in other interceptive tasks [71] and in other sporting tasks (e.g. basketball [23], golf [24]). One interpretation of such findings, and of ours, is that while good or excellent vision may be desirable for elite sports, it may not be essential. Another possibility is that a deficit in basic visual abilities might be overcome by adopting different visual strategies or by gathering the critical information from different cues. An example of the latter is that depth information is recoverable from retinal disparity but may also be available via different means if the disparity signal is reduced (see the 'Is 'Excellent' Vision a Prerequisite for Participation in Elite Cricket/Rugby League?' section). Investigating whether different visual strategies (e.g. where the eyes are looking, stability of fixation) protect against visual loss due to, for example, uncorrected myopia can be carried out by artificially degrading the retinal image quality in visual normal (e.g. [25, 26]). However, given that it may take time for the visual system to adapt to the deficit it is experiencing, it is likely to prove more informative to conduct such studies in elite-sporting individuals who have been unable to adapt following an acute reduction in vision (e.g. following an accident, [72]) or conversely in those who have reached elite levels in their sports despite habitual, sub-optimal vision. Only a small number of such studies have previously been conducted [21, 22].

To fully understand the nature of the relationship between vision and elite sports, it is important to determine the visual demands during play. Given the dynamic environment of many sports, clinical visual measures gathered in static testing conditions do not reflect the visual demands experienced during play. Hence, researchers have measured performance on non-standard vision tasks (e.g. dynamic VA [4, 12, 36, 73]) and other visual-mediated, cognitive tasks (e.g. [74]). However, different sports can have very different visual demands (e.g. golf versus squash), and even within the same sports, the demands can differ markedly (e.g. bowling versus batting). Identifying the visual demands of different sporting tasks presents a challenge in understanding how vision could limit or enhance the potential for sporting 'eliteness'. While there have been attempts to study this topic [15, 59, 75, 76], it deserves considerably more research attention. Indeed, it is notable that while there is a growing number of online, web-based training programmes claiming to improve on-field performance (e.g. 'EyeGym', 'Nike Sparq', 'Neurotracker'), for the most part, the literature to support their use is scarce [77].

A different, though not incompatible view of the contribution of good vision to eliteness is that visual abilities as measured during standard, clinical testing play a lesser role and that the contribution of vision is to facilitate perceptual-cognitive expertise that emerges via information pickup from anticipatory cues [18]. This is apparent from differences in where and when elite players and elite-sports officials look during play (e.g. [39–43, 78, 79]), in the ability to recall patterns of play (e.g. [80]), and to perform successfully with limited information (e.g. [81]). There is a large volume of literature to support the contribution of perceptual-cognitive expertise to elite sports; specifically, there may not be better vision in elites, just better use of vision (reviewed in [39]). This is compatible with our findings and those of others (e.g. [61–63]) who have concluded that, for the most part, vision as measured in clinical settings is not superior in elite-level sports individuals. However, the importance of optimising vision in elite sportspeople is far from settled because there have been positive outcomes from recent vision training studies, as well as claims that the benefits transfer to better performance on the field [20]. One area of study that is notably missing from the literature concerns intra-individual improvements in performance following the correction of visual anomalies. Such studies need to be carefully designed because of the risk of contamination from placebo effects, but they may provide a more direct answer to the question concerning the importance of optimum vision for elite sporting performance. Other studies that may also prove useful, and which are similarly absent from the literature, would involve comparing visual strategies in those with different habitual levels of basic visual abilities (e.g. due to uncorrected refractive error). Studies of this nature may reveal the extent to which visual deficits might be fully or partially compensated for through the use of different visual strategies.

Conclusions

With the exception of near stereoacuity (which was superior in our elite cricketers), vision was not superior in our modestly sized sample of high-level, sports players when compared to published values for young adults, and for some measures, it was slightly worse. Moreover, since 20–25% of our sample had non-optimal vision, our findings suggest it is not critical to have the clearest possible vision for high-level sports. In cross-sectional studies like this, it is not possible to say that on-field performance would not be better if vision was improved. Studies of change in performance following the optimization of vision in those with correctable visual anomalies would be useful and would help to better characterise the nature of the relationship between vision and elite sports performance.

Acknowledgements

We are grateful to the players and officials associated with the Huddersfield Giants, Leeds/Bradford MCC Universities, and the England national women's cricket team. The assistance of Nathan Beebe is also gratefully acknowledged.

Funding

This study was funded by grants BB/J018163/1, BB/J016365/1, and BB/J018872/1 from the UK's Biotechnology and Biological Sciences Research Council (BBSRC).

Authors' Contributions

BTB designed the study, gathered some of the data, analysed the data, wrote the first draft of the manuscript, and modified it in light of comments received from the other authors. JMH, JCF, AGC, SJB and JGB helped to design the study, contributed to the analysis of the data, and commented on the drafts of the manuscript. AM gathered some of the clinical data and commented on earlier drafts of the manuscript. All authors read and approved the final manuscript.

Authors' Information

N/A

Competing Interests

Brendan T. Barrett: none, Jonathan C. Flavell: none, Simon J. Bennett: none, Alice G. Cruickshank: none, Alex Mankowska: none, Julie M. Harris: none, and John G. Buckley: none.

Author details

[1]School of Optometry and Vision Science, University of Bradford, Bradford, UK. [2]Department of Psychology, University of York, York, UK. [3]School of Sport and Exercise Science, Liverpool John Moores University, Liverpool, UK. [4]School of Psychology and Neuroscience, University of St Andrews, St Andrews, UK. [5]School of Engineering, University of Bradford, Bradford, UK.

References

1. Winograd S. The relationship of timing and vision to baseball performance. Res Q. 1942;13:481–93.2.
2. Stine CD, Arterburn MR, Stern NS. Vision and : a review of the literature. J Am Optom Assoc. 1982;53:627–33.
3. Christenson GN, Winkelstein AM. Visual skills of athletes versus non-athletes: development of a sports vision testing battery. J Am Optom Assoc. 1988;59:666–75.
4. Rouse MW, DeLand P, Christian R, et al. A comparison study of dynamic visual acuity between athletes and non-athletes. J Am OptomAssoc. 1988; 59:946–50.
5. Laby DM, Rosenbaum AL, Kirschen DG, et al. The visual function of professional baseball players. Am J Ophthalmol. 1996;122:476–85.
6. Gao Y, Chen L, Yang SN, et al. Contributions of visuo-oculomotor abilities to interceptive skills in sports. Optom Vis Sci. 2015;92:679–89.
7. Melcher MH, Lund DR. Sports vision and the high-school athlete. J Am Optom Assoc. 1992;63:466–74.
8. Boden LM, Rosengren KJ, Martin DF, et al. A comparison of static near stereo acuity in youth baseball/softball players and non-ball players. Optometry. 2009;80:121–5.
9. Savelsbergh GJ, Williams AM, Van der Kamp J, *et al.* Visual search, anticipation and expertise in soccer goalkeepers. J Sports Sci 2002;20:279-287.
10. Morgan S, Patterson J. Differences in oculomotor behaviour between elite athletes from visually and non-visually oriented sports. Int J Sport Psychol. 2009;40:489–505.
11. Laby DM, Kirschen DG, Pantall P. The visual function of olympic-level athletes-an initial report. Eye & Contact Lens. 2011;37:116–22.
12. Hoshina K, Tagami Y, Mimura O, et al. A study of static, kinetic, and dynamic visual acuity in 102 Japanese professional baseball players. Clin Ophthalmol. 2013;7:627–32.
13. Klemish D, Ramger B, Vittetoe K, et al. Visual abilities distinguish pitchers from hitters in professional baseball. J Sports Sci. 2017;15:1–9.
14. Wimshurst ZL, Sowden PT, Cardinale M. Visual skills and playing positions of Olympic field hockey players. Percept Mot Skills. 2012;114:204–16.
15. Schwab S, Memmert D. The impact of a sports vision training program in youth field hockey players. J Sports Sci Med. 2012;11:624–31.
16. Deveau J, Ozer DJ, Seitz AR. Improved vision and on-field performance in baseball through perceptual learning. Curr Biol. 2014;24:R146–7.
17. Zwierko T, Puchalska-Niedbał L, Krzepota J, et al. The effects of sports vision training on binocular vision function in female university athletes. J Hum Kinet. 2015;49:287–96.
18. The BASES expert statement on the effectiveness of vision training programmes. Available at http://www.bases.org.uk/Effectiveness-of-Vision-Training-Programmes [Accessed 16th May 2017].
19. Classé JG, Semes LP, Daum KM, et al. Association between visual reaction time and batting, fielding, and earned run averages among players of the Southern Baseball League. J Am Optom Assoc. 1997;68:43–9.
20. Clark JF, Ellis JK, Bench J, et al. High-performance vision training improves batting statistics for University of Cincinnati baseball players. PLoS One. 2012;7(1):e29109. https://doi.org/10.1371/journal.pone.0029109.
21. Downloaded from: https://sports.ndtv.com/cricket/how-i-lost-my-eye-excerpts-from-pataudis-biography-1565773 [Accessed 24th Apr 2017].
22. Voisin A, Elliott DB, Regan D. Babe Ruth: with vision like that, how could he hit the ball? Optom Vis Sci. 1997;74:144–6.
23. Bulson RC, Ciuffreda KJ, Hung GK. The effect of retinal defocus on golf putting. Ophthalmic Physiol Opt. 2008;28:334–44.
24. Bulson RC, Ciuffreda KJ, Hayes J, et al. Effect of retinal defocus on basketball free throw shooting performance. Clin Exp Optom. 2015;98:330–4.
25. Mann DL, Ho NY, De Souza NJ, et al. Is optimal vision required for the successful execution of an interceptive task? Hum Mov Sci. 2007;26:343–56.
26. Mann DL, Abernethy B, Farrow D. The resilience of natural interceptive actions to refractive blur. Hum Mov Sci. 2010a;29:386–400.
27. Mann DL, Abernethy B, Farrow D. Visual information underpinning skilled anticipation: the effect of blur on a coupled and uncoupled in situ anticipatory response. Atten Percept Psychophys. 2010b;72:1317–26.
28. Gottin M, Giacchino M, Oberto M, et al. Vision and sport: new forensic aspects. Med Sport (Roma). 1999;52:277–86.
29. Beckerman S, Hitzeman SA. Sports vision testing of selected athletic participants in the 1997 and 1998 AAU Junior Olympic Games. Optometry. 2003;74:502–16.
30. Sapkota K, Koirala S, Shakya S, et al. Visual status of Nepalese national football and cricket players. Nepal Med Coll J. 2006;8:280–3.
31. Callaghan MJ, Jarvis C. Evaluation of elite British cyclists: the role of the squad medical. Br J Sports Med. 1996;30:349–53.35.
32. D'Ath PJ, Thomson WD, Wilson CM. Seeing you through London 2012: eye care at the Olympics. Br J Sports Med. 2013;47:463–6.
33. Wood JM, Abernethy B. An assessment of the efficacy of sports vision training programs. Optom Vis Sci. 1997;74:646–59.
34. Abernethy B, Wood JM. Do generalized visual training programmes for sport really work? An experimental investigation. J Sports Sci. 2001;19:203–22.
35. Rawstron JA, Burley CD, Elder MJ. A systematic review of the applicability and efficacy of eye exercises. J Pediatr Ophthalmol Strabismus. 2005;42:82–8.
36. Muiños M, Ballesteros S. Sports can protect dynamic visual acuity from aging: a study with young and older judo and karate martial arts athletes. Atten Percept Psychophys. 2015;77:2061–73.
37. Zimmerman AB, Lust KL, Bullimore MA. Visual acuity and contrast sensitivity testing for sports vision. Eye Contact Lens. 2011;37:153–9.
38. Carkeet A, Brown B, Chan P. Spatial interference with vertical pistol sight alignment. Ophthalmic Physiol Opt. 1996;16:158–62.
39. Mann DT, Williams AM, Ward P, et al. Perceptual-cognitive expertise in sport: a meta-analysis. J Sport Exerc Psychol. 2007;29:457–78.
40. Savelsbergh GJ, Van der Kamp J, Williams AM, Ward P. Anticipation and visual search behaviour in expert soccer goalkeepers. Ergonomics. 2005; 48:1686–97.
41. Vickers JN. Gaze control in putting. Perception. 1992;21:117–32.
42. Land MF, McLeod P. From eye movements to actions: how batsmen hit the ball. Nat Neurosci. 2000;3:1340–5.
43. Mann DL, Spratford W, Abernethy B. The head tracks and gaze predicts: how the world's best batters hit a ball. PLoS One. 2013;8:e58289.
44. Elmurr P. The relationship of vision and skilled movement-a general review using cricket batting. Eye Contact Lens. 2011;37:164–6.
45. Bailey IL, Lovie JE. New design principles for visual acuity letter charts. Am J Optom Physiol Optic. 1976;53:740–5.
46. Ferris FL, Bailey IL. Standardizing the measurement of visual acuity for clinical research studies: guidelines from the eye care technology forum. Ophthalmology. 1996;103:181–2.
47. Ahn JS, Legge GE, Luebker A. Printed cards for measuring low-vision reading speed. Vis Res. 1995;35:1939–44.
48. Loewenstein JI, Palmberg PF, Connett JE, et al. Effectiveness of a pinhole method for visual acuity screening. Arch Ophthalmol. 1985; 103:222–3.
49. Elliott DB, Yang KC, Whitaker D. Visual acuity changes throughout adulthood in normal, healthy eyes: seeing beyond 6/6. Optom Vis Sci. 1995; 72:186–91.
50. Elliott DB, Flanagan JG. Assessment of visual function. In: Elliott DB, Clinical Procedures in Primary Eye Care (4th edition). Philadelphia: Elsevier Saunders; 2014:32–67.
51. Lee SY, Koo NK. Change of stereoacuity with aging in normal eyes. Korean J Ophthalmol. 2005;19:136–9.
52. Garnham L, Sloper JJ. Effect of age on adult stereoacuity as measured by different types of stereotest. Br J Ophthalmol. 2006;90:91–5.
53. Piano ME, Tidbury LP, O'Connor AR. Normative values for near and distance clinical tests of stereoacuity. Strabismus. 2016;24:169–72.
54. Yildirim C, Altinsoy HI, Yakut E. Distance stereoacuity norms for the mentor B-VAT II-SG video acuity tester in young children and young adults. J AAPOS. 1998;2:26–32.

55. Yekta AA, Pickwell LD, Jenkins TC. Binocular vision, age and symptoms. Ophthalmic Physiol Opt. 1989;9:115–20.
56. Birch J. Worldwide prevalence of red-green color deficiency. J Opt Soc Am A Opt Image Sci Vis. 2012;29:313–20.
57. Goddard N, Coull D. Colour blind cricketers and snowballs. BMJ. 1994; 309:1684–5.
58. Harris RW, Cole BL. Five cricketers with abnormal colour vision. Clin Exp Optom. 2007;90:451–6.
59. Molia LM, Rubin SE, Kohn N. Assessment of stereopsis in college baseball pitchers and batters. J AAPOS. 1998;2:86–90.
60. Sillero QM, Refoyo RI, Lorenzo CA, et al. Perceptual visual skills in young highly skilled basketball players. Percept Mot Skills. 2007;104:547–61.
61. Abernethy B, Neal RJ. Visual characteristics of clay target shooters. J Sci Med Sport. 1999;2:1–19.
62. Eccles DW. Thinking outside the box: the role of environmental adaptation in the acquisition of skilled and expert performance. J Sports Sci. 2006; 24:1103–14.
63. Beckerman SA, Hitzeman IS. The ocular and visual characteristics of an athletic population. Optometry. 2001;72:498–509.
64. Rabaei D, Huynh SC, Kilfey A, et al. Stereoacuity and ocular associations at age 12 years: findings from a population-based study. J AAPOS. 2007; 11:356–61.
65. Solomon H, Zinn WJ, Vacroux A. Dynamic stereoacuity: a test for hitting a baseball? J Am Optom Assoc. 1988;59:522–6.
66. Mazyn LI, Lenoir M, Montagne G, et al. The contribution of stereo vision to one-handed catching. Exp Brain Res. 2004;157:383–90.
67. Mazyn LI, Lenoir M, Montagne G, et al. Stereo vision enhances the learning of a catching skill. Exp Brain Res. 2007;179:723–6.
68. Tyler CW. The horopter and binocular fusion. In: Vision and visual dysfunction, vol 9, Binocular Vision (ed D Regan) MacMillan, London; 1991.
69. Nefs HT, O'Hare L, Harris JM. Two independent mechanisms for motion-in-depth perception: evidence from individual differences. Front Psychol. 2010;1:155.
70. Czuba TB, Huk AC, Cormack LK, et al. Area MT encodes three-dimensional motion. J Neurosci. 2014;34:15522–33.
71. Higgins KE, Wood JM. Predicting components of closed road driving performance from vision tests. Optom Vis Sci. 2005;82:647–56.
72. Downloaded from : https://www.theguardian.com/sport/blog/2016/oct/21/colin-milburn-play-when-the-eye-has-gone [Accessed 26th Sep 2017].
73. Uchida Y, Kudoh D, Higuchi T, et al. Dynamic visual acuity in baseball players is due to superior tracking abilities. Med Sci Sports Exerc. 2013; 45:319–25.
74. Overney LS, Blanke O, Herzog MH. Enhanced temporal but not attentional processing in expert tennis players. PLoS One. 2008;3:e2380. doi: 10.1371/journal.pone.0002380.
75. Erickson GB. Sports vision: vision care for the enhancement of sports performance. Oxford: Butterworth-Heineman; 2007.
76. Hitzeman SA, Beckerman SA. What the literature says about sports vision. Optom Clin. 1993;3:145–69.
77. Poltavski D, Biberdorf D. The role of visual perception measures used in sports vision programmes in predicting actual game performance in division I collegiate hockey players. J Sports Sci. 2015;33:597–608.
78. Spitz J, Put K, Wagemans J, et al. Visual search behaviors of association football referees during assessment of foul play situations. Cogn Res Princ Implic. 2016;1(1):12.
79. Gonzalez CC, Causer J, Miall RC, et al. Identifying the causal mechanisms of the quiet eye. Eur J Sport Sci. 2017;17(1):74–84.
80. van Maarseveen MJ, Oudejans RR, Savelsbergh GJ. Pattern recall skills of talented soccer players: two new methods applied. Hum Mov Sci. 2015; 41:59–75.
81. Stone JA, Maynard IW, North JS, et al. Temporal and spatial occlusion of advanced visual information constrains movement (re)organization in one-handed catching behaviors. Acta Psychol. 2017;174:80–8.

14

The effect of long-term confinement and the efficacy of exercise countermeasures on muscle strength during a simulated mission to Mars: data from the Mars500 study

Christopher J. Gaffney[1,2*], Elena Fomina[1], Dennis Babich[1], Vladimir Kitov[1], Konstantin Uskov[1] and David A. Green[2,3]

Abstract

Background: Isolation and long duration spaceflight are associated with musculoskeletal deconditioning. Mars500 was a unique, high-fidelity analogue of the psychological challenges of a 520-day manned mission to Mars. We aimed to explore the effect of musculoskeletal deconditioning on three outcome measures: (1) if lower limb muscle strength was reduced during the 520-day isolation; (2) if type I or II muscle fibres were differentially affected; and (3) whether any 70-day exercise interventions prevented any isolation-induced loss of strength.

Methods: Six healthy male subjects (mean ± SEM) (34 ± 3 years; 1.76 ± 0.02 metres; 83.7 ± 4.8 kg) provided written, informed consent to participate. The subjects' maximal voluntary contraction (MVC) was assessed isometrically in the calf (predominantly type I fibres), and maximal voluntary isokinetic force (MVIF) was assessed in the quadriceps/hamstrings (predominantly type II fibres) at 0.2 and 0.4 ms^{-1} using the Multifunctional Dynamometer for Space (MDS) at 35-day intervals throughout Mars500. Exercise interventions were completed 3–7 days/week throughout the 520-day isolation in a counterbalanced design excluding 142–177 days (rest period) and 251–284 days (simulated Mars landing). Exercise interventions included motorized treadmill running, non-motorized treadmill running, cycle ergometry, elastomer-based resistance exercise, whole-body vibration (WBV), and resistance exercise using MDS.

Results: Calf MVC did not reduce across the 520-day isolation and MDS increased strength by 18% compared to before that of 70-day exercise intervention. In contrast, there was a significant bilateral loss of MVIF across the 520 days at both 0.2 ms^{-1} (R^2 = 0.53; P = 0.001) and 0.4 ms^{-1} (0.4 ms^{-1}; R^2 = 0.42; P = 0.007). WBV (+ 3.7 and 8.8%) and MDS (+ 4.9 and 5.2%) afforded the best protection against isolation-induced loss of MVIF, although MDS was the only intervention to prevent bilateral loss of calf MVC and leg MVIF at 0.2 and 0.4 ms^{-1}.

Conclusions: Mars500 induced significant loss of quadriceps/hamstrings MVIF but not calf MVC. Collectively, these data suggest that muscles with predominantly type I fibres were affected less by isolation compared to type II dominant muscles. MDS and WBV afforded the best protection against isolation-induced loss of strength and thus may have virtue in exploration class missions.

Keywords: Mars500, Confinement, Muscle strength, Spaceflight, Ground-based analogue, Spaceflight analogue, Intervention

* Correspondence: chrisjamesgaffney@gmail.com
[1]Institute of Biomedical Problems (IBMP), Moscow, Russia
[2]Centre of Human & Aerospace Physiological Sciences (CHAPS), King's College London, Faculty of Life Sciences & Medicine, Guy's Campus, London SE1 1UL, UK
Full list of author information is available at the end of the article

Key points

- Mars500 was the longest isolation study ever conducted in humans and shows that despite exercising on a regular basis, crew lost significant leg strength.
- Habitual physical activity is therefore critical to strength maintenance.
- This has great implications for spaceflight and also for public health initiatives.

Background

Exploration of Mars will require astronauts to remain healthy in space for longer than previously achieved [1] as missions to Mars are proposed to be in excess of a year [1, 2]. However, astronauts must be able to perform adequately, if not optimally, on Mars, where the gravity is ≈ 38% (3.711 ms^{-2}) of that on Earth [3]. Losses in strength of up to 50% are predicted for a mission to Mars [4], which is equivalent to that associated with ageing from the second to the seventh decade of life [5, 6]. Strength loss therefore represents a serious concern for astronaut health, and intervention data are needed to determine the best protection for astronauts against microgravity.

Similarly to spaceflight, ground-based analogue studies have shown that prolonged confinement (e.g. in submariners) can result in loss of muscle strength in only 2 months [7]. Furthermore, confinement [8] and sustained operational stress is sufficient to induce muscle atrophy in young, healthy, active, and relatively well-nourished individuals [9]. It is not known, however, if a simulated Mars mission can induce muscle atrophy and associated losses in strength despite the presence of gravitational loading and whether exercise interventions can protect against any loss. It is also not known if starting strength [10] or pre-isolation training volume [11] have any affect on the strength lost during long-term isolation or spaceflight. Certainly, lack of exercise compliance has been cited as an explanation for loss of strength encountered in early ISS missions compared to previous Russian space station missions [12]. Mars500, conducted at the Institute of Biomedical Problems (IBMP) in Moscow, attempted to simulate some of the psychological and physiological challenges of a 520-day manned mission to Mars by isolating a crew in a hermetically sealed, confined, spacecraft-like environment. Whilst not simulating microgravity, Mars500 sought to emulate the isolation, boredom, controlled diet, relative inactivity, and stress managing finite resources autonomously with only limited and delayed communication with 'the ground' (mars500.ibmp.ru).

Spaceflight is associated with a preferential loss of type I muscle fibres [11, 13, 14] and muscle atrophy [15], which is associated with reduced strength (maximum voluntary contractions (MVC)) [11]. It not known if this is similar with long-term isolation. To investigate whether isolation causes preferential atrophy of type I or II fibre dominant muscles, isokinetic dynamometry can be employed to differentiate strength in muscles containing different proportions of slow and fast contracting fibres [16, 17, 18]. In the calf, there are up to double the quantity of type I muscle fibres (soleus ~ 70–80%; gastrocnemius ~ 50–57%) known to be preferentially lost in spaceflight [14] than in the thigh (vastus lateralis ~ 32–42%; biceps femoris ~ 47%) [19–22].

Despite decades of human spaceflight, optimal lower limb exercise interventions remain to be determined. Cycle ergometry with a Vibration Isolation and Stabilisation System (CEVIS) using loads of 25–350 W and treadmill running with a vibration isolation system (TVIS) (a treadmill with a harness to secure the user and mimic gravitational loading) are routinely employed but cannot prevent loss of calf and thigh muscle volume during 6-month ISS missions [23]. Resistance exercise may curtail muscle atrophy [24], thereby reducing task-specific force/power loss via changes upstream of the neuromuscular junction [16]. Resistance exercise may also alter the hormonal milieu with exercise to prevent muscle catabolism [17] and promote the maintenance of muscle protein synthesis [25]. Indeed, the advanced resistive exercise device (ARED) on the ISS appears promising [26] but it is unsuitable for exploration class missions because of size/mass. The Multifunctional Dynamometer for Application in Space (MDS) is smaller in size and mass than ARED and can be used to assess lower limb muscle strength. Furthermore, it can be used for exercise interventions including squat, bench press, dead lift, lateral pull, back extension, and rowing, in addition to calf raises and leg presses. WBV enhances motor unit recruitment promoting an efficient, specific warm-up effect that allows the muscle to produce more force and power and aids flexibility [27, 28]. Resistance exercise coupled with vibration (WBV) has prevented muscle atrophy during 56-day bed rest [29] and may provide a simple intervention [28] suitable for exploration class missions. Furthermore, elastic expanders train many muscle groups and have low mass making them viable for long-term missions [30]. It is not known, however, if these interventions can prevent isolation-induced lower-limb loss of strength. Thus, the study sought to test the hypotheses that (1) the 520-day isolation during Mars500 was sufficient to induce loss of strength in the calf and quadriceps/hamstrings muscles; (2) muscles comprising largely of type I muscle fibres were preferentially affected; (3) loss of strength was associated with strength before Mars500; and (4) the performance of 70-day exercise interventions including the MDS and WBV were able to prevent any loss of strength.

Methods

Subjects

Six healthy male participants (34 ± 3 years; 1.76 ± 0.02 metres; 83.7 ± 4.8 kg) gave written informed consent to participate in the study that conformed to the 6th revision of the *Declaration of Helsinki* and had received ethics approval from the local university and the Institutional Review Board of the Institute for Biomedical Problems (IBMP).

Three Russian, two European, and one Chinese crew member were isolated for a total of 520 days within the habitable module of the Mars500 facility located at the IBMP. The experiment was completed under normal (Earth) gravitational conditions. All subjects completed a medical screening, which included an ECG at rest and during exercise, chest and spine X-rays, ultrasound assessment of internal organs, and blood tests to test for any inability to complete the 520-day isolation experiment an exercise training during the study. Subjects were psychologically screened for social compatibility and motivation via the Minnesota Multiphasic Personality Inventory [31].

Experimental protocol

During the 520-day isolation, the subjects were instructed to follow an exercise intervention timetable to prevent loss of strength during isolation. The subjects were randomly grouped into pairs (1 and 5, 2 and 6, 3 and 4) and all pairs completed every exercise intervention but at different dates during isolation, in a counterbalanced design. The timetable can be found in [32]. Subjects 1 and 5 correspond to 'O' and 'N', 3 and 4 to 'M' and 'L', and 2 and 6 to 'I' and 'K' in [32]. The subjects completed different exercise interventions every 70 days, and these interventions comprised of active running, passive running, cycle ergometry, expanders, and WBV or MDS. Exercise interventions were not completed during 142 to 177 days (rest period) and 251 to 284 days (simulated landing activities on Mars [33]). Heart rate (Polar RS400 monitor, Kempele, Finland) was recorded throughout all training sessions to ensure participant safety.

Endurance exercises—treadmill running and cycle ergometry

Endurance exercise interventions to prevent loss of strength comprised of active (motorized) treadmill running, passive mode (non-motorized) treadmill running, and cycling, all completed 5–6 days/week for each 70-day training block. Active and passive mode treadmill running were completed on a Cybex International 750T treadmill (Medway, MA, USA) and a non-commercial treadmill (BD-1) used in the Russian module of the International Space Station, following the training protocol in Additional file 1: Figure S1 A–C.

Training on the cycle ergometer was completed on a Kettler Velergometer (Ense, Germany), following the training protocol in Additional file 1: Figure S1 D–F. Subjects were instructed to maintain a cadence of 60–70 rpm whilst cycling. All endurance mode exercises were completed as 3 days training followed by 1 day of rest (training therefore 5–6 days/week throughout the 70-day block).

Resistance exercise—expanders, WBV, and MDS

Resistance exercise interventions to prevent loss of strength comprised of expanders, WBV, and MDS. Before completing expander training (elastomer-based resistance exercise), the subjects completed a non-prescriptive 10-min warm-up comprising of low-velocity closed-chain movements (e.g. squats) and passive stretching (e.g. quadriceps, hamstrings, and calf stretches). Subjects completed three different exercise protocols using expanders weekly, throughout the 70-day training block (total training of 3–4 days/week). Protocol 1 comprised of 2 × 15–20 reps of elbow flexion, calf raises, abdominal crunches, and standing trunk extensions; protocol 2 comprised of 2 × 15–20 reps of press ups, squats, rowing, and pull downs; protocol 3 (recovery) comprised of three to five hamstring stretches in two positions. Training sessions were completed every other day during the 70-day training block (3–4 days/week).

Exercise using WBV was completed on a Galileo oscillating platform (Novotec Medical-Stratec Medizintechnik, Germany) at amplitudes of 2–6 mm depending upon foot position, and at a fixed range of frequencies from 16 to 25 Hz (Table 1). Subjects were familiarised with exercise and foot placement during WBV; however, data on foot position was not collected and foot position was not enforced during exercise. Subjects completed protocol A 5 days/week (Tuesday, Wednesday, Friday, Saturday, and Sunday), at 9.30 a.m. and 5.30 p.m., at least an hour after breakfast and dinner. Subjects completed protocol B 2 days/week on the remaining days (Monday and Thursday), in a single 11-min session (Table 1).

Exercise on MDS (Vienna University of Technology, Austria) comprised of three to five sets of 10–20 reps of squats, calf raises, sit ups, seated row, lateral pull back, bench press, and neck muscle exercises completed every other day (3–4 days/week) (Additional file 2: Table S1).

Strength assessments

Strength assessments were completed at least 24 h after the previous training session to allow sufficient rest. MVC of the calf working isometrically was determined

Table 1 Exercise protocols A and B performed during WBV

Time (min)	Frequency (Hz)	Exercise
Protocol A		
1	16–18	Warm-up
2–4	16–18	Rapid shallow sit ups
5	16–18	Squats (4 s down; 4 s up)
6	16–18	Two-footed vertical jumps on the balls of feet
7–8		*Break*
9–10	16–18	Pelvis movements (alternating hip flexion and extension)
11	16–18	Maximal hip flexion
12	16–18	Maximal hyperextension
13	16–18	Hands behind head and twist the body maximally clockwise, then anti-clockwise
14	16–18	Hip adduction reaching towards the ankle with the hand whilst the other hand reaches into the air. Movement is only in the frontal plane
Protocol B*		
1	16–18	Warm-up
2	24–25	Rapid shallow sit ups
3	24–25	Basic stance
4–6	24–25	Deep squat
7–9		*Break*
10–11	24–25	Basic stance. Deep prised (posture skier) within a maximum time
12–13	24–25	Heels keep
14–16		*Break*
17–18	24–25	Basic stance (24–25 Hz) 'Lifting the socks' action
Example warm-up		
1	16–18	Crew member stands in a vertical position (with slightly bent knees, and the feet in the basic stance)

*20 kg tabard is worn throughout all Protocol B exercises

at 90° plantar flexion whilst subjects were seated on MDS. Maximal voluntary isokinetic force (MVIF) was determined for leg press separately in the left and right legs at 0.2 and 0.4 ms^{-1}, respectively, and the mean average was calculated to determine bilateral leg strength. Isometric assessment was completed for the calf since it generates greater force [34] and isokinetic assessment was utilized for quadriceps/hamstring strength since it is the more sensitive at detecting changes in strength than isometric assessment [35]. The leg press was completed in the seated position, and the subjects were required to extend the hip and knee joints to push the resistance away from the body at either 0.2 or 0.4 ms^{-1}. Force was measured using MDS and visual data on force produced was fed back immediately to the subject via a digital transducer to assist the subjects with the maintenance of effort (Vienna University of Technology, Vienna, Austria). Subjects completed three maximal isometric (calf) or isokinetic (quadriceps/hamstrings) contractions with approximately 60 s rest between trials. The greatest was taken as the MVC or MVIF. Strength assessments (MVC and MVIF) were completed before the start of Mars500, the day of entering isolation, and every 35 days throughout the 520-day isolation, capturing the period immediately before and at the end of each 70-day exercise intervention.

Previous work has shown that the proportion of type II (fast twitch) muscle fibres (determined by mATPase staining) shows a moderate-high correlation with MVIF at medium contractile velocities (r^2 = 0.75) and a high correlation with MVIF at high contraction velocities (r^2 = 0.89; [36]). The assessment of MVIF using isokinetic dynamometry on MDS at both 0.2 and 0.4 ms^{-1} can therefore be used to non-invasively determine changes in type II muscle fibres over the Mars500 study.

Data analysis

A power calculation was completed using data from a previous long-term spaceflight experiment [37]. Data demonstrated that long-term spaceflight (6 months) induced a loss of strength of 31% in the lower limb muscles, the same muscle group we are studying. Given that loss of strength and muscle mass in spaceflight is roughly three times greater than in ground-based analogues, we used these data to estimate the potential loss of strength during 18 months confinement, for which there are no data to base a power calculation. Using these data [37] to calculate an effect size (dz) of 1.63 and using an alpha of 0.05 and a power of 0.95, we get a minimum sample required of n = 6 for detecting a difference in strength, which was the primary outcome of our study. Indeed, in our regression analysis, we have shown significant loss of strength over the 520-day isolation (P = 0.001 for 0.2 ms^{-1} and P = 0.007 for 0.4 ms^{-1}), and therefore, our study was appropriately powered.

Training volume on MDS was calculated to investigate the effect of total training volume on the preservation of strength during 70-day training with MDS. Force and position data was recorded continuously at 50 Hz during calf and leg press training sessions on MDS. Data were processed using customized scripts in MATLAB® (R2010b, The MathWorks, Inc.®, Natick, MA, USA) that calculated total training volume from number of repetitions and force per repetition.

Data were checked to ensure no statistical assumptions were violated (autocorrelation assessed using scatter plot of residuals), and linear regression was used to determine the change in calf MVC and bilateral leg MVIF from 0 day and every 35 days throughout the 520-

day isolation. Paired *t* tests were also completed between MVC/MVIF at 0 and 520 days, and 35 and 520 days to determine whether isolation significantly reduced strength. To determine whether starting strength determined change in strength during isolation, linear regression was completed between starting MVC/MVIF and change in MVC/MVIF throughout the 520-day isolation. All data were analysed using GraphPad Prism (USA) with statistical significance defined as $P < 0.05$ although due to the low *n* number, changes in MVC/MVIF > ± 10% were deemed functionally significant.

Results

Effect of Mars500 upon calf raise MVC and leg press MVIF

Calf raise MVC did not reduce across isolation but rather increased non-significantly (0 vs. 520 days; $P > 0.05$) by 7.6% from 1641 ± 113 N to 1766 ± 82 N. In contrast, there was a bilateral and relatively linear significant loss of strength at both low (0.2 ms^{-1}; $R^2 = 0.53$; $P = 0.001$) and high velocity (0.4 ms^{-1}; $R^2 = 0.42$; $P = 0.007$) isokinetic leg presses across 520 days (Fig. 1a). The change in strength at 0.2 and 0.4 ms^{-1} did not reach statistical significance using a pre- vs. post-*t* test (0 vs. 520 days; $P > 0.05$). However, 0 day is not representative of normal strength, for example, due to detraining pre-spaceflight that occurs during the quarantine period, hence the significant increase in strength at 35 days (Fig. 1c, d). A *t* test between 35 and 520 days did confirm a significant reduction in strength across time at 0.2 ms^{-1} ($P = 0.001$) and 0.4 ms^{-1} ($P = 0.02$).

Relationship between pre-isolation MVC and changes induced by Mars500

Pre-isolation calf MVC was significantly negatively correlated ($R^2 = 0.684$; $P = 0.042$) with change in MVC across the 520 days (Fig. 2), although this includes four subjects whom increased calf MVC. In contrast, reductions in MVC at 0.2 ms^{-1} ($R^2 = 0.237$; $P = 0.327$) and 0.4 ms^{-1} ($R^2 = 0.061$; $P = 0.637$) did not correlate with pre-isolation values.

Intervention efficacy in ameliorating Mars500-induced loss of calf MVC

There was no significant reduction in calf MVC across the 520 days ($R^2 = 0.04$; $P = 0.46$), although there were moderate increases observed (with respect to 0 day) following 70 days use of expanders (2.2 ± 1.7%) and MDS (17.8 ± 10.6) (Fig. 2). Moreover, a 12.7% increase was observed during 35 days of no exercise intervention (Fig. 2). Seventy days of active running (− 7.1 ± 5.5%), passive running (− 2.4 ± 3.7), cycle ergometry (− 3.0 ± 5.2%), and WBV (− 1.5 ± 6.0%) failed to protect against loss of MVC during the 70-day exercise intervention.

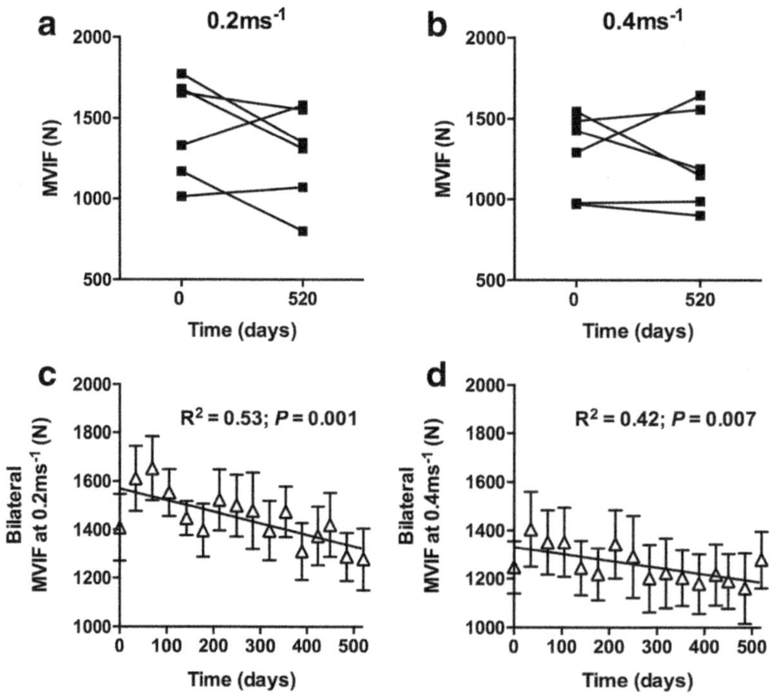

Fig. 1 Mean (±SEM) bilateral leg press maximal voluntary isokinetic force (MVIF) at 0.2 and 0.4 ms^{-1} reduced with time during Mars500. Bilateral MVIF was measured every 35 ± 3.6 days in each subject during the 520-day isolation period at 0.2 and 0.4 ms^{-1} contraction rates. Individual (**a**, **b**) and mean (±SEM) (**c**, **d**) MVIF forces at 0.2 and 0.4 ms^{-1} are shown respectively

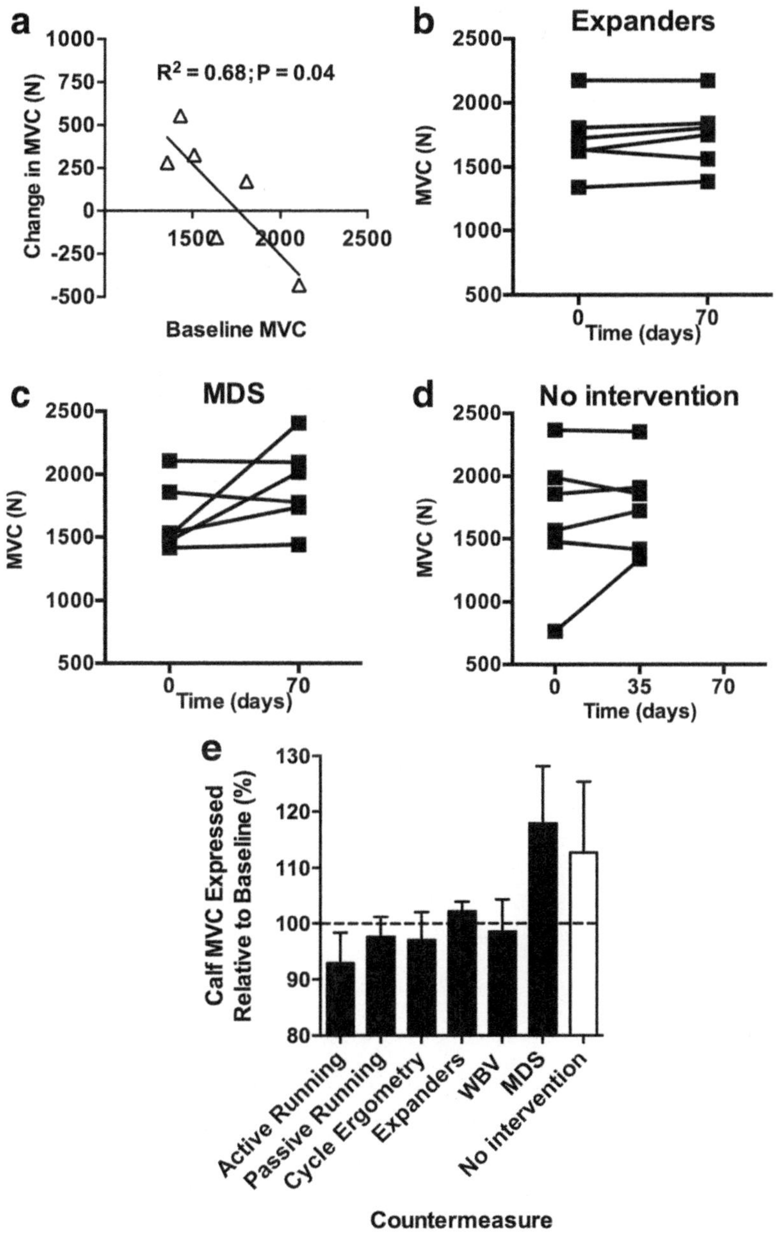

Fig. 2 a Change in calf MVC across Mars500 was significantly associated with starting calf MVC. Calf MVC was measured every 35 ± 3.6 days in each subject during the 520-day isolation period. **b**, **c** Individual changes in MVC where the intervention on average protected against loss of strength and **d** where no exercise intervention was completed. **e** Mean (±SEM) calf MVC was increased relative to baseline (day 0) following candidate 70-day exercise interventions

Intervention efficacy in ameliorating Mars500-induced loss of leg press MVIF

The 35-day time point of no exercise intervention was associated with a 4.0 ± 4.1% loss of MVIF at 0.2 ms^{-1} (Fig. 3). At 0.2 ms^{-1}, active running, passive running, and cycle ergometry all failed to protect against loss of MVIF (Fig. 3). Expanders (8.0 ± 5.5%), WBV (3.7 ± 3.1%), and MDS (4.9 ± 10.0%) protected against loss of strength and increased strength (albeit < 10%) vs. before the 70-day exercise intervention. The 35-day time point of no exercise intervention was associated with a 1.1 ± 5.0% loss of MVIF (Fig. 4). At 0.4 ms^{-1}, MVIF was not protected by active running or expanders. WBV (8.8 ± 5.4%) and MDS (5.2 ± 7.0%) were the most effective interventions at 0.4 ms^{-1} (Fig. 4).

Discussion

The main findings of this study were that the 520-day Mars500 isolation mission did not induce loss of calf MVC. In contrast, significant reductions in bilateral

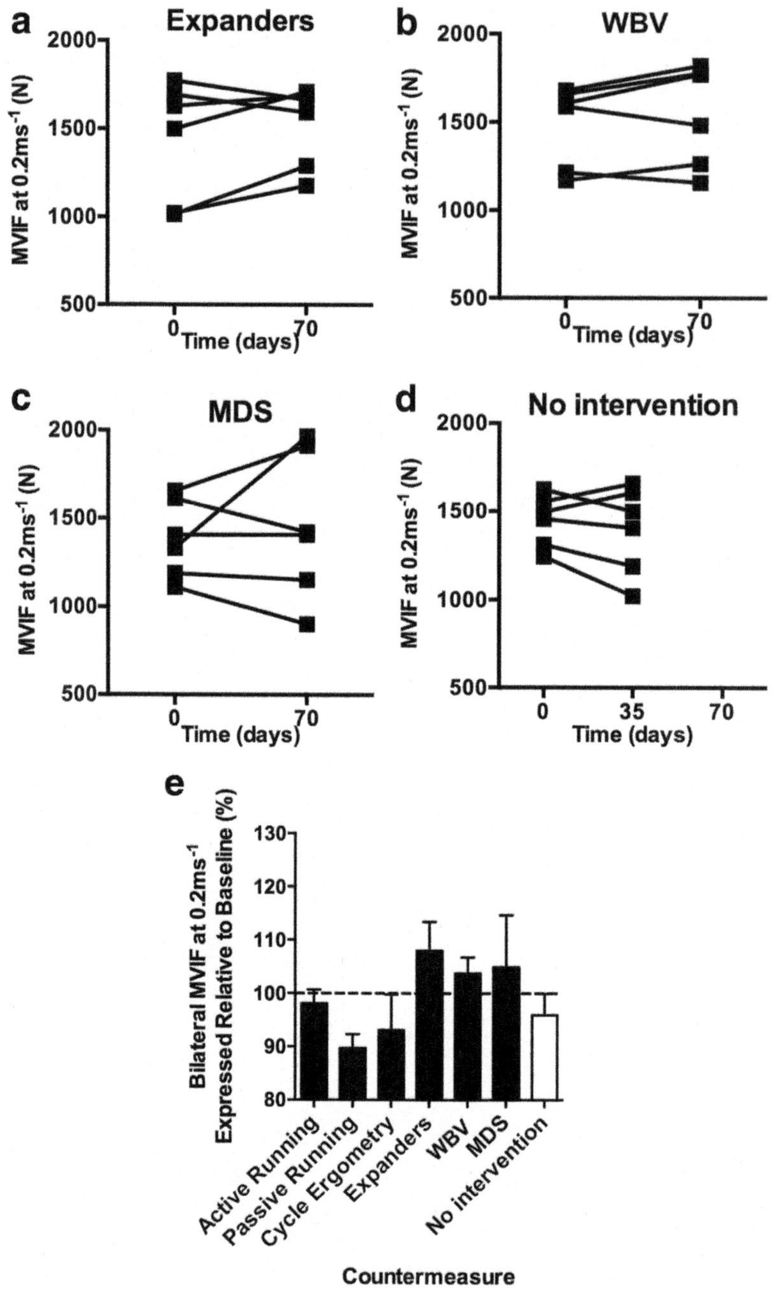

Fig. 3 a–c Individual data from exercise interventions that on average protected against loss of strength at 0.2 ms^{-1} and **d** where no exercise intervention was completed. **e** Mean (±SEM) bilateral leg MVIF at 0.2 ms^{-1} change following candidate 70-day exercise interventions

MVIF at both 0.2 and 0.4 ms^{-1} were observed that were not related to pre-isolation MVIF. At 0.2 ms^{-1}, expanders were the most effective intervention, inducing increased MVIF along with WBV and MDS. WBV and MDS were also the most effective interventions to prevent loss of MVIF at 0.4 ms^{-1}.

Significant reductions in MVIF were observed at 0.2 and 0.4 ms^{-1} across Mars500 that were not evident for calf MVC. This contrasts with calf MVC reductions being frequently associated with long-term spaceflight [11, 13]. Indeed, during 35 days of no intervention, calf MVC actually increased (+ 12.7%). Mars500, however, involved postural loading unlike microgravity, which perhaps provided sufficient stimulus to prevent loss of strength, although interpretation of data from so few subjects is challenging.

Preferential type I muscle fibre atrophy is associated with microgravity and disuse [38]. Data from this study show that strength was lost in the quadriceps/hamstrings but not the calf muscles. The calf contains

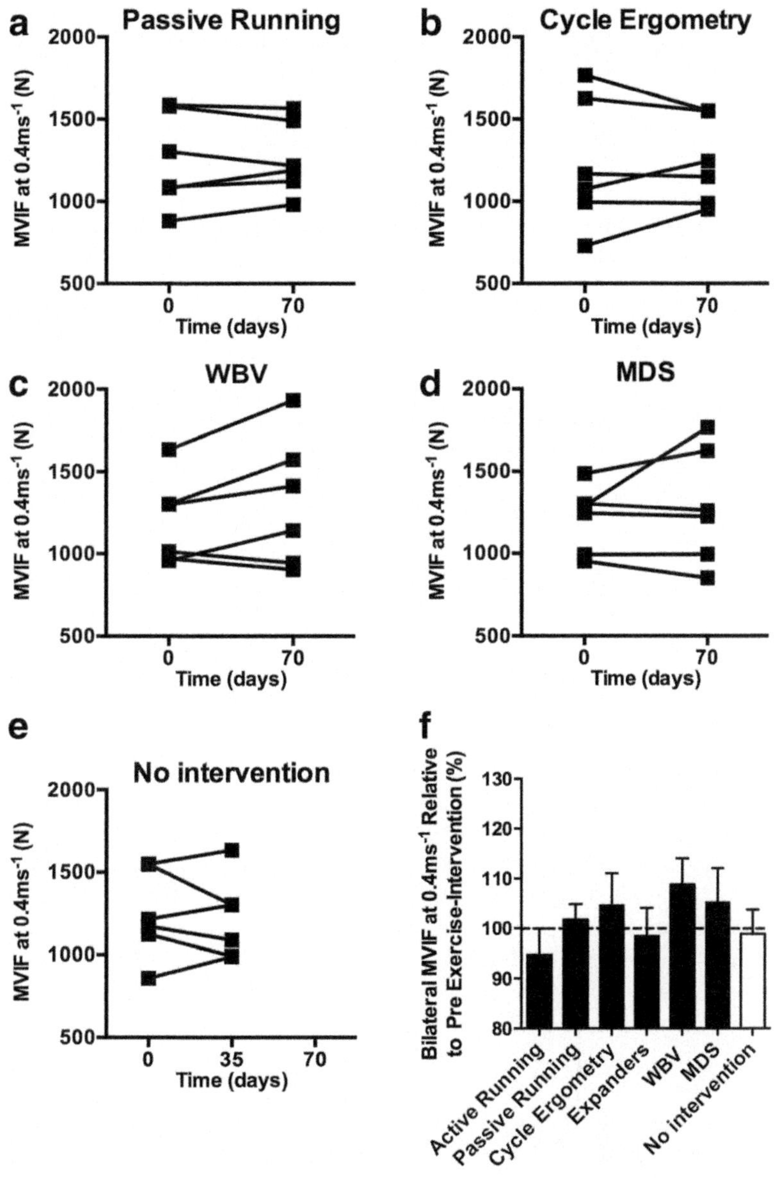

Fig. 4 **a**–**d** Individual data from exercise interventions that on average protected against loss of strength at 0.4 ms^{-1} and **e** where no exercise intervention was completed. **f** Mean (±SEM) bilateral leg MVIF at 0.4 ms^{-1} change following candidate 70-day exercise interventions

a high proportion of type I fibres and the vastus lateralis (quadriceps) and biceps femoris (hamstrings) contain a higher proportion of type II fibres [19–22]. Furthermore, determination of MVIF using MDS is a high-fidelity assessment of type II muscle fibres [36]. Collectively, the preservation of MVC in the calf and the loss of MVIF across the 520 days in the quadriceps/hamstrings suggest loss of strength in type II but not type I muscle fibres.

If the magnitude of losses observed during Mars500 is representative of strength losses on the Martian surface, they could have a significant negative impact upon mission success. Whilst not assessed in this study, on Earth, leg strength is positively correlated with walking speed [39], mobility [40], and reduced lower muscle strength; in particular, the calf is associated with increased falls [41] and subsequent hip fracture risk [42]. Thus, mechanistic understanding to inform effective interventions are required for Earth and exploration missions such as to Mars [1, 12].

Such strength losses, observed despite periodic intervention performance comparable to those employed on-board the ISS, suggests that the effect of isolation is substantial and warrants further investigation to determine the role of isolation itself [8], nutrition [7], and operational stress [9].

Nevertheless, the loss of MVIF in otherwise healthy individuals suggests that Mars500 was a valid isolation model comparable to other spaceflight analogues [7] and may have implications for long-term spaceflight recommendations that previously focused on microgravity as the cause of muscle atrophy [43]. Prolonged confinement may reduce exercise motivation [8] over time, which could be exaggerated as a crew reduces contact with mission control and the apparent 'need' to exercise in microgravity is unclear. Indeed, substantial negative changes in body composition, cardiovascular de-conditioning, bone, and strength losses have been observed in submarine and Antarctic overwinter crews [44]. The Mars500 participants were provided with an artificial light-dark cycle comparable to the ISS which itself can reduce vitamin D levels [45], which is associated with lower isometric leg strength [46].

Interestingly, the loss of leg press MVIF was not related to initial MVIF. One subject lost 369 N (– 22%) in strength vs. 0 day, and this loss of strength was equivalent to ageing from the second to seventh decade of life [6]. However, given the low *n* number and the potential differential sensitivity to isolation vs. unloading in a given individual, further investigation is warranted to determine whether pre-mission physical training is advantageous for long-term space missions [10]. Indeed, further studies should also examine the relationship between the familiarity with exercise pre-isolation/spaceflight and the individual response to particular exercises during isolation/spaceflight.

The failure to observe a significant reduction in calf MVC over the 520-day mission may relate to the subjects' ability to ambulate and weight-bear but could also reflect, at least in part, effective engagement in exercise interventions. As a result, whilst potentially ethically challenging, a control group that do not participate in any exercise throughout the 520 days is warranted to enable further comparison with bed rest studies [47], although not spaceflight studies. It must also be noted that calf strength was determined isometrically and quadriceps/hamstring strength isokinetically. Not determining strength in an identical mode is a study limitation and perhaps contributes to the differences observed in different muscle groups.

During Mars500, a range of current and candidate exercise interventions for an exploration class mission were employed for 70-day periods at training volumes considered in excess of those required to have a positive effect. This appears the case as moderate increments in calf MVC were noted following use of expanders and MDS. MDS [48] produced the greatest protection against loss of lower-limb strength but whether its employment is warranted in addition to, or instead of running [49] or cycling [23], currently key components of the astronaut health maintenance system needs to be tested.

In contrast, 70 days active running, passive running, and cycle ergometry failed to protect against Mars500-induced reduction in 0.2 ms^{-1} MVIF. However, the use of expanders, WBV, and MDS were not only protective but induced small increases in MVIF. The better protection afforded by WBV at 0.4 ms^{-1} complements the shift in the velocity-force curve [50] to the right (i.e. faster) [27] previously observed. In fact, all exercise interventions with the exception of active running (– 5.3 ± 5.4%) and expanders (– 1.6 ± 5.8%) were able to protect against loss of strength during the 70-day exercise intervention. Some differences in exercise efficacy were perhaps attributable to total training volume. The more effective exercise interventions such as MDS (3–4 days/week) and WBV (7 days/week) had higher training volumes, whereas the less effective exercises had lower training volumes in some instances (e.g. expanders 3 days/week) but not others (e.g. active running 5–6 days/week). Future isolation and spaceflight studies should match exercise interventions for total energy expenditure to increase comparability and remove this limitation.

Taken together, data from within our unique, but small cohort, provides evidence to support the proposition that the MDS [48] and exercise during WBV [29] are the most promising interventions for maintenance of calf and leg strength [30]. However, neither should be viewed as replacements for resistance exercise (via advanced resistive exercise device (ARED)) [24], currently considered the optimal ISS countermeasure [26]. ARED is impractical for exploration class missions due to its mass and volume, but similar equipment capable of multi-muscle comparison and the determination of optimal training volume should be tested in future studies.

Conclusions

Despite not unloading participants, the Mars500 analogue induced significant loss of MVIF in the legs, which were unrelated to pre-isolation MVIF with little evidence for preferential type I fibre loss. Investigation of the factors that induce such losses is warranted. No significant losses in calf MVC were observed, but this presumably relates to continued weight-bearing activity. MDS and WBV were the most effective candidate interventions in ameliorating strength loses and thus may have virtue in exploration class missions as they are less complex and resource-intensive than ARED, although optimal training volume and adherence remain to be determined.

Acknowledgements

The Russian, European, and Chinese space agencies were involved in the design of the Mars500 study, and data collection was conducted by the staff at the IBMP of the Russian space agency in Moscow, Russia.

Authors' contributions

The Mars500 study was conducted by the staff at the IBMP in Moscow, Russia. EF conceived the experiment, and EF, DB, and KU supported the experiment. CJG, VK, and DAG analysed the data. The paper was written and edited by CJG, EF, and DAG.

Funding

The Mars500 study was funded by the Russian, European, and Chinese space agencies. CJG conducted the data analysis as part of the Space Physiology & Health MSc (King's College London) at the IBMP in Moscow and was funded by King's College London. The funders had no direct role in the interpretation of the data, writing of the manuscript, or decision to publish.

Authors' information

Christopher J. Gaffney is currently a postdoctoral research fellow at the University of Exeter, UK. Elena Fomina, Dennis Babich, Vladimir Kitov, and Konstantin Uskov are researchers at the Institute of Biomedical Problems of the Russian Federal Space Agency, Moscow. David A. Green is a senior lecturer at King's College London and a member of staff at the European Astronaut Centre, Cologne, Germany.

Competing interests

Christopher J. Gaffney, Elena Fomina, Dennis Babich, Vladimir Kitov, Konstantin Uskov, and David A. Green declare that they have no conflict of interest.

Author details

[1]Institute of Biomedical Problems (IBMP), Moscow, Russia. [2]Centre of Human & Aerospace Physiological Sciences (CHAPS), King's College London, Faculty of Life Sciences & Medicine, Guy's Campus, London SE1 1UL, UK. [3]KBRwyle, European Astronaut Centre, Linder Höhe, D-51147 Cologne, Germany.

References

1. Basner M, Dinges DF, Mollicone D, Ecker A, Jones CW, Hyder EC, et al. Mars 520-d mission simulation reveals protracted crew hypokinesis and alterations of sleep duration and timing. Proc. Natl. Acad. Sci. U. S. A. [Internet]. National Academy of Sciences; 2013 [cited 2017 Jan 15];110:2635–40. Available from: http://www.ncbi.nlm.nih.gov/pubmed/23297197
2. Grigoriev AI, Kozlovskaya IB, Potapov AN. Goals of biomedical support of a mission to Mars and possible approaches to achieving them. Aviat. Space. Environ. Med. [Internet]. 2002 [cited 2016 Feb 21];73:379–84. Available from: http://www.ncbi.nlm.nih.gov/pubmed/11952060
3. Dorais GA. An artificial-gravity space-settlement ground-analogue design concept. AIAA Sp. 2016 [Internet]. Reston, Virginia: American Institute of Aeronautics and Astronautics; 2016 [cited 2017 Jan 13]. Available from: http://arc.aiaa.org/doi/10.2514/6.2016-5388
4. Carpenter R, Lang T, Bloomfield S. Effects of long-duration spaceflight, microgravity, and radiation on the neuromuscular, sensorimotor, and skeletal systems. J. [Internet]. 2010 [cited 2017 Jan 15]; Available from: http://journalofcosmology.com/Mars147.html
5. Berger MJ, Doherty TJ. Sarcopenia: prevalence, mechanisms, and functional consequences. Interdiscip. Top. Gerontol. [Internet]. 2010 [cited 2016 Feb 20]; 37:94–114. Available from: http://www.ncbi.nlm.nih.gov/pubmed/20703058
6. Frontera WR, Hughes VA, Fielding RA, Fiatarone MA, Evans WJ, Roubenoff R. Aging of skeletal muscle: a 12-yr longitudinal study. J. Appl. Physiol. [Internet]. 2000 [cited 2015 Dec 21];88:1321–6. Available from: http://www.ncbi.nlm.nih.gov/pubmed/10749826
7. Nguyen A, Medee B, Guegan C, Remy-Neris O, Verret C. Aerobic performance and isokinetic assessement of submariners before and after patrol [Internet]. Elsevier Masson; 2013 [cited 2016 Feb 21]. Available from: http://www.em-consulte.com/en/article/833472
8. Convertino VA, Bloomfield SA, Greenleaf JE. An overview of the issues: physiological effects of bed rest and restricted physical activity. Med. Sci. Sports Exerc. [Internet]. 1997 [cited 2016 Feb 21];29:187–90. Available from: http://www.ncbi.nlm.nih.gov/pubmed/9044221
9. Henning PC, Park B-S, Kim J-S. Physiological decrements during sustained military operational stress. Mil. Med. [Internet]. 2011 [cited 2016 Feb 21];176: 991–7. Available from: http://www.ncbi.nlm.nih.gov/pubmed/21987955
10. Ploutz-Snyder L. Prevention of muscle atrophy with exercise countermeasures. ntrs.nasa.gov [Internet]. 2015 [cited 2016 Mar 12]; Available from: http://www.ntrs.nasa.gov/archive/nasa/casi.ntrs.nasa.gov/20090007465_2009005538.pdf
11. Trappe S, Costill D, Gallagher P, Creer A, Peters JR, Evans H, et al. Exercise in space: human skeletal muscle after 6 months aboard the International Space Station. J. Appl. Physiol. [Internet]. 2009 [cited 2016 Feb 21];106:1159–68. Available from: http://jap.physiology.org/content/106/4/1159
12. Kozlovskaya IB, Yarmanova EN, Yegorov AD, Stepantsov VI, Fomina EV, Tomilovaskaya ES. Russian countermeasure systems for adverse effects of microgravity on long-duration ISS flights. Aerosp. Med. Hum. Perform. [Internet]. 2015 [cited 2017 Jan 14];86:24–31. Available from: http://www.ingentaconnect.com/content/asma/amhp/2015/00000086/A00112s1/art00006
13. Fitts RH, Trappe SW, Costill DL, Gallagher PM, Creer AC, Colloton PA, et al. Prolonged space flight-induced alterations in the structure and function of human skeletal muscle fibres. J. Physiol. [Internet]. 2010 [cited 2016 Feb 22]; 588:3567–92. Available from: http://www.pubmedcentral.nih.gov/articlerender.fcgi?artid=2988519&tool=pmcentrez&rendertype=abstract
14. Fitts RH, Trappe SW, Costill DL, Gallagher PM, Creer AC, Colloton PA, et al. Prolonged space flight-induced alterations in the structure and function of human skeletal muscle fibres. J. Physiol. [Internet]. 2010 [cited 2016 Aug 8];588: 3567–92. Available from: http://www.ncbi.nlm.nih.gov/pubmed/20660569
15. Convertino VA. Physiological adaptations to weightlessness: effects on exercise and work performance. Exerc. Sport Sci. Rev. [Internet]. 1990 [cited 2016 Feb 21];18:119–66. Available from: http://www.ncbi.nlm.nih.gov/pubmed/2192891
16. Nishimune H, Stanford JA, Mori Y. ROLE of exercise in maintaining the integrity of the neuromuscular junction. Muscle Nerve [Internet]. 2014 [cited 2017 Jan 14];49:315–24. Available from: http://doi.wiley.com/10.1002/mus.24095
17. Yamada M, Nishiguchi S, Fukutani N, Aoyama T, Arai H. Mail-based intervention for sarcopenia prevention increased anabolic hormone and skeletal muscle mass in community-dwelling Japanese older adults: the INE (intervention by nutrition and exercise) study. J Am Med Dir Assoc. 2015;16:654–60.
18. Thorstensson A, Grimby G, Karlsson J. Force-velocity relations and fiber composition in human knee extensor muscles. J. Appl. Physiol. [Internet]. 1976 [cited 2016 Mar 14];40:12–6. Available from: http://www.ncbi.nlm.nih.gov/pubmed/1248977
19. Edgerton VR, Smith JL, Simpson DR. Muscle fibre type populations of human leg muscles. Histochem. J. [Internet]. Kluwer Academic Publishers; 1975 [cited 2016 Oct 7];7:259–66. Available from: http://link.springer.com/10.1007/BF01003594
20. Staron RS, Hagerman FC, Hikida RS, Murray TF, Hostler DP, Crill MT, et al. Fiber type composition of the vastus lateralis muscle of young men and women. J. Histochem. Cytochem. [Internet]. 2000 [cited 2016 Dec 24];48: 623–9. Available from: http://www.ncbi.nlm.nih.gov/pubmed/10769046
21. Gollnick PD, Sjödin B, Karlsson J, Jansson E, Saltin B. Human soleus muscle: A comparison of fiber composition and enzyme activities with other leg muscles. Pflugers Arch. Eur. J. Physiol. [Internet]. Springer-Verlag; 1974 [cited 2016 Dec 24];348:247–55. Available from: http://link.springer.com/10.1007/BF00587415
22. Evangelidis PE, Massey GJ, Ferguson RA, Wheeler PC, Pain MTG, Folland JP. The functional significance of hamstrings composition: is it really a "fast" muscle group? Scand. J. Med. Sci. Sports [Internet]. 2016 [cited 2017 Apr 13]; Available from: http://doi.wiley.com/10.1111/sms.12786
23. Gopalakrishnan R, Genc KO, Rice AJ, Lee SMC, Evans HJ, Maender CC, et al. Muscle volume, strength, endurance, and exercise loads during 6-month missions in space. Aviat. Space. Environ. Med. [Internet]. 2010 [cited 2016 Jan 18];81:91–102. Available from: http://www.ncbi.nlm.nih.gov/pubmed/20131648
24. Miokovic T, Armbrecht G, Felsenberg D, Belavý DL. Differential atrophy of the postero-lateral hip musculature during prolonged bedrest and the influence of exercise countermeasures. J Appl Physiol. 2011;110
25. English KL, Paddon-Jones D. Protecting muscle mass and function in older adults during bed rest. Curr. Opin. Clin. Nutr. Metab. Care [Internet]. NIH Public Access; 2010 [cited 2017 Jan 14];13:34–9. Available from: http://www.ncbi.nlm.nih.gov/pubmed/19898232
26. Loehr JA, Lee SMC, English KL, Sibonga J, Smith SM, Spiering BA, et al. Musculoskeletal adaptations to training with the advanced resistive exercise

device. Med. Sci. Sport. Exerc. [Internet]. 2011 [cited 2015 Oct 21];43:146–56. Available from: http://www.ncbi.nlm.nih.gov/pubmed/20473227
27. Bosco C, Colli R, Introini E, Cardinale M, Iacovelli' M, Tihanyi J, et al. Adaptive responses of human skeletal muscle to vibration exposure. Clin Physiol. 1999;19:183–7.
28. Rittweger J. Vibration as an exercise modality: how it may work, and what its potential might be. Eur. J. Appl. Physiol. [Internet]. 2010 [cited 2016 Oct 7];108: 877–904. Available from: http://www.ncbi.nlm.nih.gov/pubmed/20012646
29. Armbrecht G, Belavý D, Gast U. Resistive vibration exercise attenuates bone and muscle atrophy in 56 days of bed rest: biochemical markers of bone metabolism. Osteoporos. … [Internet]. 2010 [cited 2016 Mar 12]; Available from: http://link.springer.com/article/10.1007/s00198-009-0985-z
30. Schneider SM, Amonette WE, Blazine K, Bentley J, Lee SMC, Loehr JA, et al. Training with the International Space Station interim resistive exercise device. Med. Sci. Sports Exerc. [Internet]. 2003 [cited 2016 Mar 3];35:1935–45. Available from: http://europepmc.org/abstract/med/14600562
31. Schiele BC, Baker AB, Hathaway SR. The Minnesota multiphasic personality inventory. Lancet. 1943;63:292–7.
32. Schneider S, Abeln V, Popova J, Fomina E, Jacubowski A, Meeusen R, et al. The influence of exercise on prefrontal cortex activity and cognitive performance during a simulated space flight to Mars (MARS500). Behav. Brain Res. [Internet]. 2013 [cited 2016 Feb 21];236:1–7. Available from: http://www.ncbi.nlm.nih.gov/pubmed/22944515
33. Meigal A, Fomina E. Electromyographic evaluation of countermeasures during the terrestrial simulation of interplanetary spaceflight in Mars500 project. Pathophysiology [Internet]. 2016 [cited 2017 Feb 27];23:11–8. Available from: http://linkinghub.elsevier.com/retrieve/pii/S0928468015300146
34. Trappe SW, Trappe TA, Lee GA, Costill DL. Calf muscle strength in humans. Int J Sport Med. 2001;22:186–91.
35. Nunn KD, Mayhew JL. Comparison of three methods of assessing strength imbalances at the knee. J Orthop Sport Phys Ther. 1988;10:134–7.
36. Back C, Oliveira P, Mattiello-Rosa S, Sobreira C, Martinez E, Mattiello-Sverzut A. Correlation between the proportion of fast fibers in the biceps brachii muscle and the relative torque during elbow flexion in subjects with clinical hypothesis of myopathy. Brazilian J. Phys. Ther. [Internet]. Brazilian Journal of Physical Therapy; 2008 [cited 2017 Jan 15];12:107–12. Available from: http://www.scielo.br/scielo.php?script=sci_arttext&pid=S1413-35552008000200006&lng=pt&nrm=iso&tlng=pt
37. Shackelford LC. Musculoskeletal response to space flight. In: Barratt MR, Pool SL, editors. Princ. Clin. Med. Sp. flight. Springer US; 2008. p. 293–306.
38. Ciciliot S, Rossi AC, Dyar KA, Blaauw B, Schiaffino S. Muscle type and fiber type specificity in muscle wasting. Int J Biochem Cell Biol. 2013;45:2191–9.
39. Hayashida I, Tanimoto Y, Takahashi Y, Kusabiraki T, Tamaki J, Lindle R, et al. Correlation between muscle strength and muscle mass, and their association with walking speed, in community-dwelling elderly Japanese individuals. Macaluso A, editor. PLoS One [Internet]. Public Library of Science; 2014 [cited 2017 Jan 14];9:e111810. Available from: http://dx.plos.org/10.1371/journal.pone.0111810
40. Reid KF, Pasha E, Doros G, Clark DJ, Patten C, Phillips EM, et al. Longitudinal decline of lower extremity muscle power in healthy and mobility-limited older adults: influence of muscle mass, strength, composition, neuromuscular activation and single fiber contractile properties. Eur. J. Appl. Physiol. [Internet]. Springer Berlin Heidelberg; 2014 [cited 2017 Jan 14];114: 29–39. Available from: http://link.springer.com/10.1007/s00421-013-2728-2
41. Balogun S, Winzenberg T, Wills K, Scott D. Prospective associations of low muscle mass and function with 10-year falls risk, incident fracture and mortality in community-dwelling older adults. J. Nutr. [Internet]. 2016 [cited 2017 Jan 14]; Available from: http://link.springer.com/article/10.1007/s12603-016-0843-6
42. Choi WJ, Cripton PA, Robinovitch SN. Effects of hip abductor muscle forces and knee boundary conditions on femoral neck stresses during simulated falls. Osteoporos. Int. [Internet]. Springer London; 2015 [cited 2017 Jan 14];26:291–301. Available from: http://link.springer.com/10.1007/s00198-014-2812-4
43. Loehr JA, Guilliams ME, Petersen N, Hirsch N, Kawashima S, Ohshima H. Physical training for long-duration spaceflight. Aerosp. Med. Hum. Perform. [Internet]. 2015 [cited 2016 Aug 8];86:A14–23. Available from: http://www.ncbi.nlm.nih.gov/pubmed/26630191
44. Luria T, Matsliah Y, Adir Y, Josephy N, Moran DS, Evans RK, et al. Effects of a prolonged submersion on bone strength and metabolism in young healthy submariners. Calcif. Tissue Int. [Internet]. 2010 [cited 2016 Feb 21];86:8–13. Available from: http://www.ncbi.nlm.nih.gov/pubmed/19882096
45. Smith SM, Heer MA, Shackelford LC, Sibonga JD, Ploutz-Snyder L, Zwart SR. Benefits for bone from resistance exercise and nutrition in long-duration spaceflight: evidence from biochemistry and densitometry. J. Bone Miner. Res. [Internet]. Wiley Subscription Services, Inc., A Wiley Company; 2012 [cited 2017 Jan 14];27:1896–906. Available from: http://doi.wiley.com/10.1002/jbmr.1647
46. Grimaldi AS, Parker BA, Capizzi JA, Clarkson PM, Pescatello LS, White MC, et al. 25(OH) vitamin D is associated with greater muscle strength in healthy men and women. Med. Sci. Sports Exerc. [Internet]. 2013 [cited 2016 Feb 21];45:157–62. Available from: http://www.pubmedcentral.nih.gov/articlerender.fcgi?artid=3544152&tool=pmcentrez&rendertype=abstract
47. Nielsen RO, Schjerling P, Tesch P, Stål P, Langberg H. Collagen content in the vastus lateralis and the soleus muscle following a 90-day bed rest period with or without resistance exercises. Muscles. Ligaments Tendons J. [Internet]. CIC Edizioni Internazionali; 2015 [cited 2017 Jan 14];5:305–9. Available from: http://www.ncbi.nlm.nih.gov/pubmed/26958541
48. Angeli T, Talla R, Fomina E, Barta N, Tschan H, Bachl N, et al. Mars 500: Training and diagnostic with a multifunctional dynamometer for application in space. Life Sp. Life Earth [Internet]. 2013 [cited 2016 Mar 12];706. Available from: http://adsabs.harvard.edu/abs/2013ESASP.706E..14A
49. Lee S, DeWitt J, Smith C, Laughlin M, Loehr, J.A., Norcross, J., & Hagan, R.D. Physiologic responses and biomechanical aspects of motorized and non-motorized treadmill exercise: a ground-based evaluation of treadmills for. Natl. Aeronaut. … [Internet]. 2006 [cited 2016 Mar 14]; Available from: https://www.researchgate.net/profile/Stuart_Lee/publication/315378966_Physiologic_Responses_and_Biomechanical_Aspects_of_Motorized_and_Nonmotorized_Treadmill_Exercise_A_Ground-based_Evaluation_of_Treadmills_for_Use_on_the_International_Space_Station/links/58cdb763a6fdcc5cccbbe798/Physiologic-Responses-and-Biomechanical-Aspects-of-Motorized-and-Nonmotorized-Treadmill-Exercise-A-Ground-based-Evaluation-of-Treadmills-for-Use-on-the-International-Space-Station.pdf
50. Wilkie DR. The relation between force and velocity in human muscle. J. Physiol. [Internet]. 1949 [cited 2016 Feb 21];110:249–80. Available from: http://www.pubmedcentral.nih.gov/articlerender.fcgi?artid=1392741&tool=pmcentrez&rendertype=abstract

Physiological and Biomechanical Responses of Highly Trained Distance Runners to Lower-Body Positive Pressure Treadmill Running

Kyle R. Barnes[1*] and Jessica N. Janecke[2]

Abstract

Background: As a way to train at faster running speeds, add training volume, prevent injury, or rehabilitate after an injury, lower-body positive pressure treadmills (LBPPT) have become increasingly commonplace among athletes. However, there are conflicting evidence and a paucity of data describing the physiological and biomechanical responses to LBPPT running in highly trained or elite caliber runners at the running speeds they habitually train at, which are considerably faster than those of recreational runners. Furthermore, data is lacking regarding female runners' responses to LBPPT running. Therefore, this study was designed to evaluate the physiological and biomechanical responses to LBPPT running in highly trained male and female distance runners.

Methods: Fifteen highly trained distance runners (seven male; eight female) completed a single running test composed of 4 × 9-min interval series at fixed percentages of body weight ranging from 0 to 30% body weight support (BWS) in 10% increments on LBPPT. The first interval was always conducted at 0% BWS; thereafter, intervals at 10, 20, and 30% BWS were conducted in random order. Each interval consisted of three stages of 3 min each, at velocities of 14.5, 16.1, and 17.7 $km{\cdot}h^{-1}$ for men and 12.9, 14.5, and 16.1 $km{\cdot}h^{-1}$ for women. Expired gases, ventilation, breathing frequency, heart rate (HR), rating of perceived exertion (RPE), and stride characteristics were measured during each running speed and BWS.

Results: Male and female runners had similar physiological and biomechanical responses to running on LBPPT. Increasing BWS increased stride length ($p < 0.02$) and flight duration ($p < 0.01$) and decreased stride rate ($p < 0.01$) and contact time ($p < 0.01$) in small-large magnitudes. There was a large attenuation of oxygen consumption (VO_2) relative to BWS ($p < 0.001$), while there were trivial-moderate reductions in respiratory exchange ratio, minute ventilation, and respiratory frequency ($p > 0.05$), and small-large effects on HR and RPE ($p < 0.01$). There were trivial-small differences in V_E, respiratory frequency, HR, and RPE for a given VO_2 across various BWS ($p > 0.05$).

Conclusions: The results indicate the male and female distance runners have similar physiological and biomechanical responses to LBPPT running. Overall, the biomechanical changes during LBPPT running all contributed to less metabolic cost and corresponding physiological changes.

Keywords: AlterG, Lower-body positive pressure, Body weight support, Anti-gravity, Running, Stride characteristics, Physiological characteristics, Metabolic demand, Oxygen demand, Oxygen cost

* Correspondence: barnesk@gvsu.edu
[1]Department of Movement Science, Grand Valley State University, 1 Campus Drive, Allendale, MI 49401, USA
Full list of author information is available at the end of the article

Key Points

- Well-trained male and female distance runners have similar physiological and biomechanical responses while running with body weight support on a lower-body positive pressure treadmill.
- When considering the global unweighing effects on stride parameters during running, its major influence was the large increase in flight time, which contrasted the disproportional decrease in contact time resulting in overall longer stride length and reduction in stride rate.
- There was a disproportionate decrease in oxygen consumption relative to body weight support which led to an attenuation of heart rate and rating of perceived exertion and, to a lesser degree, respiratory exchange ratio, minute ventilation, and respiratory frequency between each level of body weight support and running speed.

Background

Body weight support and running velocity both affect the physiological and biomechanical responses of human running [1]. Previous studies show that when running at normal body weight, metabolic demand increases with velocity [2, 3]. The greater metabolic demand of faster running speeds has been attributed to increases in stride frequency, increases in mechanical power, and generation of greater ground reaction forces over shorter periods of ground contact [2, 4, 5]. Coaches and athletes have used the increased metabolic demand associated with faster running velocities as a means of enhancing aerobic capacity and running performance [6, 7]. However, running at fast velocities cannot be sustained over extended durations and greatly increases the risk of overuse and orthopedic injury [8]. Thus, as a way to train at faster running speeds, to add training volume, or when people may not be able to run safely at their full body weight after orthopedic injury and/or surgery, lower-body positive pressure treadmills (LBPPT), such as the AlterG Anti-Gravity Treadmill® (AlterG, Inc., Menlo Park, CA) (Fig. 1) that supports the user's body weight, have become increasingly commonplace among highly trained athletes [9, 10].

Originally, LBPPT were designed to simulate the musculoskeletal and cardiovascular deconditioning experienced by astronauts during prolonged exposure to microgravity environment [11]. The commercially available LBPPT now have a simple interface that allows the user to select a desired percentage of body weight at which to run. The device then uses small increases in air pressure around the user's lower body to create a lifting force near the subject's mass center in order to reduce body weight (Fig. 1) [12]. Compared to the other rehabilitation training options that simulate unloaded running such as harness systems and underwater immersion [13–15], LBPPT are more comfortable and therefore allow for extended usage time. Additionally, LBPPT have relatively less impedance compared to other options, thus simulating normal overground running kinematics and gait patterns [10]. LBPPT also allow for running velocities that exceed the capabilities of even the best distance runners in the world [10, 16], therefore making it an effective training and rehabilitation tool for highly trained and elite athletes. Furthermore, providing body weight support (BWS) allows for attenuation of the biomechanical risks of running so that movements can safely be repeated and improved, potentially allowing athletes to increase training volume or return to running sooner following injury or surgery. However, athletes using LBPPT may experience a cardiovascular fitness decline because of the task's decreased aerobic demands without modifying the treadmill velocity at which they run [9, 10, 12, 16–24].

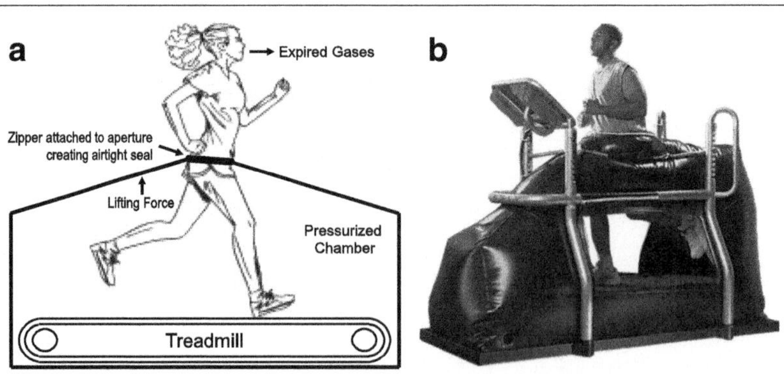

Fig. 1 **a** Schematic depictions of the lower-body positive pressure treadmill (AlterG Anti-Gravity Treadmill® P200) used during testing. **b** AlterG Anti-Gravity Treadmill® P200. The lower-body positive pressure treadmill uses an enclosed treadmill body weight support system that makes use of the ability to increase air pressure around the user's lower body to create a lifting force near the person's center of mass. The pressurized chamber contains an aperture surrounding the subject's waist. Each subject wore a pair of flexible neoprene shorts that included a kayak-style spray skirt and a zipper attached to the aperture allowing for an airtight seal around the waist. Expired gases were continuously collected and measured using a metabolic cart, and biomechanical measures were assessed using high-speed video analysis

Previous research has shown that equivalent maximal and submaximal oxygen consumption (VO_2) can be achieved while running on LBPPT by increasing the running speed to offset the reduction in oxygen consumption associated with running with BWS [12, 20, 22, 25]. When observed VO_2 values were compared with predicted values [9, 23, 24], the coefficient of determination (R^2 = 0.69–0.88) was large to very large, indicating the derived equation in their samples was a good fit and it is feasible to derive similar equations in highly trained populations [1]. All studies that showed reduction in VO_2 also showed corresponding reductions in heart rate (HR) [9, 12, 18, 22–24, 26, 27]. McNeil et al. [9] also reported decreased respiratory exchange ratio (RER). Raffalt et al. [12] reported decreased minute ventilation (V_E) during unweighted submaximal running, despite unchanged respiratory rate, whereas Gojanovic et al. [22] reported no change in V_E. Both Ruckstuhl et al. [18, 27] and McNeil et al. [9] reported decreased rating of perceived exertion (RPE) with unweighted submaximal running, whereas Sainton et al. [26] reported no changes in RPE and Gojanovic et al. [22] reported an increase in RPE during unweighted maximal running. However, rather than comparing changes in RPE across unweighted levels, Hoffman and Donaghe [23] showed that RPE and HR remained the same for a given VO_2 across various body weight settings. Studies have also found a decrease [22] and no change [12] in blood lactate concentration during unweighted maximal running.

Results are also conflicting regarding stride characteristics while running on LBPPT [10, 12, 22, 26, 28, 29]. Several studies have reported stride rate decreased with unweighting [10, 12, 26, 29], whereas Gojanovic et al. [22] found stride rate increased in males and remained unchanged in females at different absolute velocities. Grabowski and Kram [10] reported an increase in contact time, whereas Raffalt et al. [12] and Neal et al. [29] reported decreased contact time, and Sainton et al. [26] reported no change in contact time. However, studies are in agreement that stride length and flight time increase with unweighting [12, 13, 22, 28, 29]. Sometimes, runners may do a portion of their run on LBPPT and the remainder overground. In studies examining the effects of reloading at 100% body weight after previous unweighting, stride rate decreased in one study [26], whereas it was unchanged in another [10]. Grabowski and Kram [10] found contact time increased, and Sainton et al. [26] found flight time increased following unweighted running, which partially explains the anecdotal heavy-feeling athlete's experience after prolonged periods on LBPPT.

Unfortunately, while these studies provide valuable insight into the physiological and biomechanical demands of running on LBPPT among healthy and recreational runners, there are conflicting evidence and a paucity of data indicating how these results might apply to highly trained or elite caliber runners at the running speeds they habitually train at, which are considerably faster than those of recreational runners [9]. Of the ten studies that met the inclusion criteria for evaluation of physiologic and stride characteristic parameters in a recent systematic review [1], only two studies included highly trained or elite caliber distance runners [9, 12], neither of which included female runners. Previous research has established that differences in physiological and biomechanical characteristics exist between highly trained male and female runners during submaximal normal body weight running [3, 30]. However, data is limited regarding female athlete's physiological and biomechanical responses to LBPPT running. Lastly, a comprehensive examination of physiological and biomechanical responses to LBPPT running in the same population is lacking. Therefore, this study was designed to evaluate the physiological and stride characteristic responses to LBPPT running in highly trained male and female distance runners.

Methods

Subjects

Fifteen highly trained distance runners (seven male; eight female) participated in this study (Table 1). Not all subjects met the criteria to be classified as "elite" according to Barnes and Kilding [2]; therefore, subjects in the present study were considered "highly trained." Inclusion criteria were to have 1-mile personal best under 4 min and 10 s or 5 min, 5-km personal best under 14 min and 30 s or 17 min, or 10-km personal best under 30 or 35 min for men and women, respectively. Eight of the subjects (four male; four female) were heel strikers, and seven were mid-forefoot strikers. Foot strike was verified by high-speed video analysis. All subjects had prior experience running on LBPPT and refrained from any activities they were unaccustomed to in the 3 days prior to testing. The study was approved by the Grand Valley State University Human Research Review Committee (Reference No. 14–176-H) and performed in accordance with the

Table 1 Subject and training characteristics

	N	Age (years)	Body mass (kg)	Height (m)	Training history (years)	Training volume (km·wk^{-1})	IAAF score[a]
Male	7	22.1 ± 0.9	68.4 ± 2.2	1.67 ± 0.07	8.1 ± 1.2	135 ± 21	943 ± 46
Female	8	21.4 ± 2.1	54.3 ± 5.0	1.79 ± 0.03	7.3 ± 2.1	84 ± 19	996 ± 60

Data are mean ± SD

[a]International Association of Athletics Federations (IAAF) 2015 scoring tables [37]

standards of ethics outlined in the Declaration of Helsinki. All participants provided informed written consent to participate.

Experimental Testing

The subjects completed a single running test composed of 4 × 9-min interval series at fixed percentages of body weight ranging from 0 to 30% BWS in 10% increments on the AlterG Anti-Gravity P200 Treadmill® (AlterG®, Inc., Fremont, CA) (Fig. 1) set at a 1.0% gradient [31]. Prior to experimental testing, subjects performed a 5-min warmup on the LBPPT (0% BWS) at their own self-selected pace, but below that of the first experimental testing velocity. The first interval was always conducted at 0% BWS; thereafter, intervals at 10, 20, and 30% BWS were conducted in random order. Each interval consisted of three stages of 3 min each (9 min total), at velocities of 14.5, 16.1, and 17.7 $km{\cdot}h^{-1}$ (4.03, 4.47, and 4.92 $m{\cdot}s^{-1}$, respectively) for men and 12.9, 14.5, and 16.1 $km{\cdot}h^{-1}$ (3.58, 4.03, and 4.47 $m{\cdot}s^{-1}$, respectively) for women, always progressing from the slowest to fastest pace with 10-min recovery between intervals. The treadmill was calibrated before each testing session. The decision to take measurements with 10 to 30% BWS was based on previous research, indicating the actual amount of support provided by LBPPT is the most accurate between 10 and 40% BWS [32], as well as anecdotal observation that 30% BWS tends to be the maximum amount of support prescribed for athletes during training and rehabilitation. Furthermore, we took a capillary blood lactate samples (Lactate Pro, Arkray, KDK, Japan) from the fingertip at the conclusion of each interval and determined blood lactate concentrations remained below 4 $mmol{\cdot}L^{-1}$ (range 1.9 to 3.4 $mmol{\cdot}L^{-1}$ at the fastest running velocity), indicating the paces were within normal training paces for these athletes.

Throughout the running test, heart rate (Polar RS800sd, Polar Electro, Kempele, Finland) and expired gases were continuously collected and measured using a metabolic cart (ParvoMedics TrueOne 2400, Salt Lake City, UT) to determine VO_2, carbon dioxide production (VCO_2), V_E, and RER. RPE was determined during each stage using a standard Borg RPE scale upon completion of each interval [33]. Biomechanical measures (stride rate, stride length, contact time, and flight time) were determined using high-speed video analysis (240 $frames{\cdot}s^{-1}$) while running at each velocity and BWS [30]. The average physiological and biomechanical parameters during the final minute of each running speed and BWS were used for analysis.

Statistical Analyses

Data analyses were performed using SPSS, version 20.0 (SPSS Inc., Chicago, IL), and customized spreadsheets. Means ± standard deviations were calculated for physiological and biomechanical characteristics using the last minute of data collection for each speed and BWS. Comparisons of the differences between genders were made using a spreadsheet for comparing two groups [34]. The effects of BWS on physiological and biomechanical measures were analyzed with a spreadsheet for post-only crossovers [35]. The value at 0% BWS of the dependent variable was included as a covariate to improve precision of the estimate of the effects. Effects were estimated in percent units via log transformation, and uncertainty in the estimate was expressed as 90% confidence limits. The effect size (ES), which represents the magnitude of the difference between the two conditions in terms of SD, was calculated from the log-transformed data by dividing the change in the mean by the average SD of the two conditions. Magnitudes of effects on all measures were evaluated non-clinically: if the confidence interval overlapped thresholds for small positive and negative values, the effect was deemed unclear; all other effects were reported as the magnitude of the observed value and were evaluated probabilistically as described above, except that threshold values for trivial, small, moderate, large, very large, and extremely large effects were < 0.2, 0.2, 0.6, 1.2, 2.0, and 4.0 of the between-subject standard deviation in the control condition [36]. Linear regression analysis performed on the mean values defined the linear relationship (linear equation and Pearson correlation coefficients) between VO_2 and running speed.

Results

Descriptive characteristics of the runners are presented in Table 1. There were trivial differences between men and women in age (p = 0.07), training history (p = 0.23), and personal bests at racing distances between 1 mile and 10 km as represented by IAAF scores [37] (p = 0.82). However, males were moderately taller (p = 0.005), very largely heavier (p < 0.001), and trained at a very large-amount higher volume than females (p = 0.001).

Biomechanical Responses

Biomechanical responses of male and female athletes to BWS across three running velocities are presented in Tables 2 and 3, respectively. Overall, in both men and women, stride rate and contact time decreased with increasing BWS, while stride length and flight duration increased with increasing levels of BWS. There were small-moderate decreases in stride rate (p < 0.01) and moderate-very large decreases in contact time (p < 0.01) with increases in BWS for both men and women. Stride length ($p \le 0.02$) and flight duration (p < 0.01) increased in small-large magnitudes with increasing BWS in both males and females. The largest increases or decreases in biomechanical characteristics tended to occur between 10 and 20% BWS or between 20 and 30% BWS.

Table 2 Biomechanical characteristics of male runners by velocity and different levels of body weight support

	14.5 km·h^{-1} (4.03 m·s^{-1})	Difference between 0% BWS ± 90 CL (ES)[a]	Difference between BWS ± 90 CL (ES)[b]	16.1 km·h^{-1} (4.47 m·s^{-1})	Difference between 0% BWS ± 90 CL (ES)	Difference between BWS ± 90 CL (ES)	17.7 km·h^{-1} (4.92 m·s^{-1})	Difference between 0% BWS ± 90 CL (ES)	Difference between BWS ± 90 CL (ES)
				Stride length (m)					
0% BWS	1.53 ± 0.07			1.66 ± 0.07			1.75 ± 0.06		
10% BWS	1.57 ± 0.06	2.9 ± 2.3 (0.52)		1.70 ± 0.07	2.7 ± 1.2 (0.53)		1.77 ± 0.06	1.0 ± 0.8 (0.23)	
20% BWS	1.66 ± 0.06	8.5 ± 2.7 (1.46)	5.4 ± 0.8 (0.94)	1.74 ± 0.06	4.8 ± 1.1 (0.94)	2.1 ± 0.9 (0.42)	1.81 ± 0.07	3.3 ± 0.4 (0.76)	2.2 ± 0.9 (0.53)
30% BWS	1.70 ± 0.09	11.1 ± 2.0 (1.89)	2.4 ± 2.1 (0.43)	1.80 ± 0.09	8.5 ± 0.8 (1.63)	3.5 ± 1.5 (0.69)	1.87 ± 0.08	6.4 ± 0.8 (1.48)	3.1 ± 0.7 (0.72)
				Stride rate (steps·min^{-1})					
0% BWS	179.7 ± 2.8			181.4 ± 3.0			182.6 ± 2.6		
10% BWS	178.6 ± 2.8	− 0.6 ± 0.4 (0.35)		179.6 ± 2.8	− 1.0 ± 0.4 (0.35)		181.4 ± 3.2	− 0.6 ± 0.4 (0.38)	
20% BWS	175.7 ± 1.8	− 2.2 ± 0.9 (1.24)	− 1.6 ± 0.8 (0.89)	177.9 ± 1.7	− 2.0 ± 1.0 (1.24)	− 0.9 ± 0.8 (0.89)	179.7 ± 2.5	− 1.6 ± 0.5 (0.94)	− 0.9 ± 0.5 (0.56)
30% BWS	172.9 ± 1.4	− 3.8 ± 1.0 (2.14)	− 1.6 ± 0.6 (0.90)	174.8 ± 1.9	− 3.6 ± 1.0 (2.14)	− 1.7 ± 0.5 (0.90)	177.0 ± 2.1	− 3.0 ± 0.8 (1.85)	− 1.5 ± 0.5 (0.91)
				Contact time (ms)					
0% BWS	209.4 ± 7.2			197.7 ± 7.2			184.4 ± 6.8		
10% BWS	204.9 ± 8.0	− 2.2 ± 2.0 (0.56)		192.1 ± 7.6	− 2.8 ± 0.9 (0.68)		179.0 ± 6.5	− 2.9 ± 0.7 (0.70)	
20% BWS	197.1 ± 6.9	− 5.9 ± 1.1 (1.52)	− 3.8 ± 1.2 (0.96)	185.6 ± 7.2	− 6.1 ± 1.4 (1.51)	− 3.4 ± 1.8 (0.83)	172.7 ± 7.7	− 6.4 ± 1.0 (1.55)	− 3.5 ± 1.1 (0.85)
30% BWS	185.1 ± 8.7	− 11.6 ± 1.9 (3.12)	− 6.1 ± 1.8 (1.59)	175.9 ± 9.1	− 11.1 ± 2.2 (2.80)	− 5.3 ± 1.6 (1.29)	167.7 ± 7.9	− 9.1 ± 1.2 (2.25)	− 2.9 ± 0.8 (0.69)
				Flight duration (ms)					
0% BWS	139.6 ± 12.3			144.6 ± 12.0			155.7 ± 11.6		
10% BWS	147.9 ± 11.8	5.9 ± 1.2 (0.62)		152.4 ± 12.3	5.4 ± 0.8 (0.55)		163.3 ± 10.0	4.9 ± 3.7 (0.56)	
20% BWS	167.4 ± 10.6	20.1 ± 2.5 (1.96)	13.4 ± 1.9 (1.35)	173.1 ± 10.2	19.9 ± 3.6 (1.89)	13.7 ± 3.8 (1.34)	175.4 ± 12.3	12.9 ± 1.3 (1.41)	7.6 ± 3.6 (0.85)
30% BWS	185.9 ± 10.4	33.4 ± 3.0 (3.09)	11.0 ± 1.5 (1.12)	189.7 ± 9.7	31.5 ± 3.9 (2.85)	9.6 ± 1.1 (0.95)	192.7 ± 10.2	23.9 ± 2.3 (2.49)	9.8 ± 1.9 (1.08)

Data are means ± SD

BWS body weight support, *CL* confidence limits, *ES* effect size

[a]Represents the difference as percent ± 90 CL and the effects between levels of BWS and 0% BWS (e.g., 0% BWS and 10% BWS; 0% BWS and 20% BWS; 0% BWS and 30% BWS)

[b]Represents the difference as percent ± 90 CL and the effects between 10% BWS and 20% BWS or between 20% BWS and 30% BWS

Table 3 Biomechanical characteristics of female runners by velocity and different levels of body weight support

	12.9 km·h^{-1} (4.03 m·s^{-1})	Difference between 0% BWS ± 90 CL (ES)[a]	Difference between BWS ± 90 CL (ES)[b]	14.5 km·h^{-1} (4.47 m·s^{-1})	Difference between 0% BWS ± 90 CL (ES)	Difference between BWS ± 90 CL (ES)	16.1 km·h^{-1} (4.92 m·s^{-1})	Difference between 0% BWS ± 90 CL (ES)	Difference between BWS ± 90 CL (ES)
				Stride length (m)					
0% BWS	1.33 ± 0.08			1.55 ± 0.07			1.65 ± 0.08		
10% BWS	1.49 ± 0.07	12.4 ± 1.4 (1.74)		1.60 ± 0.09	3.2 ± 1.5 (0.64)		1.69 ± 0.08	2.3 ± 0.4 (0.45)	
20% BWS	1.52 ± 0.07	14.8 ± 1.6 (2.05)	2.2 ± 0.3 (0.31)	1.65 ± 0.08	6.2 ± 0.9 (1.24)	2.9 ± 1.0 (0.59)	1.73 ± 0.08	4.6 ± 0.5 (0.87)	2.2 ± 0.5 (0.43)
30% BWS	1.62 ± 0.08	22.2 ± 1.7 (2.98)	6.5 ± 0.8 (0.93)	1.71 ± 0.09	10.4 ± 1.0 (2.05)	4.0 ± 0.7 (0.81)	1.77 ± 0.08	7.2 ± 0.5 (1.34)	2.5 ± 0.5 (0.47)
				Stride rate (steps·min^{-1})					
0% BWS	182.4 ± 3.3			183.9 ± 3.0			186.1 ± 3.9		
10% BWS	181.6 ± 2.8	− 0.4 ± 0.6 (0.20)		182.9 ± 2.8	− 0.5 ± 0.6 (0.21)		184.5 ± 3.4	− 0.9 ± 0.5 (0.37)	
20% BWS	177.9 ± 2.5	− 2.5 ± 0.7 (1.21)	− 2.1 ± 0.5 (1.01)	179.0 ± 1.7	− 2.6 ± 0.8 (1.20)	− 2.2 ± 0.7 (0.99)	181.8 ± 2.7	− 2.3 ± 0.8 (0.99)	− 1.5 ± 0.5 (0.63)
30% BWS	174.6 ± 2.4	− 4.2 ± 0.9 (2.10)	− 1.8 ± 0.5 (0.89)	176.5 ± 1.9	− 4.0 ± 1.1 (1.83)	− 1.4 ± 0.5 (0.63)	178.6 ± 2.3	− 4.0 ± 1.1 (1.72)	− 1.7 ± 0.6 (0.73)
				Contact time (ms)					
0% BWS	224.0 ± 8.2			210.8 ± 6.6			197.1 ± 6.7		
10% BWS	215.6 ± 6.1	− 3.8 ± 1.3 (1.32)		205.1 ± 7.2	− 2.7 ± 0.9 (0.77)		188.3 ± 7.1	− 4.5 ± 1.1 (1.22)	
20% BWS	204.0 ± 6.8	− 8.9 ± 1.9 (3.22)	− 5.4 ± 1.4 (1.90)	187.6 ± 6.2	− 11.0 ± 0.8 (3.31)	− 8.5 ± 0.9 (2.54)	177.8 ± 6.3	− 9.8 ± 0.4 (2.73)	− 5.6 ± 1.3 (1.51)
30% BWS	191.5 ± 8.5	− 14.5 ± 1.4 (5.40)	− 6.1 ± 1.7 (2.18)	180.5 ± 6.3	− 14.4 ± 1.3 (4.42)	− 3.8 ± 0.6 (1.11)	171.1 ± 6.7	− 13.2 ± 0.5 (3.74)	− 3.7 ± 0.5 (1.01)
				Flight duration (ms)					
0% BWS	127.5 ± 8.2			130.6 ± 7.7			137.8 ± 7.9		
10% BWS	138.8 ± 6.1	8.9 ± 4.5 (1.15)		143.1 ± 7.1	9.6 ± 2.3 (1.36)		152.8 ± 7.9	10.9 ± 1.0 (1.57)	
20% BWS	160.5 ± 6.8	26.0 ± 2.9 (3.10)	15.7 ± 2.9 (1.64)	169.1 ± 8.8	29.5 ± 1.9 (3.84)	18.1 ± 3.4 (2.48)	173.1 ± 8.0	25.7 ± 1.5 (3.47)	13.4 ± 1.2 (1.90)
30% BWS	181.4 ± 8.5	42.4 ± 2.9 (4.74)	13.0 ± 1.2 (1.96)	185.5 ± 8.0	42.1 ± 2.7 (5.22)	9.7 ± 1.3 (1.38)	190.3 ± 9.1	38.2 ± 1.3 (4.90)	9.9 ± 1.2 (1.43)

Data are means ± SD

BWS body weight support, *CL* confidence limits, *ES* effect size

[a]Represents the difference as percent ± 90 CL and the effects between levels of BWS and 0% BWS (e.g., 0% BWS and 10% BWS; 0% BWS and 20% BWS; 0% BWS and 30% BWS)

[b]Represents the difference as percent ± 90 CL and the effects between 10% BWS and 20% BWS or between 20% BWS and 30% BWS

Physiological Responses

Physiological responses of male and female athletes to BWS across three running velocities are presented in Tables 4 and 5, respectively. There were large-extremely large effects on running economy (VO_2) at each speed and between all BWS for men ($p \leq 0.001$) and moderate-large effects for women ($p < 0.001$). There were trivial differences between the first 15 s and the last 15 s of the last minute analyzed at each running speed and BWS, indicating our subjects did achieve a steady state during each interval series. Equations from linear regression analyses defining VO_2 ($ml{\cdot}kg^{-1}{\cdot}min^{-1}$) as functions of running speed ($m{\cdot}s^{-1}$) at each BWS are presented in Table 6. There was increased variability with additional BWS (from 0.993 to 0.973 in men and 0.985 to 0.929 in women); however, coefficients of determinations (R^2) were nearly perfect between 0 and 30% BWS [36]. For both men and women, effects on RER were trivial-small with only significant differences between 0 and 10% BWS at 16.1 $km{\cdot}h^{-1}$ ($p = 0.02$) for men and 20 and 30% BWS at 16.1 $km{\cdot}h^{-1}$ ($p = 0.04$) for women. Minute ventilation and respiratory frequency decreased in trivial-moderate magnitudes with BWS ($p > 0.05$). Heart rate decreased with increasing BWS at moderate-large magnitudes ($p < 0.01$) in men except between 20 and 30% BWS at 16.1 and 17.7 $km{\cdot}h^{-1}$ ($p = 0.14$ and 0.08, respectively). In females, HR decreased significantly ($p < 0.05$) at 14.5 and 16.1 $km{\cdot}h^{-1}$ with increasing BWS, but not 12.9 $km{\cdot}h^{-1}$ ($p > 0.08$). Rating of perceived exertion went down in mostly small-moderate magnitudes with increasing BWS across all speeds ($p < 0.01$). There were trivial-small differences in V_E, respiratory frequency, HR, and RPE for a given VO_2 across various BWS ($p > 0.05$).

Discussion

This is the first study to assess the physiological and biomechanical responses of running on a LBPPT among highly trained female distance runners across typical training speeds and different levels of BWS, while it adds to the body of literature regarding highly trained male distance runners. The most important finding of the current study is that male and female runners had similar physiological and biomechanical responses to running on LBPPT. In general, we found that increasing BWS on a LBPPT increased stride length and flight duration and decreased stride rate and contact time while attenuating a variety of physiological characteristics at a range of treadmill velocities.

Biomechanical changes to LBPPT running are not well defined and, in the case of stride characteristics, are inconsistent. When considering the global unweighing effects on stride parameters during running, its major influence was the large increase in flight time, which contrasted the disproportional decrease in contact time resulting in overall longer stride length and reduction in stride rate. Sainton et al. [26] described this pattern of movement as similar to the gait patterns adopted by astronauts on the Moon as defined by Minetti et al. [38]. Studies are in agreement that unweighing-induced changes in flight time increase with increasing levels of BWS [12, 13, 26, 29]. In our study, flight time was less affected by higher running speeds but was significantly affected by BWS. Presumably, the BWS provides a longer swing phase and theoretically lowers the working demand of the hip flexion muscles [12].

Both the current data and those of previous studies [12, 22, 28, 29] are in disagreement with the work of Mercer and Chona [39] who reported no effects on stride length with increased BWS. We found small to moderate increases in stride length with each 10% incremental increase in BWS. These findings support our observation that flight time increases with BWS, in line with others' observations of increased flight times and stride durations [12, 13, 26, 29]. The effect of BWS on stride length seems to be less when running at faster speeds. There was a 22% increase in stride length at 12.9 $km{\cdot}h^{-1}$ from 0 to 30% BWS compared to only 7% increase at 16.1 $km{\cdot}h^{-1}$ in females. Raffalt et al. [12] reported similar phenomena in stride rate and stride length. In this study, flight time was also affected less at faster running velocities, indicating that the running pattern was less affected by BWS at higher running speeds.

There is a natural reciprocal relationship between stride length and stride rate [30]; therefore, it is not surprising then to find reductions in stride rate, considering the increases in stride length in the present study and others with increasing BWS [10, 12, 26, 29]. Only Gojanovic et al. [22, 25] have reported increases in stride rate during BWS running, but that was only in male runners during maximal or supramaximal running velocities. Mercer and Chona [39] and Gojanovic et al. [22] reported no change in stride rate with BWS in males and females during maximal or supramaximal running speeds. An increase in stride rate has been reported to reduce the risk of chronic knee injuries by reducing joint loading and increasing gluteal activation [40]. Conversely, decreasing stride rate may place the knee joint under greater load and potentially increase the risk of injury [29]. Given that LBPPT are intended for rehabilitating injured athletes, preventing injuries, and enhancing performance, it is important that training benefits achieved on LBPPT translate to overground running too [1]. Our results and others support that running on a LBPPT at submaximal running speeds promotes a decrease in stride rate [10, 12, 26, 29], which may not be beneficial for athletes trying to add training volume, prevent injury, or rehabilitate an injury. However, there is no evidence suggesting the effects of LBPPT running persist for a long term after returning to overground running.

Table 4 Physiological characteristics of male runner by velocity and different levels of body weight support

	14.5 km·h^{-1} (4.03 m·s^{-1})	Difference between 0% BWS ± 90 CL (ES)[a]	Difference between BWS ± 90 CL (ES)[b]	16.1 km·h^{-1} (4.47 m·s^{-1})	Difference between 0% BWS ± 90 CL (ES)	Difference between BWS ± 90 CL (ES)	17.7 km·h^{-1} (4.92 m·s^{-1})	Difference between 0% BWS ± 90 CL (ES)	Difference between BWS ± 90 CL (ES)
Running economy (VO_2 ml·kg^{-1}·min^{-1})									
0% BWS	45.4 ± 2.4			50.6 ± 2.4			57.8 ± 2.9		
10% BWS	39.6 ± 2.7	− 12.8 ± 4.1 (2.29)		44.6 ± 2.1	− 11.9 ± 2.5 (2.39)		49.8 ± 3.4	− 13.9 ± 3.2 (2.57)	
20% BWS	30.9 ± 1.3	− 31.9 ± 4.2 (6.45)	− 21.9 ± 4.0 (4.16)	36.9 ± 1.3	− 27.2 ± 4.8 (6.00)	− 17.4 ± 4.9 (3.61)	41.3 ± 2.6	− 28.6 ± 5.5 (5.78)	− 17.0 ± 6.1 (3.21)
30% BWS	28.1 ± 1.6	− 38.1 ± 7.8 (8.04)	− 9.0 ± 4.6 (1.59)	33.9 ± 1.7	− 33.1 ± 3.5 (7.61)	− 8.1 ± 2.7 (1.60)	37.2 ± 2.5	− 35.8 ± 5.8 (7.61)	− 10.1 ± 1.6 (1.83)
Respiratory exchange ratio (VCO_2/VO_2)									
0% BWS	0.82 ± 0.04			0.84 ± 0.03			0.86 ± 0.04		
10% BWS	0.83 ± 0.04	1.9 ± 1.2 (0.29)		0.83 ± 0.03	− 1.2 ± 0.9 (0.24)		0.85 ± 0.03	− 1.6 ± 0.7 (0.28)	
20% BWS	0.83 ± 0.04	0.1 ± 1.4 (0.02)	0.9 ± 1.6 (0.22)	0.83 ± 0.04	− 1.9 ± 1.9 (0.38)	− 1.1 ± 2.5 (0.21)	0.84 ± 0.04	− 1.3 ± 1.3 (0.21)	− 0.1 ± 2.0 (0.01)
30% BWS	0.83 ± 0.04	0.2 ± 1.5 (0.03)	− 1.4 ± 1.4 (0.14)	0.83 ± 0.04	− 2.6 ± 2.4 (0.51)	0.0 ± 1.0 (0.00)	0.84 ± 0.03	− 1.2 ± 2.2 (0.20)	− 0.4 ± 2.4 (0.06)
Minute ventilation (L·min^{-1})									
0% BWS	52.3 ± 5.8			56.8 ± 5.7			60.4 ± 7.8		
10% BWS	50.1 ± 4.6	− 5.2 ± 4.4 (0.38)		53.3 ± 4.6	− 5.7 ± 4.4 (0.51)		59.5 ± 6.0	− 1.3 ± 9.6 (0.09)	
20% BWS	48.6 ± 4.1	− 6.2 ± 5.3 (0.46)	− 4.3 ± 5.6 (0.32)	51.3 ± 6.3	− 9.8 ± 4.3 (0.90)	− 5.5 ± 7.7 (0.50)	55.4 ± 4.8	− 8.0 ± 8.4 (0.56)	− 6.8 ± 6.6 (0.47)
30% BWS	46.2 ± 2.6	− 11.3 ± 10.9 (0.86)	− 3.7 ± 5.4 (0.27)	49.9 ± 4.7	− 12.0 ± 8.8 (1.12)	− 2.5 ± 9.5 (0.22)	54.9 ± 5.0	− 8.7 ± 8.4 (0.61)	− 0.7 ± 2.2 (0.05)
Respiratory frequency (breathes·min^{-1})									
0% BWS	34.4 ± 4.6			35.6 ± 4.7			37.0 ± 5.1		
10% BWS	34.0 ± 5.1	2.2 ± 13.0 (0.12)		34.9 ± 5.0	− 2.2 ± 9.2 (0.13)		36.1 ± 4.6	− 2.8 ± 4.2 (0.20)	
20% BWS	33.4 ± 3.5	− 0.7 ± 10.1 (0.04)	1.3 ± 8.3 (0.07)	32.7 ± 5.7	− 7.8 ± 8.9 (0.49)	− 8.3 ± 9.9 (0.52)	33.8 ± 5.0	− 6.1 ± 4.9 (0.45)	− 6.4 ± 11.6 (0.47)
30% BWS	29.4 ± 4.2	− 12.3 ± 19.0 (0.74)	− 13.0 ± 15.6 (0.78)	31.2 ± 2.7	− 11.3 ± 14.1 (0.71)	− 4.1 ± 16.2 (0.25)	33.6 ± 4.2	− 8.5 ± 9.4 (0.64)	1.0 ± 12.9 (0.07)
Heart rate (BPM)									
0% BWS	143 ± 5			150 ± 6			157 ± 8		
10% BWS	135 ± 6	− 5.0 ± 2.6 (1.33)		143 ± 5	− 4.8 ± 2.7 (0.99)		150 ± 6	− 4.7 ± 2.8 (0.87)	
20% BWS	126 ± 3	− 11.7 ± 3.3 (3.21)	− 7.0 ± 1.9 (1.88)	132 ± 5	− 11.9 ± 3.5 (2.52)	− 7.4 ± 2.1 (1.53)	141 ± 5	− 10.0 ± 3.9 (1.92)	− 5.6 ± 2.0 (1.05)
30% BWS	121 ± 5	− 15.1 ± 4.9 (4.23)	− 3.9 ± 2.2 (1.03)	129 ± 7	− 14.3 ± 3.5 (3.08)	− 2.8 ± 3.2 (0.56)	137 ± 8	− 12.7 ± 4.8 (2.46)	− 2.9 ± 4.1 (0.54)
RPE (6–20 AU)									
0% BWS	13.7 ± 1.3			14.7 ± 1.1			15.6 ± 1.3		
10% BWS	11.9 ± 0.7	− 13.4 ± 6.9 (1.39)		12.6 ± 0.8	− 14.5 ± 4.7 (1.88)		13.6 ± 0.8	− 12.7 ± 6.7 (1.49)	
20% BWS	10.6 ± 0.8	− 22.8 ± 4.8 (2.51)	− 10.9 ± 4.7 (1.12)	11.4 ± 0.8	− 22.3 ± 9.4 (3.03)	− 9.1 ± 5.6 (0.45)	12.4 ± 1.0	− 20.2 ± 9.5 (2.46)	− 8.5 ± 5.5 (0.98)
30% BWS	9.9 ± 0.9	− 28.1 ± 7.4 (3.19)	− 6.9 ± 5.0 (0.69)	11.0 ± 0.6	− 25.2 ± 9.3 (3.48)	− 3.7 ± 4.8 (1.15)	11.7 ± 0.8	− 24.7 ± 10.5 (3.10)	− 5.7 ± 4.1 (0.64)

Data are means ± SD

AU arbitrary units, *BPM* beats per minute, *BWS* body weight support, *CL* confidence limits, *ES* effect size, *RPE* rating of perceived exertion, VO_2 oxygen consumption

[a]Represents the difference as percent ± 90 CL and the effects between levels of BWS and 0% BWS (e.g., 0% BWS and 10% BWS; 0% BWS and 20% BWS; 0% BWS and 30% BWS)

[b]Represents the difference as percent ± 90 CL and the effects between 10% BWS and 20% BWS or between 20% BWS and 30% BWS

Table 5 Physiological characteristics of female runners by velocity and different levels of body weight support

	12.9 km·h^{-1} (3.58 m·s^{-1})	Difference between 0% BWS ± 90 CL (ES)[a]	Difference between BWS ± 90 CL (ES)[b]	14.5 km·h^{-1} (4.03 m·s^{-1})	Difference between 0% BWS ± 90 CL (ES)	Difference between BWS ± 90 CL (ES)	16.1 km·h^{-1} (4.47 m·s^{-1})	Difference between 0% BWS ± 90 CL (ES)	Difference between BWS ± 90 CL (ES)
				Running economy (VO_2 ml·kg^{-1}·min^{-1})					
0% BWS	43.5 ± 3.6			48.3 ± 4.0			55.6 ± 4.8		
10% BWS	37.2 ± 4.0	− 14.7 ± 3.5 (1.66)		41.1 ± 5.0	− 15.3 ± 4.4 (1.70)		48.7 ± 5.5	− 13.1 ± 4.1 (2.29)	
20% BWS	29.1 ± 3.3	− 33.2 ± 4.2 (4.22)	− 21.7 ± 2.2 (2.56)	32.0 ± 3.9	− 34.0 ± 5.0 (4.24)	− 22.1 ± 2.5 (2.55)	38.0 ± 4.4	− 31.8 ± 5.1 (6.45)	− 21.6 ± 3.0 (4.16)
30% BWS	26.5 ± 2.9	− 39.2 ± 4.3 (5.21)	− 9.0 ± 2.7 (0.99)	28.7 ± 3.4	− 40.8 ± 5.0 (5.35)	− 10.3 ± 2.5 (1.11)	34.8 ± 4.4	− 37.6 ± 6.4 (8.04)	− 8.5 ± 3.5 (1.59)
				Respiratory exchange ratio (VCO_2/VO_2)					
0% BWS	0.83 ± 0.06			0.84 ± 0.06			0.86 ± 0.06		
10% BWS	0.82 ± 0.05	− 0.6 ± 6.6 (0.22)		0.81 ± 0.05	− 3.9 ± 5.3 (0.53)		0.84 ± 0.05	− 1.6 ± 6.9 (0.22)	
20% BWS	0.82 ± 0.05	− 0.6 ± 9.0 (0.40)	0.0 ± 2.7 (0.18)	0.83 ± 0.05	− 1.0 ± 7.4 (0.14)	3.0 ± 4.3 (0.39)	0.83 ± 0.04	− 3.0 ± 6.9 (0.40)	− 1.4 ± 2.2 (0.18)
30% BWS	0.81 ± 0.04	− 2.0 ± 8.0 (0.09)	− 1.4 ± 3.6 (0.31)	0.85 ± 0.04	0.4 ± 7.7 (0.06)	1.5 ± 1.8 (0.20)	0.85 ± 0.04	− 0.7 ± 7.6 (0.09)	2.4 ± 2.6 (0.31)
				Minute ventilation (L·min^{-1})					
0% BWS	44.7 ± 3.7			50.8 ± 6.0			57.0 ± 7.0		
10% BWS	42.2 ± 5.5	− 6.0 ± 7.3 (0.63)		45.0 ± 6.0	− 11.6 ± 5.8 (0.87)		52.4 ± 6.5	− 8.2 ± 7.3 (0.59)	
20% BWS	38.3 ± 6.8	− 15.2 ± 13.3 (1.69)	− 9.8 ± 7.3 (1.05)	42.3 ± 6.9	− 17.2 ± 6.4 (1.33)	− 6.3 ± 7.7 (0.46)	46.7 ± 6.2	− 18.1 ± 7.9 (1.38)	− 10.8 ± 5.3 (0.79)
30% BWS	36.0 ± 5.3	− 19.9 ± 10.4 (2.28)	− 5.6 ± 8.9 (0.59)	41.1 ± 6.9	− 19.5 ± 7.8 (1.54)	− 2.9 ± 4.6 (0.21)	45.0 ± 7.9	− 21.7 ± 11.1 (1.69)	− 4.4 ± 6.5 (0.31)
				Respiratory frequency (breathes·min^{-1})					
0% BWS	38.0 ± 4.6			38.8 ± 4.4			41.2 ± 6.4		
10% BWS	35.9 ± 9.7	− 7.9 ± 21.2 (0.63)		38.3 ± 8.3	− 2.6 ± 14.1 (0.20)		38.7 ± 5.6	− 5.8 ± 16.9 (0.20)	
20% BWS	33.7 ± 4.7	− 11.6 ± 10.6 (0.94)	− 4.0 ± 14.7 (0.31)	34.9 ± 5.4	− 10.4 ± 14.3 (0.84)	− 8.0 ± 13.6 (0.63)	37.1 ± 3.9	− 9.2 ± 14.7 (0.84)	− 3.6 ± 8.4 (0.63)
30% BWS	30.5 ± 4.1	− 19.9 ± 3.8 (1.70)	− 9.4 ± 9.6 (0.76)	32.7 ± 2.9	− 15.7 ± 12.4 (1.30)	− 5.9 ± 8.6 (0.46)	35.8 ± 3.7	− 12.5 ± 17.5 (1.30)	− 3.7 ± 8.4 (0.46)
				Heart rate (BPM)					
0% BWS	151 ± 14			161 ± 14			168 ± 14		
10% BWS	142 ± 13	− 5.5 ± 4.3 (0.57)		151 ± 13	− 6.7 ± 4.2 (0.73)		156 ± 15	− 7.4 ± 5.2 (0.88)	
20% BWS	133 ± 16	− 12.0 ± 7.5 (1.27)	− 6.8 ± 7.8 (0.70)	142 ± 15	− 12.1 ± 4.8 (1.37)	− 5.8 ± 4.4 (0.55)	148 ± 13	− 12.2 ± 5.3 (1.49)	− 4.3 ± 5.1 (0.61)
30% BWS	129 ± 18	− 14.7 ± 8.6 (1.58)	− 3.1 ± 13.2 (0.31)	135 ± 15	− 16.6 ± 6.3 (1.92)	− 5.1 ± 9.0 (0.64)	142 ± 15	− 15.9 ± 4.8 (2.00)	− 4.3 ± 5.7 (0.50)
				RPE (6–20 AU)					
0% BWS	13.3 ± 1.8			14.4 ± 1.9			15.1 ± 1.7		
10% BWS	11.9 ± 1.6	− 10.4 ± 3.8 (0.70)		13.0 ± 1.5	− 9.5 ± 3.1 (0.66)		13.8 ± 1.6	− 9.2 ± 3.8 (0.73)	
20% BWS	11.0 ± 1.3	− 16.8 ± 5.2 (1.18)	− 7.2 ± 3.2 (0.48)	11.9 ± 1.6	− 17.5 ± 4.1 (1.28)	− 8.9 ± 3.8 (0.62)	12.6 ± 1.7	− 16.7 ± 4.4 (1.39)	− 8.3 ± 3.0 (0.81)
30% BWS	9.8 ± 1.4	− 26.5 ± 6.6 (1.98)	− 11.6 ± 5.3 (0.79)	10.6 ± 1.5	− 26.2 ± 5.2 (2.02)	− 10.6 ± 3.9 (0.74)	11.4 ± 1.6	− 25.1 ± 6.8 (2.19)	− 10.1 ± 8.2 (0.66)

Data are means ± SD

AU arbitrary units, *BPM* beats per minute, *BWS* body weight support, *CL* confidence limits, *ES* effect size, *RPE* rating of perceived exertion, VO_2 oxygen consumption

[a]Represents the difference as percent ± 90 CL and the effects between levels of BWS and 0% BWS (e.g., 0% BWS and 10% BWS; 0% BWS and 20% BWS; 0% BWS and 30% BWS)

[b]Represents the difference as percent ± 90 CL and the effects between 10% BWS and 20% BWS or between 20% BWS and 30% BWS

Table 6 Equations from linear regression analyses defining oxygen consumption (VO_2 ml·kg^{-1}·min^{-1}) as functions of running speed (m·s^{-1}) at each BWS for male and female runners

% body weight support	Regression equations	R^2
Male runners		
0% BWS	VO_2 (ml·kg^{-1}·min^{-1}) = 12.807 × speed (m·s^{-1}) − 10.204	0.993
10% BWS	VO_2 (ml·kg^{-1}·min^{-1}) = 10.493 × speed (m·s^{-1}) − 5.8871	0.999
20% BWS	VO_2 (ml·kg^{-1}·min^{-1}) = 10.706 × speed (m·s^{-1}) − 14.521	0.992
30% BWS	VO_2 (ml·kg^{-1}·min^{-1}) = 9.2819 × speed (m·s^{-1}) − 11.185	0.973
Female runners		
0% BWS	VO_2 (ml·kg^{-1}·min^{-1}) = 9.8994 × speed (m·s^{-1}) − 4.2691	0.985
10% BWS	VO_2 (ml·kg^{-1}·min^{-1}) = 9.336 × speed (m·s^{-1}) − 6.6136	0.967
20% BWS	VO_2 (ml·kg^{-1}·min^{-1}) = 7.3159 × speed (m·s^{-1}) − 5.2166	0.957
30% BWS	VO_2 (ml·kg^{-1}·min^{-1}) = 6.8762 × speed (m·s^{-1}) − 5.6689	0.929

BWS body weight support, *VO_2* oxygen consumption, *R^2* proportion of explained variability

In contrast to Grabowski and Kram [10] and Farley and McMahon [41] who reported an increase in contact time and Sainton et al. [26] who found no change in contact time, we found significant decreases in contact time with increased BWS across all speeds. Several other studies also found decreases in contact time with BWS [12, 29]. Sainton et al. [26] suggest that this is a result of greater knee extension and ankle plantar flexion while running on a LBPPT because the aperture (Fig. 1) provides progressively more lifting force with increased BWS. Furthermore, as BWS is increased, a shift in regional loading of the shoe towards the forefoot occurs due to this lifting force that may result in reduced contact time and altered running patterns, particularly at ≥ 20% BWS [42]. The study of Raffalt et al. [12] is one of the few other studies using high-trained runners and suggests this could simply be explained by the participant's better ability to apply force to the treadmill belt due to their experience with LBPPT running and training background. However, running at the same speed with increased BWS has also been shown to decrease the vertical ground reaction force impulse [13, 15] which can be achieved either by lower peak vertical ground reaction forces or by shorter contact times.

The conflicting findings in biomechanical responses, particularly contact time, between studies may depend on a number of factors, including the magnitude of unloading (e.g., 20% BWS may produce different results than 60% BWS), accuracy of unloading, running speed, fitness levels of subjects, treadmill running experience, and more specifically, LBPPT running experience [1, 32]. According to a recent systematic review, the current LBPPT literature suggests that there are non-linear changes in muscle activity with different increments of BWS [1]. Some data indicate certain muscles are not affected until significant increases in BWS occur (e.g., significant differences present at 40% BWS but not 20% BWS) [26]. However, other data suggest some muscles experience changes with minimal BWS (i.e., 10% BWS) but not with further unweighting (i.e., 30% BWS), while some muscle experience consistent changes with incremental increases in BWS [39, 43]. Additionally, there is evidence of an accommodation effect, such that previous research has shown multiple trials of unweighted running are necessary for reliable measures of metabolic cost to be made [21], and this may be the case with biomechanical characteristics too.

The biomechanical changes in the present study with LBPPT running contribute to less metabolic cost and corresponding physiological changes. Specifically, if less force needs to be produced to support body weight, neuromuscular activation is reduced, and therefore, there is a decreased need for energy production [1, 2]. Accordingly, it is not surprising that, as BWS increased within a given running velocity, running economy was improved (metabolic demand is decreased), and thus, HR, respiratory frequency, and minute ventilation were also reduced. Our results support a growing body of literature that metabolic cost is reduced with BWS [9, 10, 12, 18, 20–23, 26]. In the present study, we saw very large to extremely large reductions in VO_2 from 0 to 10% BWS and from 10 to 20% BWS; however, the effect, while still moderate to large in magnitude, was attenuated with additional BWS between 20 and 30% BWS. Kline et al. [20] reported that a proportion of metabolic demand to BWS was nearly equivalent between 10 and 30% BWS; however, with additional BWS, the proportion of metabolic demand differed significantly from the proportion of BWS. Here, the proportional reduction in metabolic cost was greater than that of BWS, particularly between 10 and 20% BWS and between 20 and 30% BWS. Fortunately, previous research has shown that equivalent maximal and submaximal VO_2 can be achieved while running on LBPPT by increasing the running speed to offset the reduction in oxygen consumption associated with running with BWS [12, 20, 22, 25].

It is important to note that the metabolic demands of running at 0% BWS on a LBPPT are lower than those of running on a regular treadmill [32]. McNeill et al. [9] showed that standing weight on a LBPPT was on average 7% lower than predicted body weight which according to Kline et al. [20] resulted in a 3–9% lower metabolic cost at running velocities between 8.0 and 17.7 km·h^{-1} [32]. The reductions in weight and metabolic demand have been attributed to the inflation of the chamber, which provides additional vertical and horizontal support in the mediolateral direction and reduces the need to propel in the anterior-posterior direction [1, 32, 44]. Thus, in the present study, the proportional decreases in metabolic demand are likely greater than that presented when compared to regular treadmill running. Similar to previous research reporting increased variability in metabolic demand with increased BWS [9], we also found increased variability (from 0.999 down to 0.929) from 0 and 30% BWS; however, our coefficients of determinations (R^2) were substantially higher than those of previous studies [9, 23, 24]. The differences could be attributed to differences in methodology between studies. Multiple studies have implemented multiple day testing protocols to assess the effects of LBPPT running [9, 10, 12, 20, 21, 23] which may be warranted during long duration or maximal running protocols where the slow drift of VO_2 may be present. However, Barnes and Kilding [2] reported that the intraindividual variation (typical error) in metabolic cost is attributable to a number of factors and is between 1.3 and 5% at speeds between 12 and 18 km·h^{-1} in well-trained and elite caliber athletes. Thus, we utilized a randomized single-session approach, thus reducing the day-to-day variability possibly seen in other studies. Additionally, our subjects were highly trained distance runners who were used to running 12–20 km during a typical training session; thus, the demand to run 36 min on a LBPPT is relatively negligible to their typical training regimen. This is supported by the fact that RER values did not exceed 1.0 and blood lactate samples at the conclusion of each 9-min interval series were < 4 mmol·L^{-1} (range 1.9 to 3.4 mmol·L^{-1} at the fastest running velocity). Only one other study has reported changes in RER during submaximal LBPPT running [9]. Our results agree with McNeill et al. [9] in that there were no significant effects on RER with BWS at slower running velocities; however, at faster speeds, a significant reduction occurred in both men and women. It should be noted, however, that the 3-min intervals used in this study represent a relatively short time period to reach a physiological steady state and, in a lesser-trained population, would not be appropriate for analysis. However, our data indicated there was no difference between the first 15 s and the last 15 s of the last minute analyzed, indicating our subjects did achieve a steady state.

In addition to the reduction in oxygen consumption, we also found a significant decrease in HR and RPE during unweighted running. Studies are in agreement that there are concomitant decreases in HR and VO_2 during BWS running [9, 12, 18, 22, 23, 26, 28, 45]. Changes in HR tended to be similar across running speeds; however, the magnitude of effects was attenuated with increases in BWS. Gojanovic et al. [22] suggest that the decrease in HR might be linked to a positive effect of lower-body positive pressure on venous return, which, in turn, might be compensated adequately by an increase in stroke volume. However, we observed that HR was similar at that same VO_2 independent of BWS, indicating that LBPP on its own did not affect blood flow, stroke volume, and subsequently, HR. In contrast to several studies that reported no significant change in RPE with BWS [23, 26, 45], the reduction in RPE in our study agrees with McNeill et al. [9] and Ruckstuhl et al. [18] who also reported significant reductions in perception of effort at fixed running speeds with increasing BWS. The findings of this study and other studies suggest that BWS does not alter the relationship between HR and VO_2 or RPE and VO_2, which indicates that using HR or RPE to prescribe training intensities does not require adjustment when running on a LBPPT with BWS [9, 18, 23].

In addition to examining changes in physiological characteristics across levels of BWS, we found that when compared at the same VO_2 across various BWS, minute ventilation, respiratory frequency, HR, and RPE were similar. Hoffman and Donaghe [23] also showed that HR and RPE remained the same for a given VO_2 (25 ml·kg^{-1}·min^{-1}) across various BWS in healthy untrained subjects. Because the speed necessary to achieve a given VO_2 must be increased with BWS [12, 20, 22, 25], the unaltered relationship between RPE and VO_2 suggests that the stimulus for perceived effort is related more to aerobic demand than actual running speed [23]. The other physiological responses (HR, ventilation, respiratory frequency) are consistent with other studies describing physiologic correlates with steady-state oxygen consumption at specific running velocities [2, 3].

Conclusions

In conclusion, our results indicate the male and female distance runners have similar physiological and biomechanical responses to LBPPT running. When considering the overall effects of BWS on stride parameters, its major influence was the large increase in flight time, which contrasted the smaller decrease in contact time resulting in overall longer stride length and reduction in stride rate. There was a disproportionate decrease in oxygen consumption relative to BWS which led to an attenuation of all other physiological characteristics measured to varying magnitudes between each level of BWS and running speed. The rationale for the disproportional decrease in VO_2 has not been fully elucidated but may be related to biomechanical changes leading to reduced neuromuscular activation at a given running velocity and, therefore, a decreased need for energy production resulting in less metabolic cost and corresponding physiological changes.

Abbreviations

AU: Arbitrary units; BPM: Beats per minute; BWS: Body weight support; CL: Confidence limits; ES: Effect size; HR: Heart rate; IAAF: International Association of Athletics Federations; LBPPT: Lower-body positive pressure treadmill; RER: Respiratory exchange ratio; RPE: Rating of perceived exertion; V_E: Minute ventilation; VO_2: Oxygen consumption

Acknowledgements

The authors would like to thank all of the athletes for participating in the study. Funding for this study was received through the Student Summer Scholars program at Grand Valley State University. The authors have no professional relationship or affiliation with AlterG, Inc.

Funding

This study was funded by the Office of Undergraduate Research and Scholarship's Student Summer Scholars program at the Grand Valley State University.

Authors' Contributions

KRB conceived and designed the study, assisted with the data collection, analyzed the data, and wrote the paper. JNJ collected the data and assisted with the data analysis and writing of the paper. Both authors read and approved the final manuscript.

Authors' Information

KRB is an Assistant Professor in the Department of Movement Science at the Grand Valley State University in Allendale, Michigan, USA.

Competing Interests

Kyle Barnes and Jessica Janecke declare that they have no competing interests.

Author details

[1]Department of Movement Science, Grand Valley State University, 1 Campus Drive, Allendale, MI 49401, USA. [2]Office of Undergraduate Research and Scholarship, Grand Valley State University, 1 Campus Drive, Allendale, MI 49401, USA.

References

1. Farina KA, Wright AA, Ford KR, Wirfel LA, Smoliga JM. Physiological and biomechanical responses to running on lower body positive pressure treadmills in healthy populations. Sports Med. 2017;47:261–75.
2. Barnes KR, Kilding AE. Running economy: measurement, norms and determining factors. Sports Med-Open. 2015;1
3. Daniels JT, Daniels N. Running economy of elite male and elite female runners. Med Sci Sports Exerc. 1992;24:483–9.
4. Kram R. Muscular force or work: what determines the metabolic energy cost of running? Exerc Sport Sci Rev. 2000;28:138–43.
5. Nilsson J, Thorstensson A. Ground reaction forces at different speeds of human walking and running. Acta Physiol Scand. 1989;136:217–27.
6. Costill D. A scientific approach to distance running. Mountain View: Tafnews; 1979.
7. Daniels JT. Daniels' running formula. Champaign: Human Kinetics; 2013.
8. Hoeberigs JH. Factors related to the incidence of running injuries. A review. Sports Med. 1992;13:408–22.
9. McNeill DK, Kline JR, de Heer HD, Coast JR. Oxygen consumption of elite distance runners on an anti-gravity treadmill. J Sports Sci Med. 2015;14:333–9.
10. Grabowski AM, Kram R. Effects of velocity and weight support on ground reaction forces and metabolic power during running. J Appl Biomech. 2008;24:288–97.
11. Schlabs T, Rosales-Velderrain A, Ruckstuhl H, Stahn AC, Hargens AR. Comparison of cardiovascular and biomechanical parameters of supine lower body negative pressure and upright lower body positive pressure to simulate activity in 1/6 G and 3/8 G. J Appl Physiol. 1985;115:275–84.
12. Raffalt PC, Hovgaard-Hansen L, Jensen BR. Running on a lower-body positive pressure treadmill: VO2max, respiratory response, and vertical ground reaction force. Res Q Exerc Sport. 2013;84:213–22.
13. Chang YH, Huang HW, Hamerski CM, Kram R. The independent effects of gravity and inertia on running mechanics. J Exp Biol. 2000;203:229–38.
14. Reilly T, Dowzer CN, Cable NT. The physiology of deep-water running. J Sports Sci. 2003;21:959–72.
15. Teunissen LP, Grabowski A, Kram R. Effects of independently altering body weight and body mass on the metabolic cost of running. J Exp Biol. 2007;210:4418–27.
16. Grabowski AM. Metabolic and biomechanical effects of velocity and weight support using a lower-body positive pressure device during walking. Arch Phys Med Rehabil. 2010;91:951–7.
17. Grabowski A, Farley CT, Kram R. Independent metabolic costs of supporting body weight and accelerating body mass during walking. J Appl Physiol. 2005;98:579–83.
18. Ruckstuhl H, Schlabs T, Rosales-Velderrain A, Hargens AR. Oxygen consumption during walking and running under fractional weight bearing conditions. Aviat Space Environ Med. 2010;81:550–4.
19. Figueroa M, Wicke J, Manning J, Escamilla P, Santillo N, Wolkstein J, et al. Validation of ACSM metabolic equations in an anti-gravity environment: a pilot study. Int J Appl Sci Technol. 2012;2:204–10.
20. Kline JR, Raab S, Coast JR, Bounds R, McNeill D, de Heer HDA. Conversion table for running on lower body positive pressure treadmills. J Strength Cond Res. 2015;29:854–62.
21. McNeill DK, de Heer HD, Williams CP, Coast JR. Metabolic accommodation to running on a body weight-supported treadmill. Eur J Appl Physiol. 2015;115:905–10.
22. Gojanovic B, Cutti P, Shultz R, Matheson GO. Maximal physiological parameters during partial body-weight support treadmill testing. Med Sci Sports Exerc. 2012;44:1935–41.
23. Hoffman M, Donaghe H. Physiological responses to body weight-supported treadmill exercise in healthy adults. Arch Phys Med Rehabil. 2011;92:960–6.
24. Lee KY, Han JY, Kim JH, Kim DJ, Choi IS. Physiological responses during the lower body positive pressure supported treadmill test. Ann Rehabil Med. 2016;40:915–23.
25. Gojanovic B, Shultz R, Feihl F, Matheson G. Overspeed HIIT in lower-body positive pressure treadmill improves running performance. Med Sci Sports Exerc. 2015;47:2571–8.
26. Sainton P, Nicol C, Cabri J, Barthelemy-Montfort J, Berton E, Chavet P. Influence of short-term unweighing and reloading on running kinetics and muscle activity. Eur J Appl Physiol. 2015;115:1135–45.
27. Ruckstuhl H, Kho J, Weed M, Wilkinson MW, Hargens AR. Comparing two devices of suspended treadmill walking by varying body unloading and Froude number. Gait Posture. 2009;30:446–51.
28. Cutuk A, Groppo ER, Quigley EJ, White KW, Pedowitz RA, Hargens AR. Ambulation in simulated fractional gravity using lower body positive pressure: cardiovascular safety and gait analyses. J Appl Physiol (1985). 2006;101:771–7.
29. Neal M, Fleming N, Eberman L, Games K, Vaughan J. Effect of body-weight-support running on lower-limb biomechanics. J Orthop Sports Phys Ther. 2016;46:784–93.
30. Barnes KR, McGuigan MR, Kilding AE. Lower-body determinants of running economy in male and female distance runners. J Strength Cond Res. 2014;28:1289–97.
31. Jones AM, Doust JH. A 1% treadmill grade most accurately reflects the energetic cost of outdoor running. J Sports Sci. 1996;14:321–7.
32. McNeill DK, de Heer HD, Bounds RG, Coast JR. Accuracy of unloading with the anti-gravity treadmill. J Strength Cond Res. 2015;29:863–8.
33. Borg G. Perceived exertion as an indicator of somatic stress. Scand J Rehab Med. 1970;2:92–8.
34. Hopkins WG. A spreadsheet to compare means of two groups. Sportscience. 2007;11:22–3.
35. Hopkins WG. Spreadsheets for analysis of controlled trials, with adjustment for a subject characteristic. Sportscience. 2006;10:46–50.
36. Hopkins WG, Marshall SW, Batterham AM, Hanin J. Progressive statistics for studies in sports medicine and exercise science. Med Sci Sports Exerc. 2009;41:3–13.
37. Spiriev B. International Association of Athletics Federations Scoring Tables of Athletics. Monaco: International Association of Athletics Federations; 2011. https://www.iaaf.org/news/iaaf-news/scoring-tables-2017.

38. Minetti A, Pavei G, Biancardi C. The energetics and mechanics of level and gradient skipping: preliminary results for a potential gair of choice in low gravity enviroments. Planet Space Sci. 2012;74:142–5.
39. Mercer J, Chona C. Stride length-velocity relationship during running with body weight support. J Sport Health Sci. 2015;4:391–5.
40. Ivanenko YP, Grasso R, Macellari V, Lacquaniti F. Control of foot trajectory in human locomotion: role of ground contact forces in simulated reduced gravity. J Neurophysiol. 2002;87:3070–89.
41. Farley CT, McMahon TA. Energetics of walking and running: insights from simulated reduced-gravity experiments. J Appl Physiol. 1992;73:2709–12.
42. Smoliga JM, Wirfel LA, Paul D, Doarnberger M, Ford KR. Effects of unweighting and speed on in-shoe regional loading during running on a lower body positive pressure treadmill. J Biomech. 2015;48:1950–6.
43. Hunter I, Seeley MK, Hopkins JT, Carr C, Franson JJ. EMG activity during positive-pressure treadmill running. J Electromyogr Kinesiol. 2014;24:348–52.
44. Chang YH, Kram R. Metabolic cost of generating horizontal forces during human running. J Appl Physiol. 1999;86:1657–62.
45. Yates J, Mohney L, Abel M, Shapiro R. Effect of unweighting using the Alter-G trainer on VO2, heart rate and perceived exertion. Med Sci Sports Exerc. 2011;43:779.

16

Hypothalamic-Pituitary-Adrenal (HPA) Axis Functioning in Overtraining Syndrome: Findings from Endocrine and Metabolic Responses on Overtraining Syndrome (EROS)—EROS-HPA Axis

Flavio A. Cadegiani* and Claudio E. Kater

Abstract

Background: Overtraining syndrome (OTS) results from excessive training load without adequate recovery and leads to decreased performance and fatigue. The pathophysiology of OTS in athletes is not fully understood, which makes accurate diagnosis difficult. Previous studies indicate that alterations in the hypothalamus-pituitary-adrenal (HPA) axis may be responsible for OTS; however, the data is not conclusive. This study aimed to compare, through gold standard and exercise-independent tests, the response of the HPA axis in OTS-affected athletes (OTS group) to healthy physically active subjects (ATL group) and healthy non-active subjects (NCS group).

Methods: Selected subjects were evaluated for cortisol response to a 250-μg cosyntropin stimulation test (CST), cortisol and adrenocorticotropic hormone (ACTH) responses during an insulin tolerance test (ITT), and salivary cortisol rhythm (SCR).

Results: A total of 51 subjects were included (OTS, $n = 14$; ATL, $n = 25$; and NCS, $n = 12$). Cortisol response in the CST was similar among the three groups. Conversely, mean cortisol response during an ITT was significantly higher in ATL (21.7 μg/dL; increase = 9.2 μg/dL) compared to OTS (17.9 μg/dL; 6.3 μg/dL) and NCS (16.9 μg/dL; 6.0 μg/dL) ($p \leq 0.001$; $p = 0.01$). Likewise, median ACTH response during an ITT was significantly higher in ATL (91.4 pg/mL; increase = 45.1 pg/mL) compared to OTS (30.3 pg/mL; 9.7 pg/mL) and NCS (51.4 pg/mL; 38.0 pg/mL) ($p = 0.006$; $p = 0.004$). For SCR, mean cortisol 30 min after awakening was significantly higher in ATL (500 ng/dL) compared to OTS (323 ng/dL) and NCS (393 ng/dL) ($p = 0.004$). We identified the following cutoffs that could help exclude or confirm OTS: cortisol level at 30 min after awakening (exclusion = > 530 ng/dL); cortisol response to ITT (exclusion = > 20.5 μg/dL; confirmation = < 17 μg/dL or increase < 9.5 μg/dL); and ACTH response (exclusion = > 106 pg/mL or increase > 70 pg/mL; confirmation = < 35 pg/mL and increase < 14.5 pg/mL).

Conclusion: The findings of the present study showed that healthy athletes disclose adaptions to exercises that helped improve sport-specific performance, whereas this sort of hormonal conditioning was at least partially lost in OTS, which may explain the decrease in performance in OTS.

Keywords: Overtraining syndrome, Sports endocrinology, Hypothalamus-pituitary-adrenal axis, Hormones

* Correspondence: superendocrinology@gmail.com
Adrenal and Hypertension Unit, Division of Endocrinology and Metabolism, Department of Medicine, Escola Paulista de Medicina, Universidade Federal de São Paulo (EPM/UNIFESP), R. Pedro de Toledo 781 – 13th floor, São Paulo, SP 04039-032, Brazil

Key-points

- The hypothalamus-pituitary-adrenal (HPA) axis response to ITT are exacerbated in healthy athletes, compared to sedentary healthy subjects. ITT may be a tool to evaluate whether the athlete is well-conditioned and to predict performance, once the exacerbation of the HPA axis responses may play an important role in the progressive improvement in sports performance.
- There are intrinsic dysfunctions of the HPA axis response to a stress situation in OTS-affected athletes, compared to healthy athletes, in an independent way from exercise-induced stimulation; the dysfunctions of the HPA axis are located in the hypothalamus and the pituitary, and not the adrenals. In case an athlete is suspected for OTS, an ITT stimulation test may be performed. In the absence of confounding diseases, blunted cortisol and ACTH responses most likely confirm the diagnosis of OTS, with accurate cutoffs.
- Two new concepts were unprecedentedly demonstrated by the study. The first new concept is that physical activity, at least moderate-to-intense, elicits conditioning effects of hormonal responses to stimulation that goes beyond exercise, which we called as "hormonal conditioning of the athlete". Besides helping explain the improvement in the sports performance, the novel conditioning process found by our study may be the missing link for the understanding of the underlying mechanisms of the improvement observed in several responses to harmful situations, such as infections, neoplasms, traumas, inflammations, and psychiatric conditions that are observed in athletes, and which were not fully understood so far. The second concept is that whereas healthy athletes seem to present hormonal conditioning adaptions, those affected by overtraining seem to have impaired or maladapted hormonal conditioning, as over-trained athletes have a blunted optimized hormone response to stress that seem to be acquired by athletes; as a sort of deconditioning process, which indicates that the decreased performance and the reduced time-to-fatigue observed during OTS; these two key features of OTS, not yet fully understood, may be at least partly explained by the present findings.

Despite these unprecedented findings, further studies are recommended to confirm our results.

Background

The combination of excessive training load and lack of adequate recovery can lead to a decrease in sport-specific performance associated with fatigue, termed overtraining syndrome (OTS). Similar states that are related to OTS include functional overreaching (FOR) and non-functional overreaching (NFOR), which differ in terms of the duration of the signs and symptoms and in performance after recovery [1].

Improper recovery, low calorie intake, social problems, and excessive progression in training volume and intensity are the key triggers of OTS and correlate states. An inhospitable environment resulted from the inability to recover from intense energy demands induced an extensive dysfunctional adaption (maladaptation) with consequent abnormal responses of multiple markers [1].

As OTS and related states can affect 15–60% of elite athletes [1], and there are a growing number of high performance athletes, understanding the pathophysiology of OTS is essential [1–3]. As OTS is a diagnosis of exclusion, it is important to screen for inflammatory, metabolic, hormonal, psychiatric, and infectious conditions that could be the primary reason of decrease in sports performance [1–4].

Among some proposed biomarkers for diagnosis of OTS, impaired hormonal responses to stressful tests induced by maximal exercise have been reported [1–9], although further reproduction of the findings is recommended. With regard to the likely cause of the impaired hormonal responses, chronic exposure to stress could decrease the responsiveness of hypothalamic pituitary adrenal (HPA) axis [1, 4, 7–12]. Other alterations of the HPA axis were related to fatigue states and could be helpful for the diagnosis of OTS, such as a decreased cortisol awakening response (CAR) [13–17], which is an expected physiological increase in cortisol levels upon waking, and altered salivary cortisol rhythm [13, 14]. A decrease in CAR does not necessarily indicate impaired HPA axis function, but more likely worsened sleep, which is one of the features of OTS [1, 3, 12–30].

The impaired hormonal response to exercise-induced stress reported in previous studies [7–9] may result from impaired signaling from the musculoskeletal and cardiovascular systems to the HPA axis, rather than a decreased responsiveness of the glands. Moreover, in a recent systematic review [3], we learned that none of the previous studies were performed with gold standard functional tests, which are standardized to identify hormones at the primary site of the dysfunction caused by OTS (that is, the changes are not due to a lack of external signaling).

In this study, we performed a complete evaluation of the HPA axis at different levels by employing gold standard stimulation tests that are independent of exercises to ensure the hormone findings are the primary responses. The present study also aimed to correlate other cortisol findings [18–27] with OTS and to find new criteria for OTS.

Methods

A detailed description of the materials and methods and the raw data can be found elsewhere [31], but the inclusion and exclusion criteria, study design, questionnaire, and tests performed in this study are described below.

Inclusion and Exclusion Criteria

Subjects were recruited through social media (Facebook and Instagram) and contacted by the main researcher (FAC) and were required to be male, have present body mass index (BMI) of 20.0–32.9 kg/m^2 (for athletes) and 20.0–30.0 kg/m^2 (for non-athletes), and be 18–50 years old, who do not present previous psychiatric disorders, do not use any centrally acting drugs, or have not used any hormonal therapy in the previous 6 months. This was phase 1 of the inclusion criteria.

A minimum amount of physical activity was required from athletes, as specified in the EROS study methodology manuscript [31]. In particular, a minimum of four sessions and 300 min of moderate-to-intensive training per week was required, at a training level typical for professional competition, and at least 6 months of continuous training. In addition, the subject must be referred to as an athlete by a professional coach.

Volunteers suspected of OTS were required to disclose underperformance of at least 10% of reduction of the previous performance, as confirmed by a sports-related coach that regularly follows the athlete, unexplained by conditions that could lead to reduction in performance including infections (particularly Epstein-Barr), inflammation, overt hormonal dysfunctions (that would be the primary cause of the decreased performance), and psychosocial or psychiatric conditions, whose exclusion of the confounding conditions was performed by the main researcher (FAC). For inclusion in the OTS group, athletes must show persistent fatigue, an increased sense of effort in trainings that required less effort prior to the OTS, worsening in sleep quality (this criteria was not obligatory), and fulfill the recommended protocol for diagnosis of OTS proposed by the most recent guidelines on OTS [1].

Remaining subjects then underwent biochemical examination (phase 2 of the inclusion process). Subjects were to show levels within the normal range to be included in this study, in order to prevent confounding diagnosis.

Design of the Study

All selected subjects signed a written informed consent for participation in the study, approved by the ethics committee of the Federal University of São Paulo.

In the EROS-HPA axis arm of the study, we evaluated peripheral and central components of the HPA axis (primary or peripheral: adrenal; central: pituitary and hypothalamus), with cosyntropin stimulation test, that directly evaluates adrenal responses to synthetic ACTH [32], insulin tolerance test (ITT), which evaluates the integrity of the HPA axis [33], and salivary cortisol rhythm, to identify patterns of the circadian rhythm of the cortisol [13–17].

Questionnaire

After the selection criteria, an initial private interview about training patterns was performed with the selected athletes (sedentary subjects were not assessed at this moment), as part of the EROS study (for all arms). The interview included questions regarding training intensity (self-evaluation and evaluation by a professional coach, on a scale from 0 to 10 compared to athletes of the same level of training) and time since starting training. Other questions asked in the interview included whether they worked or studied besides training, and if they did, how many hours they worked or studied per day (on average); self-referred libido (on a scale from 0 to 10 compared to libido 1 year prior to the questionnaire); details of food ingestion each day in the 7 days prior to the questionnaire (including number of calories per kilogram per day, grams of carbohydrates, proteins and fats per kilogram per day); and sleeping patterns (average duration of sleep, self-referred sleep quality on a scale from 0 to 10, and presence or absence of initial insomnia and terminal insomnia). For all athletes affected by OTS, questions regarding the average number of days to overcome the underperformance state and changes in sensitivity to heat or to coldness or in sleep quality was performed.

Testing of the HPA Axis

A sequence of tests was then performed in all subjects, including the cosyntropin stimulation test (CST), the insulin tolerance test (ITT), and the salivary cortisol rhythm (SCR).

Cosyntropin Stimulation Test (CST)

The cosyntropin (synthetic adrenocorticotropic hormone [ACTH]) stimulation test is performed with a synthetic ACTH in high doses (250 μg) in order to directly stimulate the adrenal glands.

For the CST, blood was collected (time 0) from the antecubital vein of all subjects at 8.00 AM, after 30 min of resting and 8 h of fasting, and 250 μg of cosyntropin was infused. Blood was then collected at 30 min (time 1) and 60 min (time 2) for analysis of cortisol response (that is, the cortisol increase in absolute levels [μg/dL] in response to the infusion of 250 μg of cosyntropin stimulation).

Insulin Tolerance Test (ITT)

We used a gold standard ITT to evaluate the intrinsic responsiveness and integrity of the HPA axis, since a normal response required absence of dysfunctions in all levels (hypothalamus, pituitary, and adrenals) of the HPA axis. With a normal CST response, any abnormality found in the ITT is located either in the hypothalamus or in the pituitary. Unlike exercise stimulation tests, whose hormone responses depend on external neuromuscular and cardiovascular signaling, an impaired hormone response to ITT means the dysfunction is truly located in the HPA axis.

Subjects performed the ITT 48 h after the CST, following the same protocol of fasting, arrival time, and resting period prior to the beginning of the ITT. Blood was initially collected (time 0), a dose of 0.1 IU/kg of regular insulin was infused intravenously and new blood was collected during hypoglycemia (time 1) and 30 min after (time 2). After the blood collection during hypoglycemia, 10 mL of 50% glucose solution was given intravenously, and high-glycemic index food was offered ad libitum. At all times, cortisol (μg/dL), ACTH (pg/mL), and glucose (mg/dL) were assessed, and absolute ACTH/cortisol ratio was calculated.

Due to the risk of ITT-induced severe hypoglycemia (unconsciousness), three doses of subcutaneous glucagon were available (GlucaGen HypoKit, 1 μg, NovoNordisk), as well as syringes containing 20 mL of 50% glucose solution and an automated external defibrillator (AED).

Salivary Cortisol Rhythm

After stimulation tests, we assessed salivary cortisol rhythm (SCR) as an attempt to reproduce previous findings in fatigue-related states studies [3, 15], as a potential marker of fatigue.

From 2 to 7 days after ITT, saliva was collected at the time of awakening, at 30 min after awakening, at 4 PM, and at 11 PM, and specific recommendations were provided. Saliva samples were collected by the subjects themselves, using laboratory kits provided by the researcher (FAC).

All hormones of the present study (salivary cortisol, serum cortisol, and serum ACTH) were analyzed by specific electrochemiluminescence assays using specific commercial kits at a laboratory, whereas serum glucose levels were analyzed by an enzymatic assay of hexokinase. Importantly, the 8 AM serum cortisol was collected at the same time, while salivary cortisol was collected at the awakening moment and 30 min later, regardless if, and for this reason, salivary and serum cortisol levels are not comparable.

Statistical Analysis

Statistical analysis was performed using IBM SPSS statistics 24 software (IBM, USA). Each parameter was compared among the three groups (OTS, ATL, and NCS), and pairwise tests were performed between OTS and ATL, OTS and NCS, and ATL and NCS, whenever $p < 0.05$. As none of the variables depend on other variables, main and interaction effects were not evaluated (cortisol levels at a certain time do not reflect the ACTH levels at the same time).

Criteria for normal distribution was evaluated using Kolgomogorov–Sminorv test. Whenever normal distribution criteria were met, one-way ANOVA tests were performed, whereas when results were not normally distributed, Kruskal-Wallis tests (nonparametric ANOVA tests) were performed. Adjusted Dunn's test, Dunnett's T3, and Tukey analyses were performed when differences were statistically significant between the three groups ($p < 0.05$), according to the normality criteria.

Results

Baseline Characteristics and Training Patterns of the Study Participants

From the 146 initially recruited subjects, 51 subjects were included in the study (34.2%), and divided in three different groups, of OTS-affected athletes (OTS group; $n = 14$), healthy athletes (ATL group; $n = 25$), and healthy but physically non-active control subjects (normal control subjects [NCS]; $n = 12$). All athletes performed both resistive and endurance exercises, and all the training patterns were similar between OTS and ATL. All OTS were classified as OTS (and not FOR or NFOR) due to their prolonged recovery time.

Regarding the baseline characteristics, the average age (OTS = 30.6 years, ATL = 32.7 years, and NCS = 33.2 years) and average BMI (OTS = 26.7 kg/m^2, ATL = 24.9 kg/m^2, and NCS = 33.2 kg/m^2) were statistically similar among the groups. In addition, the average number of minutes of training per week (OTS = 574.3 min and ATL = 550.0 min), mean training intensity (OTS = 8.79 and ATL = 8.76, on a scale from 0 to 10), and number of training days per week (OTS = 5.36 days and ATL = 5.46 days) were similar between the two groups of athletes.

Basal Hormone Levels

As summarized in Tables 1, 2, and 3, basal serum hormone levels of OTS are within the normal range, and similar to ATL and to NCS, as previously observed [1–4, 6–9, 17–29, 34–36].

Evaluation of the Adrenal Gland—Cosyntropin Stimulation Test (CST)

As summarized in Table 1, cortisol response to 250 μg cosyntropin stimulation disclosed a normal and comparable responses between OTS, ATL, and NCS. The normal cortisol responses observed in the OTS-affected athletes confirm that adrenals are unimpaired in the OTS [33].

Table 1 Mean (±SD) basal serum cortisol and response to a cosyntropin stimulation test (CST) with 250 μg of synthetic ACTH

Cortisol response to CST (μg/dL)	OTS athletes	Healthy athletes	Sedentary
Basal	13.1 (± 4.1)	12.1 (± 3.2)	12.1 (± 5.7)
30	19.1 (± 1.9)	19.7 (± 2.4)	19.7 (± 3.2)
60′	21.9 (± 2.4)	22.2 (± 2.9)	22.9 (± 4.4)

All comparison/analyses were not significant
SD = Standard deviation

Evaluation of the HPA Axis—ITT

While basal cortisol levels were similar among the three groups, cortisol levels were higher in the ATL during and 30 min after hypoglycemia compared to the OTS and NCS. The mean cortisol increase was higher in the ATL compared to the OTS and NCS (Table 2 and Fig. 1).

At 30 min after hypoglycemia, seven (85.7%) OTS, five (20%) ATL, and nine (75%) NCS showed cortisol levels < 18 μg/dL. A cortisol peak of < 17 μg/dL in response to hypoglycemia was reached by four (28.6%) OTS, none of ATL, and eight (66.7%) NCS. Cortisol levels of > 20.5 μg/dL in response to hypoglycemia were found in none of OTS, 15 (60%) ATL, and three (25%) NCS. A cutoff of 19.1 μg/dL disclosed the highest accuracy (84.6%) to distinct ATL from OTS, although was not precise for neither confirmation nor exclusion of OTS. Furthermore, a cortisol increase of > 9.5 μg/dL was not observed in any OTS, but was found in 15 (60%) ATL and two (16.7%) NCS. A cortisol response of < 17.0 μg/dL at 30 min after the peak of hypoglycemia in the ITT seems to be a reliable cutoff to help confirm the diagnosis of OTS with a likely high positive predictive value when evaluated in athletes. Conversely, a cortisol response of > 20.5 μg/dL and a cortisol increase of > 9.5 μg/dL during the ITT seems to have a high negative predictive value (100%) according to our findings. Whereas ATL displayed a prompt cortisol response to hypoglycemia, OTS and NCS exhibited a delayed cortisol response.

Basal ACTH and ACTH during hypoglycemia were similar between the three groups (Table 3). However, the late increase of ACTH was higher in the ATL compared to the OTS (Fig. 2). Meanwhile, the median ACTH levels 30 min after hypoglycemia in the NCS were lower than in the ATL and higher than in the OTS, although the differences were not statistically significant, whereas ACTH increase was higher in the ATL than the OTS (Fig. 3).

An ACTH peak of > 46 pg/mL was observed in three OTS (21.4%), in 18 ATL (72%), and in eight NCS (66.7%); there is a cluster of blunted ACTH response to ITT among OTS including 78.6% of subjects. ACTH were < 35 pg/mL in nine (57.1%) OTS, in three (12%) ATL, and in four (33.3%) NCS, with an accuracy of 80% to distinct OTS. Conversely, ACTH peak > 106 pg/mL was observed in only one OTS (an outlier) whereas it was observed in eight ATL (32%).

Two (14.3%) OTS, 14 (56%) ATL, and seven (58.3%) NCS showed a > 34 pg/mL increase in absolute ACTH levels. Meanwhile, no OTS, 10 (40%) ATL, and three (25%) NCS showed a > 70 pg/mL increase in ACTH. The highest accuracy was found for a cutoff of 20 pg/mL (77.0%), although imprecise to determine the absence or presence of OTS.

Based on our results, an ACTH response of > 106 pg/mL seems to be highly predictive of exclusion of OTS, whereas an ACTH response of < 35 pg/mL increases the likelihood of the diagnosis of OTS. Despite the highly variable ACTH increase levels, an increase of > 70 μg/dL could be useful to exclude OTS, whereas blunted ACTH increase was only observed in OTS and NCS.

In a subgroup of the ATL, ACTH and cortisol were also performed 60 min after hypoglycemia, and disclosed lower levels than 30 min, and therefore were not measured in the remaining subjects.

During the ITT, ACTH/cortisol ratio was similar between groups basally and during hypoglycemia, but was significantly lower in the OTS group compared to the ATL ($p = 0.024$) and NCS ($p = 0.018$) groups (Table 4).

Table 2 Mean (±SD) basal serum cortisol and response to insulin tolerance test (ITT)

Cortisol response to ITT (μg/dL)	OTS athletes (OTS) ($n = 14$)	Healthy athletes (ATL) ($n = 25$)	Non-active subjects (NCS) ($n = 12$)
Basal	11.6 (± 2.5)	12.5 (± 3.1)	10.9 (± 2.8)
During hypoglycemia	12.4* (± 3.3)	15.9$^{\&}$ (± 5.3)	11.8 (± 3.1)
30′ after hypoglycemia	17.9*** (± 2.9)	21.7$^{\&\&\&\&}$ (± 3.1)	16.9 (± 4.1)
Absolute increase from basal to 30 min after hypoglycemia	6.3** (± 2.3)	9.2$^{\&}$ (± 3.7)	5.9 (± 3.9)

Differences between OTS and ATL: $^{*}p < 0.05$; $^{**}p < 0.01$; $^{***}p < 0.005$
Differences between ATL and NCS: $^{\&}p < 0.05$; $^{\&\&\&\&}p < 0.001$
SD standard deviation

Table 3 Median (95% CI) ACTH response to insulin tolerance test (ITT)

ACTH response to ITT (pg/mL)	OTS athletes (OTS) ($n = 14$)	Healthy athletes (ATL) ($n = 25$)	Non-active subjects (NCS) ($n = 12$)	p
Basal	19.6 (11.4–32.9)	18.7 (6.5–37.8)	21.4 (8.7–37.8)	n/s
During hypoglycemia	28.2 (8.4–238.9)	57.8 (7.3–229.5)	29.5 (14.8–191.7)	n/s
30′ after hypoglycemia	30.3**** (9.8–93.7)	59.9 (22.1–195.7)	51.4 (22.7–137.5)	*0.006*
Absolute increase	9.7**** (−14.4–64.4)	45.1 (22.1–195.7)	38.0 (0.5–108.8)	*0.004*
Percentage increase (%)	52.2	266.2	200.4	– n/a

Differences between OTS and ATL: ****$p < 0.001$
Level of significance = $p < 0.05$
CI confidence interval; *n/s* = non significant; *n/a* = non appliable

Glucose levels were similar initially and during hypoglycemia between groups, reinforcing the equality of conditions of the ITT and foreclosing differences due to the intensity of hypoglycemia.

Salivary Cortisol Rhythm (SCR)

SCR was assessed in 23 of the 25 ATL and in all OTS and NCS. SCR was similar among groups, although ATL presents exacerbated and significant elevation on 30 min after awakening compared to OTS and NCS (Table 5 and Fig. 4). Conversely, CAR, awakening, 4 PM, and 11 PM salivary cortisol levels were similar between OTS, ATL, and SED. Although CAR was higher in ATL, it did not achieve statistical significance.

A cutoff of 370 ng/dL has a high accuracy (80%) but is not reliable to exclude or confirm OTS. Conversely, higher salivary cortisol levels (> 530 ng/dL) were not observed in any of the OTS and in only one NCS, whereas they were observed in majority of ATL (12 of 22; 59.1%), and therefore we suggest that a cutoff of > 530 ng/dL may be a tool to reinforce the exclusion of OTS (Fig. 4).

Discussion

Results

This study examined the role of the HPA axis in OTS. To learn whether the differences in hormone responses between OTS and ATL resulted from a physiological adaptation to sports (which has not been analyzed in previous studies) or from dysfunctional OTS responses, we included two control groups, of healthy athletes and healthy non-active subjects. Overall, we found that OTS have blunted hormonal responses compared to ATL, but not to NCS, whereas ATL showed more exacerbated responses than NCS. It means that athletes affected by OTS do not disclose actual dysfunctional responses, as hormonal responses were not different from normal non-active control subjects, but nullifies the likely adaptive hormonal responses observed in healthy athletes, as healthy athletes disclosed different responses compared to sedentary control subjects, whereas the different responses compared to NCS were not observed when compared to OTS-affected subjects. This means that the different responses, a likely adaptive process observed in healthy athletes, are nullified when OTS is present.

While CST reflects the adrenal status, ITT discloses the integrity of the entire HPA axis. As the adrenals

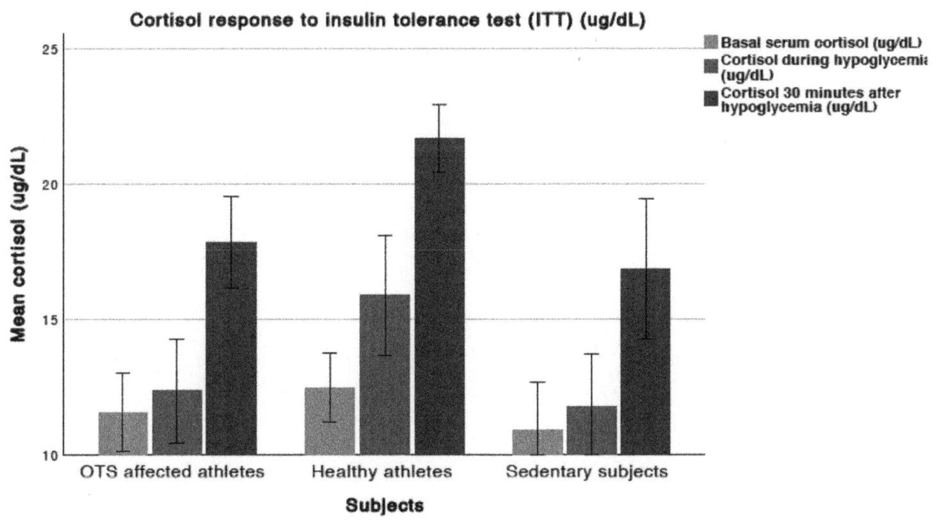

Fig. 1 Cortisol response to an ITT

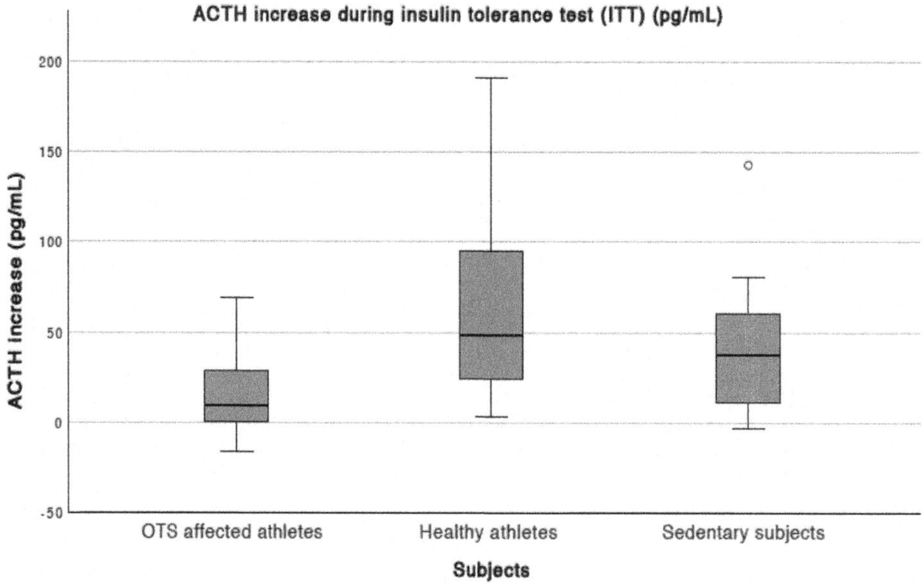

Fig. 2 Median and CI (P5-P95) ACTH increase in response to an ITT

responded normally in the abovementioned ACTH stimulation test, any abnormality found at the ITT must be located centrally (either in the hypothalamus or in the pituitary). Moreover, as the ITT directly stimulates the glands of the HPA axis (whose pathway of stimulation is the hypothalamus, then the pituitary, and then the adrenal glands, in this order), any alterations in responses due to differences in signaling coming from the neuromuscular and cardiovascular systems are abolished. Finally, the response to hypoglycemia does not depend on sports capacity and conditioning, and therefore, impaired hormone responses to ITT show a truly impaired HPA axis.

Indeed, differences in cortisol and ACTH responses were observed between groups, suggesting differences in the HPA axis responsivity to stressful situations. However, instead of the presence of dysfunctional impaired responses in OTS, exacerbated and hastened responses were observed in ATL, compared to NCS and OTS, for both ACTH and cortisol, whereas basal levels were similar among groups. Basal cortisol and ACTH levels tended to be normal in OTS, as reported by previous studies [1, 3, 6, 9–12],

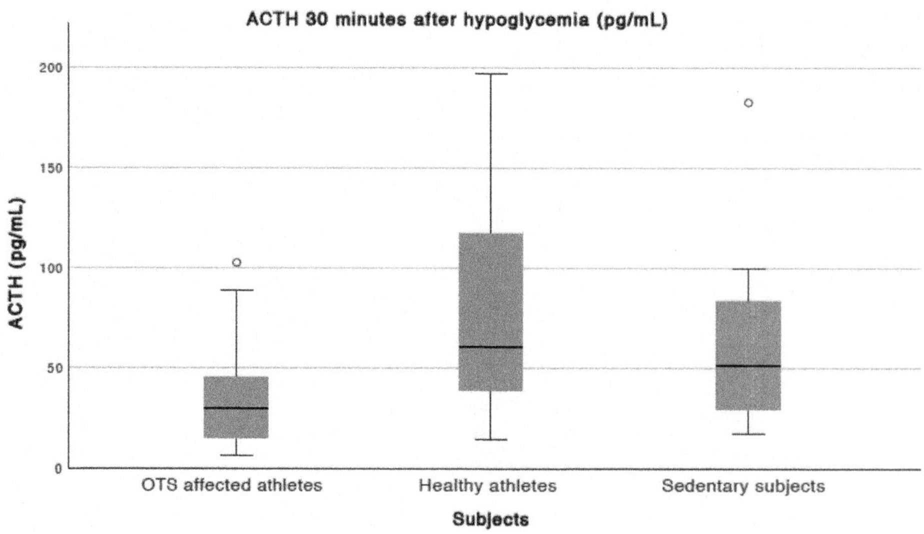

Fig. 3 Median and CI (P5-P95) plasma ACTH 30 min after hypoglycemia, in response to an ITT

Table 4 Median (p95 confidence interval) ACTH/cortisol ratios during insulin tolerance test (ITT)

ACTH/cortisol ratio	OTS athletes (OTS) ($n = 14$)	Healthy athletes (ATL) ($n = 25$)	Non-active subjects (NCS) ($n = 12$)	*p*
Basal	184.9 (90.8–332.5)	141.5 (77.4–270.1)	178.0 (91.9–347.3)	n/s
During hypoglycemia	252.3 (77.1–1312.1)	363.5 (111.3–1421.3)	332.9 (122.0–1976.3)	n/s
30′ after hypoglycemia	156.0* (60.4–598.0)	286.2& (96.6–986.5)	321.9 (146.3–723.6)	*0.03*

Differences between OTS and ATL: *$p < 0.05$
Differences between ATL and NCS: &$p < 0.05$
CI confidence interval

although some studies reported either reduced [23] or increased levels [34]; contrariwise, stimulated cortisol and ACTH levels showed predominantly reduced levels [1, 3, 7–9], which is corroborated by us.

Despite the higher cortisol in the ATL during hypoglycemia, the valuable point of cortisol is actually 30 min after the hypoglycemia event, due to the delay between ACTH stimulation and consequent cortisol release. Cortisol levels were already higher during hypoglycemia likely to the fact that the reduction in glucose levels and consequent ACTH stimulation began minutes before the hypoglycemia event. Although ACTH was not statistically higher during hypoglycemia in the ATL, the mean and median of ACTH levels were substantially increased compared to OTS and NCS. The reduced ACTH/cortisol ratio observed in the OTS group 30 min after hypoglycemia reflects the blunted ACTH levels observed in the OTS-affected athletes at this time. However, a reduced ACTH/cortisol ratio does not provide additional information in regard to a supposed level of sensitivity of the adrenal glands to the ACTH stimulation, as ACTH levels cannot be correlated with the cortisol levels of the same time [13, 32].

If we followed the adrenal criteria of < 18 μg/dL as relative adrenal insufficiency [33], the majority of OTS and NCS would be considered as affected, although we modified the ITT protocol after the hypoglycemic episode to prevent severe hypoglycemia [37, 38]. Importantly, the relative adrenal insufficiency is only found during a stimulation test and does not bring about the typical risks of the classical and frank primary adrenal insufficiency that can be diagnosed by elevated basal serum ACTH levels and reduced basal serum cortisol levels [33].

We did not perform the 60 min cortisol after hypoglycemia as we initially performed with some athletes ($n = 13$) and cortisol levels did not disclose increased responses between 30 and 60 min.

Furthermore, previous studies hypothesized that OTS was characterized by alterations in the sensitivity of the HPA axis [1, 7–11]. Therefore, the ACTH/cortisol ratio would be altered in OTS-affected athletes. We found the ACTH/cortisol ratio basally, during hypoglycemia, and 30 min after hypoglycemia was similar among the three groups at all times. While our results seem to invalidate the theory regarding the hyposensitivity of the HPA axis in OTS, an altered ACTH/cortisol ratio does not indicate a difference in response in the HPA axis, as the process of releasing ACTH to stimulate cortisol release can take a few minutes. Therefore, the cortisol level at a certain time point does not reflect the ACTH level at that same moment.

The loss of circadian rhythm of the cortisol release can be a feature of fatigue-related disorders, as previously described [13–17], although causality of adrenal impairment has not been demonstrated. However, an intact cortisol rhythm was observed in all subjects, regardless of the group. Nonetheless, an exacerbated cortisol awakening increase was observed in ATL, although CAR was not statistically significant due to high variation of the results. However, if there were three times more subjects, with the same median and confidence interval, statistical significance would be achieved for the CAR. The significant difference was found at 30 min after awakening and seemed to be a reliable marker of sports conditioning, whose adaption showed to disappear when OTS is present.

Table 5 Mean and SD of salivary cortisol rhythm

Salivary cortisol (ng/dL)	OTS athletes (OTS) ($n = 14$)	Healthy athletes (ATL) ($n = 25$)	Non-active subjects (NCS) ($n = 12$)
Awakening	329 (± 222)	337 (± 131)	266 (± 149)
30′ after awakening	324*** (± 116)	500& (± 168)	393 (± 149)
4 PM	166 (± 113)	144 (± 83)	130 (± 57)
11 PM	94 (± 39)	95 (± 38)	83 (± 11)
Cortisol awakening response (CAR) %	32.4	62.2	79.08

Differences between OTS and ATL: ***$p < 0.005$;
Differences between ATL and NCS: &$p < 0.05$
SD standard deviation

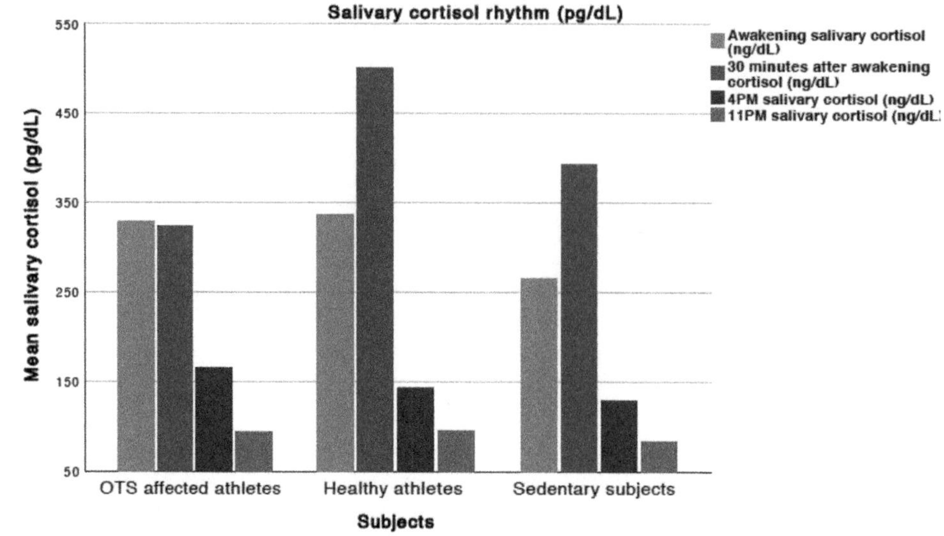

Fig. 4 Salivary cortisol rhythm

The Hormonal Deconditioning Effect of OTS

It has been previously proposed that hypersensitivity of the HPA axis (during the beginning of the overtraining state process) followed by a progression to insensitivity is involved in OTS [1, 7, 8]. However, our results suggest that the hyposensitive HPA axis is only observed when compared to healthy athletes. We found the cortisol response to hypoglycemia was significantly higher among healthy athletes than OTS and NCS. This shows that the improvement in HPA axis sensitivity in athletes is loss during OTS, and not that OTS presents any frank dysfunctions, as OTS discloses similar responses compared to the general population (i.e., non-active healthy subjects with same age, gender, and BMI). Furthermore, while cortisol response was observed 30 min after hypoglycemia in OTS, it is unlikely that any further increased cortisol levels (at any time after 30 min) would be sustained, as ACTH (the major stimulator of cortisol release) levels were reduced at 30 min after hypoglycemia at this group.

In summary, all the findings of the present study, including cortisol and ACTH responses to ITT and salivary cortisol 30 min after awakening, seemed to be positive adaptions to exercises in healthy athletes (in the absence of OTS) that helped improve sport-specific performance, and for some reason, this hormonal conditioning (which were the positive adaptions to exercises) was at least partially lost in OTS, which may explain the decrease in performance in OTS.

As healthy athletes disclosed optimized HPA axis responses to hypoglycemia compared to sedentary individuals, we suggest that there is a possible hyperresponsivity of the HPA axis in athletes (as an adaption or conditioning response) that can be expressed independently of exercise.

Correlations Between Findings with Clinical Features of OTS

Besides fatigue and underperformance, a key feature of OTS is the inability to sustain a sport-specific performance capacity throughout an intensive training session [1–4, 39, 40]. OTS-affected athletes are usually able to perform normally in the beginning of the training load, but are not able to complete at the expected pace (i.e., OTS-affected subjects tend to fatigue too early compared to healthy athletes). We found a similar early increase in ACTH levels among all three groups, but an early fall in ACTH levels among OTS-affected athletes, with especially blunted ACTH levels at 30 min after hypoglycemia. These findings (normal early ACTH increase with late blunted levels) may at least partly explain the reduced time-to-fatigue found in athletes affected by OTS. Indeed, ACTH and cortisol are two fundamental hormones required to sustain performance and pace in any sport. (Thus, as the integrity of the HPA axis is required throughout training to maintain performance, a shortened response duration of the HPA axis in OTS-affected athletes would affect sustained performance).

Suggestions of Cutoffs for Biochemical Diagnosis of OTS

While the number of subjects included in this study was small, we were able to suggest helpful cutoffs for the diagnosis or exclusion of OTS due to a number of factors. First, the number of subjects of the present study is significantly higher than previous studies [3]. Second, the diagnosis of OTS was strictly performed (without confounding bias), and therefore all 14 OTS presented real OTS. Finally, the hormone levels were markedly different between OTS and ATL, with few overlapping results in most findings. A summary of the possible cutoffs to help confirm or exclude OTS are described in Table 6.

Table 6 Proposed cutoffs for overtraining syndrome

	Suggested cutoffs	Practical application
Salivary cortisol (ng/dL) 30 min after awakening	> 530 ng/dL	Highly predictable of exclusion of OTS (93.9%).
	370 ng/dL	Highly accurate (80%), but unable to help diagnosis OTS
Serum cortisol (μg/dL) 30 min after hypoglycemia in ITT	> 20.5 μg/dL	High negative predictive value for OTS (100%)
	> 17.0 μg/dL	High positive predictive value for OTS, although not specific (28.6%)
	19.1 μg/dL	High accuracy (84.6%), but not precise for confirmation or exclusion of OTS
Cortisol increase during ITT (μg/dL)	> 9.5 μg/dL	100% specific to exclude OTS
Plasma ACTH (pg/mL) 30 min after hypoglycemia in ITT	> 106 pg/mL	High negative predictive value (92.9%) and highly accurate (80%)
ACTH increase during ITT (pg/mL)	< 35 pg/mL	80% accurate to distinguish OTS from ATL

Final Discussion

In summary, to the best of our knowledge, this is the first study on the endocrine system in OTS to (1) demonstrate that there are intrinsic dysfunctions of the HPA axis response to a stress situation in OTS-affected athletes, compared to healthy athletes; (2) demonstrate that the hypothalamus and the pituitary, and not the adrenals, are likely responsible for the changes in the cortisol response in an independent way from exercise-induced stimulation; (3) show that salivary cortisol levels 30 min after awakening are blunted in OTS-affected subjects, which may be a reliable marker of OTS; (4) propose useful cutoffs of salivary cortisol, and cortisol and ACTH responses to ITT, as an additional tool to help exclude or confirm OTS; (5) demonstrate that overtrained athletes have a blunted optimized hormone response to *training stress*; and (6) *indicate* that reduced time-to-fatigue, a key feature of OTS, not yet fully understood, seems to be at least partly explained by the present findings.

The main limitations of the present study are as follows: (1) the small number of subjects, due to the excluded subjects when strict criteria was used (but still larger compared to previous studies) and (2) a high variability and the lack of normal distribution observed in ACTH responses, which typically occurs in tests with ACTH responses, but challenges the statistical interpretation.

Moreover, the presence of outliers reinforces the individuality of overtraining syndrome presentation in each athlete, which leads to distinct responses to different tests. Also, as all athletes were considered as OTS in this study (that is, the prolonged *overtraining* state), it is unclear whether the changes could be found earlier in OTS, in the functioning and non-functioning *overreaching* states.

Conclusions

Whereas healthy athletes seem to present hormonal conditioning adaptions, those affected by overtraining seem to have impaired or maladapted hormonal conditioning, which may explain the decreased performance observed during OTS, as a sort of deconditioning process. Our findings allowed us to suggest useful cutoff values for the 30 min after awakening cortisol, cortisol and ACTH 30 min after hypoglycemia, and cortisol and ACTH increase during the ITT to help exclude or confirm diagnosis of OTS. Despite these unprecedented findings, further studies are recommended to confirm our results.

Abbreviations

ACTH: Adrenocorticotropic hormone; ATL: Healthy athletes group; CBG: Cortisol-binding globulin; CST: Cosyntropin stimulation test; EROS: Endocrine and Metabolic Responses on Overtraining Syndrome; ITT: Insulin tolerance test; NCS: Normal control subjects; OTS: Overtraining syndrome; SCR: Salivary cortisol rhythm

Acknowledgements

We acknowledge the support of the team of Sports Medicine and Endocrinology Departments of Federal University of São Paulo, who helped to design the most appropriate methods to assess OTS athletes and to improve the inclusion and exclusion criteria.
We also acknowledge the DASA Laboratórios da América that provided all the biochemical material and personal staff to help perform the tests, and Corpometria Institute, that provided all the body metabolism and composition analysis.

Authors' Contributions

FAC performed the research, selection of subjects, performance of the tests, and analysis of the results and part of the discussions and conclusions. CEK participated in the design of the study and in the discussions and conclusions. FAC and CEK performed the discussion, the conclusions, and the design of the tables. Both authors read and approved the final manuscript.

Funding

Funding was not provided for the study, although the study has been non-financially funded by DASA and by Corpometria Institute.

Competing Interests

Flavio A. Cadegiani and Claudio E. Kater declare that they have no competing interests.

References

1. Meeusen R, Duclos M, Foster C, Fry A, Gleeson M, Nieman D, Raglin J, Rietjens G, Steinacker J, Urhausen A, European College of Sport Science; American College of Sports Medicine. Prevention, diagnosis, and treatment of the overtraining syndrome: joint consensus statement of the European College of Sport Science and the American College of Sports Medicine. Med Sci Sports Exerc. 2013 Jan;45(1):186–205.
2. Le Meur Y, Hausswirth C, Natta F, et al. A multidisciplinary approach to overreaching detection in endurance trained athletes. J Appl Physiol. 1 February 2013;114(3):411–20.
3. Nederhof E, Zwerver J, Brink M, Meeusen R, Lemmink K. Different diagnostic tools in nonfunctional overreaching. Int J Sports Med. 2008 Jul;29(7):590–7.
4. Lehmann M, Foster C, Keul J. Overtraining in endurance athletes: a brief review. Med Sci Sports Exerc. 1993;25(7):854–62.
5. Cadegiani FA, Kater CE. Hormonal aspects of overtraining syndrome: a systematic review. BMC Sports Sci Med Rehabil. 2017 Aug 2;9:14.
6. Thiel C, Vogt L, Bürklein M, Rosenhagen A, Hübscher M, Banzer W. Functional overreaching during preparation training of elite tennis professionals. J Hum Kinet. 2011 Jun;28:79–89.
7. Meeusen R, Nederhof E, Buyse L, Roelands B, De Schutter G, Piacentini MF. Diagnosing overtraining in athletes using the two-bout exercise protocol. Br J Sports Med. 2010;44(9):642–8.
8. Meeusen R, Piacentini MF, Busschaert B, Buyse L, De Schutter G, Stray-Gundersen J. Hormonal responses in athletes: the use of a two bout exercise protocol to detect subtle differences in (over)training status. Eur J Appl Physiol. 2004 Mar;91(2–3):140–6.
9. Urhausen A, Gabriel HH, Kindermann W. Impaired pituitary hormonal response to exhaustive exercise in overtrained endurance athletes. Med Sci Sports Exerc. 1998 Mar;30(3):407–14.
10. Barron G, Noakes T, Levy W, Smidt C, Millar R. Hypothalamic dysfunction in overtrained athletes. J Clin Endocrinol Metab. 1985;60:803–6. Cizza G, Kvetnansky R, Tartaglia M, Blackman M, Chrousos G,
11. Gold P. Immobolisation stress rapidly decreases hypothalamic corticotropin-releasing hormone secretion in vitro in the male 344/N Fischer rat. Life Sci. 1993;53:233–40.
12. Duclos M, Corcuff J-B, Arsac L, et al. Corticotroph axis sensitivity after exercise in endurance-trained athletes. Clin Endocrinol. 1998;8:493–501.
13. Cadegiani FA, Kater CE. Adrenal fatigue does not exist: a systematic review. BMC Endocr Disord. 2016 Aug 24;16(1):48.
14. Ryan R, Booth S, Spathis A, Mollart S, Clow A. Use of salivary diurnal cortisol as an outcome measure in randomised controlled trials: a systematic review. Ann Behav Med. 2016 Apr;50(2):210–36.
15. Stalder T, Kirschbaum C, Kudielka BM. Assessment of the cortisol awakening response: expert consensus guidelines. Psychoneuroendocrinology. 2016 Jan;63:414–32.
16. Oosterholt BG, Maes JH, Van der Linden D, Verbraak MJ, Kompier MA. Burnout and cortisol: evidence for a lower cortisol awakening response in both clinical and non-clinical burnout. J Psychosom Res. 2015 May; 78(5):445–51.
17. Powell DJ, Liossi C, Moss-Morris R, Schlotz W. Unstimulated cortisol secretory activity in everyday life and its relationship with fatigue and chronic fatigue syndrome: a systematic review and subset meta-analysis. Psychoneuroendocrinology. 2013 Nov;38(11):2405–22.
18. Slivka DR, Hailes WS, Cuddy JS, Ruby BC. Effects of 21 days of intensified training on markers of overtraining. J Strength Cond Res. 2010 Oct;24(10):2604–12.
19. Rietjens GJ, Kuipers H, Adam JJ, et al. Physiological, biochemical and psychological markers of strenuous training-induced fatigue. Int J Sports Med. 2005 Jan-Feb;26(1):16–26.
20. Coutts AJ, Reaburn P, Piva TJ, Rowsell GJ. Monitoring for overreaching in rugby league players. Eur J Appl Physiol. 2007 Feb;99(3):313–24.
21. Schmikli SL, de Vries WR, Brink MS, Backx FJ. Monitoring performance, pituitary-adrenal hormones and mood profiles: how to diagnose non-functional over-reaching in male elite junior soccer players. Br J Sports Med. 2012 Nov;46(14):1019–23.
22. Tanskanen MM, Kyröläinen H, Uusitalo AL, Huovinen J, Nissilä J, Kinnunen H, Atalay M, Häkkinen K. Serum sex hormone-binding globulin and cortisol concentrations are associated with overreaching during strenuous military training. J Strength Cond Res. 2011 Mar;25(3):787–97.
23. Kraemer WJ, French DN, Paxton NJ. Changes in exercise performance and hormonal concentrations over a big ten soccer season in starters and nonstarters. J Strength Cond Res. 2004 Feb;18(1):121–8.
24. Hug M, Mullis PE, Vogt M, Ventura N, Hoppeler H. Training modalities: over-reaching and over-training in athletes, including a study of the role of hormones. Best Pract Res Clin Endocrinol Metab. 2003 Jun;17(2):191–209.
25. Steinacker JM, Lormes W, Kellmann M, et al. Training of junior rowers before world championships. Effects on performance, mood state and selected hormonal and metabolic responses. J Sports Med Phys Fitness. 2000 Dec;40(4):327–35.
26. Fry AC, Kraemer WJ, Ramsey LT. Pituitary-adrenal-gonadal responses to high-intensity resistance exercise overtraining. J Appl Physiol (1985). 1998 Dec;85(6):2352–9.
27. Fry RW, Morton AR, Garcia-Webb P, Crawford GP, Keast D. Biological responses to overload training in endurance sports. Eur J Appl Physiol Occup Physiol. 1992;64(4):335–44.
28. Lehmann M, Gastmann U, Petersen KG, Bachl SA, Khalaf AN, Fischer S, Keul J. Training-overtraining: performance, and hormone levels, after a defined increase in training volume versus intensity in experienced middle- and long-distance runners. Br J Sports Med. 1992 December;26(4):233–42.
29. O'Connor PJ, Morgan WP, Raglin JS, Barksdale CM, Kalin NH. Mood state and salivary cortisol levels following overtraining in female swimmers. Psychoneuroendocrinology. 1989;14(4):303–10.
30. Barron LJ, Noakes TD, Levy W, Smith C, Millar RP. Hypothalamic dysfunction in overtrained athletes. J Clin Endocrinol Metab. 1985;60(4):803–6.
31. Cadegiani FA, Kater CE. Rationale, design, material, methods, subject selection and baseline characteristics of the Endocrine and Metabolic Responses on Overtraining Syndrome (EROS) study. Available at: https://osf.io/bhpq9/.
32. Ospina NS, Al Nofal A, Bancos I, Javed A, Benkhadra K, Kapoor E, et al. ACTH stimulation tests for the diagnosis of adrenal insufficiency: systematic review and meta-analysis. J Clin Endocrinol Metab. 2016;101(2):427–34.
33. Bornstein SR, Allolio B, Arlt W, Barthel A, Don-Wauchope A, Hammer GD, et al. Diagnosis and treatment of primary adrenal insufficiency: an endocrine society clinical practice guideline. J Clin Endocrinol Metab. 2016;101(2):364–89.
34. Roberts AC, McClure RD, Weiner RI, Brooks GA. Overtraining affects male reproductive status. Fertil Steril. 1993 Oct;60(4):686–92.
35. Bae YJ, Kratzsch J. Corticosteroid-binding globulin: modulating mechanisms of bioavailability of cortisol and its clinical implications. Best Pract Res Clin Endocrinol Metab. 2015 Oct;29(5):761–72.
36. Perogamyros I, Aarons L, Miller AG, Trainer PJ, Ray DW. Corticosteroid-binding globulin regulates cortisol pharmacokinetics. Clin Endocrinol. 2011 Jan;74(1):30–6.
37. Brooks K, Carter J. Overtraining, exercise and adrenal insufficiency. J Nov Physiother. 2013;3(125).
38. Angeli A, Minetto M, Dovio A, Paccotti P. The overtraining syndrome in athletes: a stress-related disorder. J Endocrinol Investig. 2004;27(6):603–12.
39. Urhausen A, Gabriel H, Kindermann W. Blood hormones as markers of training stress and overtraining. Sports Med. 1995;20:251–76.
40. Budgett R, Newsholme E, Lehmann M, et al. Redefining the overtraining syndrome as the unexplained underperformance syndrome. Br J Sports Med. 2000;34:67–8.

17

A Randomised, Placebo-Controlled, Crossover Study Investigating the Effects of Nicotine Gum on Strength, Power and Anaerobic Performance in Nicotine-Naïve, Active Males

Toby Mündel*, Marine Machal, Darryl J. Cochrane and Matthew J. Barnes

Abstract

Background: Nicotine use amongst athletes is high and increasing, especially team sports, yet the limited previous studies investigating the performance consequences of this behaviour have not examined the effects of the principal active ingredient, nicotine, per se. Therefore, we determined whether nicotine gum affected muscular and anaerobic performance.

Methods: Nine active males (24 ± 3 years) completed three trials in a random order in which 20 min prior to testing they chewed 2 mg (NIC-2), 4 mg (NIC-4) nicotine or flavour-matched placebo (PLA) gum. Peak and average peak isometric, concentric and eccentric leg extensor torque was measured followed by vertical counter-movement jump height and a 30-s Wingate test. Heart rate was measured whilst capillary blood samples determined pH, HCO_3^- and venous blood confirmed the presence of nicotine.

Results: Nicotine was confirmed by the presence of its major metabolite, cotinine and participants reported no side effects with nicotine. Peak and average peak isometric and eccentric torque was significantly affected (NIC-2 > PLA; $p < 0.05$) whilst peak (NIC-2 > PLA; $p < 0.05$) but not average peak ($p > 0.05$) concentric torque was different between trials. Counter-movement jump height was similar across trials ($p > 0.05$). Anaerobic capacity during the Wingate remained similar across trials ($p > 0.05$); however, pacing strategy (peak power and rate of fatigue) was different during NIC-2 than PLA. pH was affected by nicotine (NIC-2 > PLA; $p < 0.05$) and was reduced following the Wingate in all trials. HCO_3^- showed similar responses across trials ($p > 0.05$) although it was also reduced following the Wingate ($p < 0.05$), whilst heart rate was significantly affected (NIC-2/NIC-4 > PLA; $p < 0.05$).

Conclusions: Chewing low-dose (2 mg) nicotine gum 20 min prior to exercise significantly improved leg extensor torque but did not affect counter-movement jump height or Wingate performance compared to a placebo, whilst there were minimal effects of the 4 mg nicotine gum on the performance parameters measured.

Keywords: Chewing gum, Doping, Stimulant, Performance, WADA

* Correspondence: T.Mundel@massey.ac.nz
School of Sport and Exercise, Massey University, Private bag 11 222, Palmerston North 4442, New Zealand

Key Points

- Recent monitoring (urine screening) has determined that active consumption of nicotine and nicotine-containing substances in-competition occurs in approximately 25–50% of athletes in sports that are characterised by strength, power and anaerobic capacity (cf. endurance), e.g. American football, ice hockey, wrestling, bobsleigh, gymnastics, rugby and skiing.
- Whilst the World Anti-Doping Agency placed nicotine onto its monitoring program in 2012, few studies have determined the performance effects of nicotine administration, and none without the confounders of tobacco, withdrawal and tolerance.
- The current study has demonstrated that a low-dose (2 mg) nicotine gum increases leg extensor torque but counter-movement jump height and anaerobic capacity remained unchanged when compared to a placebo gum.
- These and our previous results indicate that nicotine per se can improve exercise endurance and muscular strength, and alongside patterns of (mis)use future studies should continue to practically and mechanistically determine the full extent of this under-researched stimulant in terms of performance enhancement and athlete health.

Background

The (ab)use of nicotine and nicotine-containing substances by athletes, especially by professional and elite status, is prevalent. For example, Marclay et al. [20] reported on a one-year monitoring study of 2185 urine samples from professional athletes in 43 different sport disciplines. Traces of nicotine and/or tobacco-related alkaloids were detected in 23% of the samples, with prevalence of "active" nicotine consumption (cf. passive environmental exposure) immediately prior to and/or during sport practice determined at 15% [20]. Of note, cumulative exposure of >25% (greater than the worldwide prevalence in the general population, as reported by the World Health Organization) was reported in American football (56%), ice hockey (32%), wrestling (32%), bobsleigh (31%), gymnastics (29%), rugby (28%) and skiing (26%). These findings were preceded by the alarming observation that approximately half of the athletes at the 2009 Ice Hockey World Championships were active nicotine consumers before and/or during games [21]. Therefore, the use of nicotine by athletes, regardless of its form (e.g. snuff, snus), is frequent across many sports and countries (e.g. [8, 22]).

Athletes' beliefs are that consumption of nicotine/smokeless tobacco proves ergogenic by preventing xerostomia [6], weight control [2], improving reaction time and concentration [13], helping relaxation and desirable arousal-attention [8]. These reports are supported by a meta-analysis determining that the stimulant effects of nicotine enhance aspects of cognition and attention, namely motor abilities, attention and memory [15]. The results are noteworthy as included studies were not confounded by nicotine's withdrawal effects, lack of a placebo control, patient group deficit or elderly decline in cognition and therefore likely represent true performance enhancement. However, there are reports that a dose–response relationship exists whereby lower doses prove nootropic whilst higher doses do not [25, 26], this is perhaps due to the known pharmacological and physiological action of low-dose nicotine as a central nervous system (CNS) stimulant whilst at high doses, a depressant or relaxant effect occurs [18, 28].

As the sports and athletes with the most use of nicotine concern strength, power and anaerobic events (see above), it follows that performance and research protocols reflect this. Previous research has shown no performance enhancement with smokeless tobacco use for leg extensor force and power [12], anaerobic performance [2, 27] or handgrip strength, counter-movement jump and agility [23]. However, smokeless tobacco includes many other ingredients that might confound results and the use of participants that are habitual users is confounded by withdrawal or tolerance effects, whether acute or chronic. In an effort to determine the actual performance effects of nicotine in an acute experimental setting, in the present study, nicotine-naïve participants received acute nicotine supplementation, as using this rationale, we and others have previously demonstrated physical and cognitive performance enhancement [15, 24] *despite* the oft-reported side effects [23, 24].

Nicotine was added to the World Anti-Doping Agency (WADA) Monitoring Program in 2012, indicating that WADA wished to detect patterns of misuse [29]. Concurrently, there should be an increased investigation focusing on whether nicotine can enhance performance and/or represents a health threat to athletes in order to inform WADA on whether nicotine should remain a monitored substance or even be upgraded to the List of Prohibited Substances. Therefore, the experimental hypothesis of the present study was that through its stimulatory effect on the CNS, nicotine would prove ergogenic at the lower but not at the higher dose administered compared to a placebo for measures of leg extensor torque, muscular power and anaerobic performance.

Methods

Participants

Nine healthy, never-smoker males were recruited for the study (mean ± SD: age, 24 ± 3 years; body mass, 78 ± 15 kg; height, 179 ± 13 cm). All participants had been competitive in team sports and trained (including gym sessions) or competed regularly ≥3 times per week for at least 2 years. Each participant was fully informed of all potential risks and experimental procedures, after which informed written consent was obtained. All experimental procedures and protocols were approved by the Institutional Human Ethics Committee and performed in accordance with the latest revision of the Declaration of Helsinki.

Study Design

All testing was conducted in the same laboratory environment (~20 °C, 600 lx). Participants visited the laboratory on four occasions, one anthropometric and familiarisation session and three experimental trials separated by > 2 < 7 days. All participants had previously completed the measures of performance required for this study; however, a full familiarisation was still performed before commencing the experimental trials to minimise learning. Experimental trials were conducted at the same time of day (±1 h), and the day of and prior to any experimental trial was marked by abstinence from alcohol, any exercise and only habitual caffeine use (as abstinence would in itself confound from withdrawal effects). Additionally, participants were asked to replicate their diet during the first experimental visit for subsequent trials to ensure a similar metabolic state. For experimental trials, 30 min prior to performance testing, participants chewed 2 mg (NIC-2) or 4 mg (NIC-4) nicotine or a flavour-matched placebo (PLA) gum, the order of which was randomised using a Latin square design. Immediately following this, participants completed five voluntary maximal contractions (MVC) each of isometric (ISO), concentric (CON) and eccentric (ECC) contractions of the *quadriceps femoris* muscle of the dominant leg followed by three maximal vertical counter-movement jumps (CMJ) and a 30-s Wingate test (WAnT). A 5-min ergometer warm-up at 100 W preceded the measurement of leg extensor force and a further 1-min warm-up prior to the WAnT. This order of tests was kept constant and was <20 min in duration (Fig. 1).

Experimental Protocol and Measures

On arrival to the laboratory, participants fastened a heart rate (HR) strap and monitor (Polar, Kempele, Finland) and were seated for 5 min, after which a baseline HR measurement was taken. Participants then chewed gum for 20 min whilst seated before completing a 5-min warm-up on a cycle ergometer (Monark, Varberg, Sweden) at 100 W, during which HR measurement was taken in the final minute before removing the gum. The participant was then seated on the isokinetic dynamometer (Biodex Medical Systems, New York, USA) at the previously recorded seat adjustments so that the femoral epicondyle was aligned with the dynamometer's axis of rotation and the ankle strap positioned 5 cm proximal to the medial malleolus. Along with the ankle, straps were placed around the chest, the hips and the leg to be tested in order to isolate the *quadriceps femoris* muscle. The lower limb was weighed,

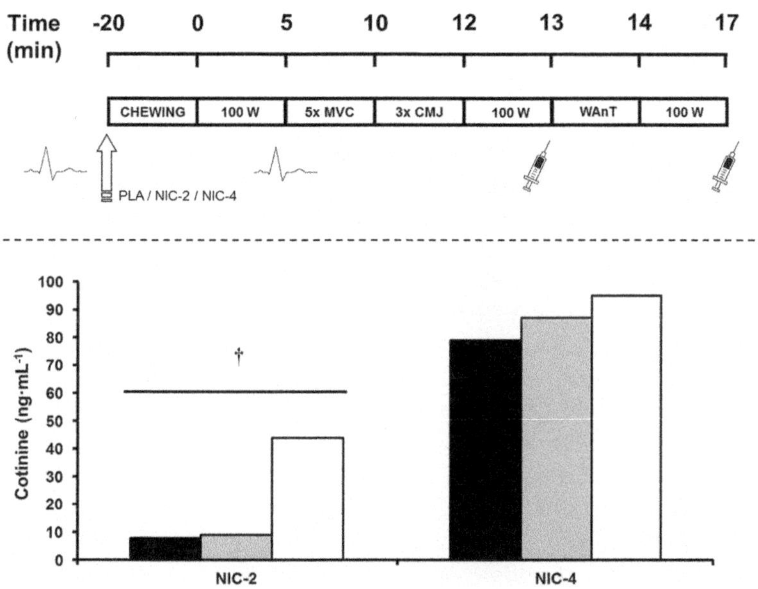

Fig. 1 *Upper panel*: Schematic of experimental protocol. Seated rest for 5 min and HR measurement followed by chewing gum for 20 min, a cycle ergometer warm-up at 100 W and another HR measurement. A set of five MVC's each for ISO, CON and ECC leg extensor force separated by a 2-min rest. Three maximal CMJ, after a further 1-min cycling at 100 W a capillary blood sample followed by the WAnT and 3-min cool-down at 100 W ending with a capillary blood sample. *Lower panel*: Individual plasma cotinine concentration in 2 mg (NIC-2) and 4 mg (NIC-4) gum trials for the third, sixth and ninth participants to start trials; none detected for PLA. †Significant difference to corresponding NIC-4 value

with the knee fully extended, to account for the action of gravity. CON and ECC contractions were performed over a 60° range of motion (from ~110° knee flexion) and ISO tension measured at 75°. The participant then performed five MVC of each type with each set separated by 2 min of passive recovery. CON and ECC torque was measured at an angular velocity of 30° s^{-1}. Peak and average peak torque for CON and ECC, and peak and average peak ISO tension (average calculated from the five contractions) were recorded.

Participants then performed three CMJ, each separated by 30 s of passive rest. Participants descended to a self-selected depth and immediately jumped upward as high as possible. To exclude the influence of arm swing, participants were instructed to keep their hands placed on their hips. Jump height was measured with an electronic jump mat (Swift Performance, NSW, Australia), and the peak and average (of three) values were recorded. Following this, participants completed a further 1-min cycling at 100 W during which a 50-μL fingertip blood sample was collected into a heparinised glass capillary tube, before completing their WAnT. The WAnT was completed on a friction-loaded ergometer (Monark, Varberg, Sweden) using a resistive load of 7.5% of body mass, where cadence was recorded every 5 s and power output calculated from friction load and flywheel velocity. The highest and lowest 5-s values were used to determine peak power (W) and rate of fatigue (%), whilst the sum of all 5-s values determined the anaerobic capacity (kJ). Finally, participants cooled down for 3 min at 100 W at which time collection of a final 50-μL fingertip blood sample occurred. The capillary blood samples were analysed immediately for determination of pH and bicarbonate (HCO_3^-) via an automated analyzer (Radiometer, Brønshøj, Denmark).

Nicotine Intervention and Verification

Participants were instructed according to the manufacturer's recommendations: one piece of gum (2 mg, 4 mg and placebo; Nicorette Icy Mint, Johnson & Johnson Pacific, Auckland, New Zealand) was introduced into the mouth followed by the instructions "chew until there is a strong taste, then place between your cheek and gums, and chew again when the taste has faded", with this encouraged for 20 min. Participants were not aware of the research hypotheses, only that on two of the three occasions they would be receiving nicotine. To verify the presence of systemic nicotine a resting (following 20-min chewing but prior to warm-up) venous blood sample was obtained from every third participant beginning the study (i.e. $n = 3$); this reduced sample was due to resource limitation. Venous blood samples were obtained from an antecubital vein into a 4-ml lithium heparin vacutainer tube (Becton–Dickinson, Plymouth, UK) then placed on ice for 10 min before being centrifuged (Eppendorf, Hamburg, Germany) at 4 °C for 10 min at 805*g*. Plasma was removed, aspirated into 500-μl aliquots and frozen at −80 °C for later analyses using high-performance liquid chromatography (HPLC). Due to nicotine's tendency to fluctuate and relatively short half-life (~2 h), cotinine, its major (~70%) metabolite with a longer retention time (~18–20 h) is preferred [11]. Sample preparation, solid phase extraction and analysis by HPLC were based on previous methodology [9] and performed in duplicate.

Statistical Analysis

All statistical analyses were performed with SPSS software for windows (IBM SPSS Statistics 20, NY, USA). Descriptive values were obtained and reported as means and standard deviation (SD) unless stated otherwise. Levene's test was used to ensure that data did not differ substantially from a normal distribution. Baseline/resting data (for physiological variables) were first analysed using one-way ANOVA. Data repeated over time (pH, HCO_3^-, HR) were analysed by two-way (trial × time) ANOVA, whilst all other (performance) data were analysed by one-way ANOVA. Sphericity was assessed and where the assumption of sphericity could not be assumed, adjustments to the degrees of freedom were made ($\varepsilon > 0.75$ = Huynh-Feldt; $\varepsilon < 0.75$ = Greenhouse-Geisser). Following a significant F test post-hoc pairwise analyses were performed using a paired samples t test (Bonferroni correction where relevant), with statistical significance set at $p \leq 0.05$. Partial eta-squared (η_p^2) is reported as a measure of effect size, with demarcations of small (<0.09), medium (>0.09 < 0.25) and large (>0.25) effects.

Results

No order effects were observed (all $p > 0.11$, $\eta_p^2 < 0.16$) and all participants completed the study without reporting negative side effects; the only comment made was that most experienced a scratchy/tickly throat during some (nicotine) trials.

Physiological Variables

Of the samples screened for blood cotinine concentration ($n = 3$; Fig. 1), none was detected during PLA whereas cotinine concentration increased as a function of dose (NIC-2: 20 ± 21 ng mL^{-1}, NIC-4: 87 ± 8 ng mL^{-1}; trial: $p = 0.01$, $\eta_p^2 = 0.97$). Resting HR was similar prior to treatment (trial: $p = 0.49$, $\eta_p^2 = 0.08$) but following treatment differed between trials as a function of time (trial × time: $p = 0.03$, $\eta_p^2 = 0.34$; Table 1) such that the increase in HR was more pronounced during NIC-2 (6 ± 7 beats · min^{-1}) and NIC-4 (7 ± 9 beats · min^{-1}) compared to PLA. HCO_3^- before the WAnT was similar

Table 1 Heart rate, venous bicarbonate and pH for placebo, 2 and 4 mg nicotine gum. Values are mean ± SD, $n = 9$

	Pre			Post		
	PLA	NIC-2	NIC-4	PLA	NIC-2	NIC-4
HR (beats min^{-1})	65 ± 11	67 ± 9	64 ± 9	117 ± 15[a]	125 ± 19[a,b]	123 ± 15[a,b]
HCO_3^- (mmol L^{-1})	25 ± 5	27 ± 2	25 ± 5	14 ± 4[a]	15 ± 3[a]	16 ± 4[a]
pH	7.46 ± 0.08	7.52 ± 0.06[b,c]	7.47 ± 0.06	7.29 ± 0.10[a]	7.35 ± 0.08[a]	7.30 ± 0.10[a]

Heart rate (HR) at rest pre-treatment (Pre) and during cycling at 100 W post-treatment (Post); bicarbonate (HCO_3^-) and pH before (Pre) and after (Post) WAnT; placebo (PLA), 2 mg (NIC-2) and 4 mg (NIC-4) trials
[a]Significant difference to corresponding Pre value
[b]Significant difference to corresponding PLA value
[c]Significant difference to corresponding NIC-4 value

between trials (trial: $p = 0.40$, $\eta_p^2 = 0.11$) but was decreased following the WAnT (time: $p < 0.01$, $\eta_p^2 = 0.97$), whilst pH was different between trials (trial: $p = 0.03$, $\eta_p^2 = 0.37$) and across time (time: $p < 0.01$, $\eta_p^2 = 0.90$).

Performance Variables

Peak and average ISO tension differed between trials (trial: $p = 0.02$, $\eta_p^2 > 0.37$; Table 2) such that NIC-2 > PLA. Peak (trial: $p = 0.05$, $\eta_p^2 = 0.30$) but not average (trial: $p = 0.28$, $\eta_p^2 = 0.15$) CON torque differed between trials such that NIC-2 > PLA. Peak (trial: $p < 0.01$, $\eta_p^2 = 0.48$) and average (trial: $p = 0.03$, $\eta_p^2 = 0.37$) ECC torque differed between trials such that NIC-2 > PLA. Peak and average CMJ height was similar between trials (trial: $p > 0.65$, $\eta_p^2 < 0.05$). During the WAnT (Fig. 2), anaerobic capacity was similar between trials (trial: $p = 0.73$, $\eta_p^2 = 0.04$) although pacing strategy seemed to differ; peak power differed between trials (trial: $p < 0.01$, $\eta_p^2 = 0.57$) such that NIC-2 < PLA by 6 ± 3% or 49 ± 24 W whilst the rate of fatigue differed between trials (trial: $p < 0.01$, $\eta_p^2 = 0.59$) such that NIC-2 (38 ± 11%) and NIC-4 (37 ± 12%) < PLA (44 ± 10%).

Discussion

This is the first study to investigate whether nicotine improves measures of leg extensor torque, muscular power and anaerobic performance. The main findings from this study were that (1) low-dose nicotine (2 mg) increased leg extensor force by ~6% compared to the placebo, whereas neither low- nor high-dose nicotine affected counter-movement jump height; (2) during the WAnT, anaerobic capacity was unchanged although low-dose nicotine altered the pacing strategy adopted; (3) physiologically, low-dose nicotine caused a relative alkalosis and both nicotine doses caused heart rate to be higher than placebo.

Low-Dose Nicotine Increases Peak and Average Leg Extensor Torque But Not Muscular Power

Overall, five out of six measures of torque were significantly improved with NIC-2 (6 ± 5%) with only the average concentric torque unaffected (4 ± 4%). To our knowledge, only one previously published study has measured leg extensor performance. Escher et al. [12] tested a greater range of flexion (90°) and angular velocity (250° s^{-1}) than in the current study using college athletes who regularly used smokeless tobacco; their participants were tested following ~12-h abstention from tobacco or having consumed smokeless tobacco 2 h and immediately prior to testing. They reported that MVC was lower when using compared to abstaining from tobacco but commented that they do not know whether it was the nicotine or any other substance within tobacco proving ergolytic. However, cotinine concentration during the tobacco trials in that study were considerably higher than in our study when using NIC-4 (~144 vs. ~87 ng mL^{-1}) and therefore it

Table 2 Peak and average leg extensor torque and counter-movement jump height for placebo, 2 and 4 mg nicotine gum. Values are mean ± SD, $n = 9$

	Peak			Average		
	PLA	NIC-2	NIC-4	PLA	NIC-2	NIC-4
Leg extensor torque (N m)						
ISO	309 ± 79	330 ± 82[a]	314 ± 79	290 ± 73	309 ± 77[a]	293 ± 71
CON	240 ± 59	258 ± 67[a]	251 ± 53	208 ± 61	218 ± 66	220 ± 59
ECC	332 ± 77	356 ± 73[a]	350 ± 75	316 ± 81	334 ± 73[a]	332 ± 76
CMJ (cm)	38 ± 8	38 ± 9	37 ± 9	37 ± 8	37 ± 9	36 ± 9

ISO isometric, *CON* concentric and *ECC* eccentric torque; *CMJ* counter-movement jump; *PLA* placebo, 2 mg (NIC-2) and 4 mg (NIC-4) trials
[a]Significant difference to corresponding PLA value

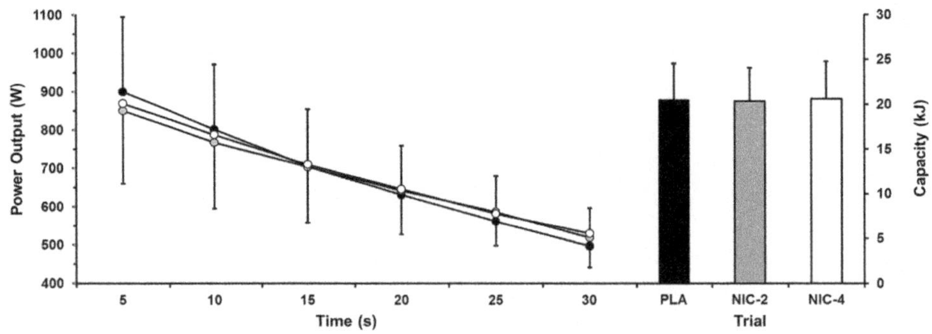

Fig. 2 Power output and anaerobic capacity during the WAnT for placebo (*filled circle*, PLA), 2 mg (*grey circle*, NIC-2) and 4 mg (*open circle*, NIC-4) nicotine gum. Values are mean ± SD, $n = 9$

remains plausible that in their participants, nicotine caused a depressant or relaxant effect [18, 28]. However, our results support those previously obtained when using another CNS stimulant, amphetamine, albeit by a smaller magnitude [5].

Given our results on leg extensor strength, it was surprising that NIC-2 did not affect CMJ performance. On the one hand, it might be argued that having produced more work during NIC-2 than PLA (141 ± 62 J, $p < 0.01$) could have produced greater fatigue that would mask any enhancement during the CMJ, or that the addition of velocity to force (i.e. power) attenuates any "true" effect (or single- vs. multi-joint movements). Previous studies have also found no improvement in CMJ [23] or rate of leg extensor force development [12] with smokeless tobacco; in fact, Escher et al. [12] noted an ergolytic effect when regular users consumed rather than abstained from tobacco, although this may be due to nicotine's biphasic effect at the neuromuscular junction whereby it exerts excitatory (acutely, when naïve or after withdrawal) then inhibitory (chronically, when tolerant) effects [1, 19]. Chandler and Blair [5] also failed to demonstrate any effect of amphetamine on leg power. It might also be that a CMJ is not sufficiently sensitive a test.

Low-Dose Nicotine Affects Pacing But Not Anaerobic Capacity During the WAnT

Previous studies have failed to detect any difference in anaerobic capacity during the WAnT when administering sublingual nicotine in naive participants [27] or smokeless tobacco in regular users [2]; therefore, in this respect, our results are in agreement. Furthermore, other CNS stimulants (caffeine, pseudoephedrine) have also failed to affect WAnT performance [7, 16]. However, that we observed a reduction in peak power yet an attenuation in fatigue when administered NIC-2 compared to PLA was surprising (Fig. 2) and difficult to explain. We observed a significant relative alkalosis immediately prior to the WAnT during NIC-2 only whereas the ~2 mmol L^{-1} higher HCO_3^- was not significant ($p = 0.2$, Table 1); thus, whilst this could provide a mechanism for reduced fatigue via improved acid–base balance, it does not explain why the rate of fatigue was equally reduced during NIC-4. Indeed, as an alkaloid, nicotine is a weak base ($pK_a = 8.0$) that in gum form, it is buffered to alkaline pH to facilitate buccal absorption [3]. The authors feel that further explanation/discussion is not possible, especially without further mechanistic insight, as this would be too speculative.

Potential Mechanism(s) of Action

That nicotine that had been sufficiently absorbed systemically within both NIC-2 and NIC-4 was confirmed by our measurement of cotinine concentration (Fig. 1), and that heart rate was elevated during both trials compared to PLA (Table 1). The sympatho-adrenal (excitatory) effects of nicotine are well known [14] although, given the ergogenic characteristics discussed here (muscular and anaerobic performance), it is most likely that nicotine is exerting its effects via stimulating cholinergic neurotransmission in the basal forebrain (cortical arousal) and/or enhanced mesolimbic dopaminergic activity (motivation and reward) [4]. Nevertheless, a hypoalgesic effect of nicotine should not be discounted as it has been experimentally demonstrated to increase the pain threshold [17], and might therefore prove ergogenic via antinociception as proposed by caffeine [10]. The possibility of a placebo effect cannot be discounted; indeed, it is difficult to mask the effects such as those from (m)any CNS stimulants. However, several steps were taken during the study design: (1) although only single-blind, participants were unaware of the study hypotheses and only told that they would be receiving nicotine on two of three occasions, (2) a flavour-matched placebo was used, and (3) although participants might have detected the portion of nicotine swallowed (first-pass metabolism) or the psychoactive/sympatho-adrenal effects, were a placebo effect is indeed evident in the current study then it would likely be seen for NIC-4 also and this was not the case.

Considerations and Future Research

It is acknowledged that a sample size of $n = 9$ is relatively small; however, clear and directional statistical results were observed even with this sample. It is also worth noting that the finding of the 4 mg gum minimally affecting the performance measures was not due to side effects masking or reducing any ergogenic effect(s), as none were reported. There are many different nicotine delivery systems commonly available (over-the-counter) including nasal spray, gum, inhaler, lozenge, sublingual tablet and transdermal patch. The different delivery systems result in different nicotine bioavailability and absorption and therefore pharmacokinetics such that, for example, peak systemic concentrations are observed whilst smoking a cigarette, followed by oral snuff and chewing tobacco with gum being the lowest, possibly due to the first-pass metabolism and nicotine being retained in the gum itself [3]. The observed cotinine concentration from chewing gum was indeed lower than that observed with oral smokeless tobacco and transdermal patch [12, 24]; therefore, it would be of interest to directly compare different delivery systems on the same experimental sample and performance protocol. There is also considerable inter-individual variability in nicotine metabolism (e.g. nutrition, age, sex, medication, ethnicity, genetics; see [3]) as we observed for NIC-2 (Fig. 1) and thus, we cannot be certain that our $n = 3$ is the representative of the whole sample. Further, dosing (e.g. absolute vs. relative) needs to be more carefully considered for future studies. Finally, as the primary outcome measure of the present study was performance, future studies should include further mechanistic insights i.e. motor unit activation (twitch interpolation, electromyography).

Conclusions

The present study has demonstrated that low-dose (2 mg) nicotine gum increases leg extensor torque, but countermovement jump and anaerobic capacity during WAnT remained unchanged when compared to a placebo, whilst there were minimal effects of the 4-mg nicotine gum on the performance parameters measured. Together with our previous observation [24], these results indicate that nicotine per se can improve exercise endurance and muscular strength, something that WADA should continue to monitor alongside patterns of (mis)use.

Acknowledgements
This study was funded in part by a grant from the World Anti-Doping Agency.

Authors' Contributions
TM contributed to the obtaining funding, conception and design of the work; data acquisition, analysis, and interpretation; drafting and critically revising important intellectual content. MM contributed to the design of the work; data acquisition and analysis. DJC contributed to the design of the work; critically revising important intellectual content. MJB contributed to the design of the work; data acquisition; critically revising important intellectual content. All authors approved the final version of the manuscript. All experimental procedures were performed in the School of Sport and Exercise, Massey University, Palmerston North.

Competing Interests
Toby Mündel, Marine Machal, Darryl Cochrane and Matthew Barnes report that they have no conflicts of interest.

References

1. Ashton H, Stepney R. Smoking psychology and pharmacology. New York: Tavistock & Methuen; 1982.
2. Baldini FD, Skinner JS, Landers DM, O'Connor JS. Effects of varying doses of smokeless tobacco at rest and during brief, high-intensity exercise. Mil Med. 1992;157(2):51–5.
3. Benowitz NL, Hukkanen J, Jacob III P. Nicotine chemistry, metabolism, kinetics and biomarkers. Handb Exp Pharmacol. 2009;192:29–60.
4. Boutrel B, Koob GF. What keeps us awake: the neuropharmacology of stimulants and wakefulness-promoting medications. Sleep. 2004;27(6):1181–94.
5. Chandler JV, Blair SN. The effect of amphetamines on selected physiological components related to athletic success. Med Sci Sports Exerc. 1980;12(1):65–9.
6. Christen AG, McDaniel RK, Doran JE. Snuff dipping and tobacco chewing in a group of Texas college athletes. Tex Dent J. 1979;97(2):6–10.
7. Collomp K, Ahmaidi S, Audran M, Chanal JL, Préfaut C. Effects of caffeine ingestion on performance and anaerobic metabolism during the Wingate Test. Int J Sports Med. 1991;12(5):439–43.
8. Connolly GN, Orleans CT, Kogan M. Use of smokeless tobacco in major-league baseball. N Engl J Med. 1988;318(19):1281–5.
9. Dams R, Benijts T, Lambert WE, De Leenheer AP. Simultaneous determination of in total 17 opium alkaloids and opioids in blood and urine by fast liquid chromatography–diode array detection–fluorescence detection, after solid-phase extraction. J Chromatogr B Analyt Technol Biomed Life Sci. 2002;773(1):53–61.
10. Davis JK, Green JM. Caffeine and anaerobic performance: ergogenic value and mechanisms of action. Sports Med. 2009;39(10):813–32.
11. Dhar P. Measuring tobacco smoke exposure: quantifying nicotine/cotinine concentration in biological samples by colorimetry, chromatography and immunoassay methods. J Pharm Biomed Anal. 2004;35(1):155–68.
12. Escher SA, Tucker AM, Lundin TM, Grabiner MD. Smokeless tobacco, reaction time, and strength in athletes. Med Sci Sports Exerc. 1998;30(10): 1548–51.
13. Glover ED, Edmundson EW, Edwards SW, Schroeder KL. Implications of smokeless tobacco use among athletes. Phys Sportsmed. 1986;14(12): 95–105.
14. Haass M, Kübler W. Nicotine and sympathetic neurotransmission. Cardiovasc Drugs Ther. 1997;10(6):657–65.
15. Heishman SJ, Kleykamp BA, Singleton EG. Meta-analysis of the acute effects of nicotine and smoking on human performance. Psychopharmacology (Berl). 2010;210(4):453–69.
16. Hodges AN, Lynn BM, Bula JE, Donaldson MG, Dagenais MO, McKenzie DC. Effects of pseudoephedrine on maximal cycling power and submaximal cycling efficiency. Med Sci Sports Exerc. 2003;35(8):1316–9.
17. Jamner LD, Girdler SS, Shapiro D, Jarvik ME. Pain inhibition, nicotine, and gender. Exp Clin Psychopharmacol. 1998;6(1):96–106.
18. Lee WE. The action of tobacco smoke, with special reference to arterial pressure and degeneration. Q J Exp Physiol. 1908;1(4):335–58.
19. Lester MJ, Jacobson BH, Edwards SW. Effect of ingestion of smokeless tobacco on motor distal latency of the median nerve. Percept Mot Skills. 1988;67(1):283–90.
20. Marclay F, Grata E, Perrenoud L, Saugy M. A one-year monitoring of nicotine use in sport: frontier between potential performance enhancement and addiction issues. Forensic Sci Int. 2011;213(1–3):73–84.
21. Marclay F, Saugy M. Determination of nicotine and nicotine metabolites in urine by hydrophilic interaction chromatography-tandem mass spectrometry: potential use of smokeless tobacco products by ice hockey players. J Chromatogr A. 2010;1217(48):7528–38.

22. Martinsen M, Sundgot-Borgen J. Adolescent elite athletes' cigarette smoking, use of snus, and alcohol. Scand J Med Sci Sports. 2014;24(2):439–46.
23. Morente-Sánchez J, Zandonai T, Mateo-March M, Sanabria D, Sánchez-Muñoz C, Chiamulera C, Zabala DM. Acute effect of Snus on physical performance and perceived cognitive load on amateur footballers. Scand J Med Sci Sports. 2015;25(4):e423–31.
24. Mündel T, Jones DA. Effect of transdermal nicotine administration on exercise endurance. Exp Physiol. 2006;91(4):705–13.
25. Perkins KA, Grobe JE, Fonte C, Goettler J, Caggiula AR, Reynolds WA, Stiller RL, Scierka A, Jacob RG. Chronic and acute tolerance to subjective, behavioral and cardiovascular effects of nicotine in humans. J Pharmacol Exp Ther. 1994;270(2):628–38.
26. Poltavski DV, Petros TV, Holm JE. Lower but not higher doses of transdermal nicotine facilitate cognitive performance in smokers on gender non-preferred tasks. Pharmacol Biochem Behav. 2012;102(3):423–33.
27. Pysny L, Petru D, Pysna J, Cihlar D. The acute effect of nicotine on anaerobic exercise performance. J Phys Ed Sport. 2015;15(1):103–7.
28. Silvette H, Hoff EC, Larson PS, Haag HB. The actions of nicotine on central nervous system functions. Pharmacol Rev. 1962;14:137–73.
29. World Anti-Doping Agency (2012), The World Anti-Doping Code, The 2012 Monitoring Program, Montreal. www.wada-ama.org, 2012 (Accessed Jan 2012).

18

The Effect of Concurrent Plyometric Training Versus Submaximal Aerobic Cycling on Rowing Economy, Peak Power, and Performance in Male High School Rowers

Julian D. Egan-Shuttler, Rohan Edmonds, Cassandra Eddy, Veronica O'Neill and Stephen J. Ives*

Abstract

Background: Plyometric training has been shown to increase muscle power, running economy, and performance in athletes. Despite its use by rowing coaches, it is unknown whether plyometrics might improve rowing economy or performance.

The purpose was to determine if plyometric training, in conjunction with training on the water, would lead to improved rowing economy and performance.

Methods: Eighteen male high school rowers were assigned to perform 4 weeks of either plyometric training (PLYO, $n = 9$) or steady-state cycling below ventilatory threshold (endurance, E, $n = 9$), for 30 min prior to practice on the water (matched for training volume) 3 days per week. Rowing performance was assessed through a 500-m rowing time trial (TT) and peak rowing power (RP), while rowing economy (RE) was assessed by measuring the oxygen cost over four work rates (90, 120, 150, and 180 W).

Results: Rowing economy was improved in both PLYO and E ($p < 0.05$). The 500-m TT performance improved significantly for PLYO (from 99.8 ± 9 s to 94.6 ± 2 s, $p < 0.05$) but not for E (from 98.8 ± 6 s to 98.7 ± 5 s, $p > 0.05$). Finally, RP was moderately higher in the PLYO group post-training (E 569 ± 75 W, PLYO 629 ± 51 W, ES = 0.66)

Conclusions: In a season when the athletes performed no rowing sprint training, 4 weeks of plyometric training improved the 500-m rowing performance and moderately improved peak power. This increase in performance may have been mediated by moderate improvements in rowing power, but not economy, and warrants further investigation.

Keywords: Rowing, Stretch shorten cycle, Oxygen consumption

Key Points

- Four weeks of plyometric training lead to increased rowing performance, which may be mediated by a moderate increase in peak power.
- Time-matched cycling exercise did not improve performance or peak power; however, rowing economy was improved similarly in both groups.
- These findings suggest that plyometric training is useful for increasing rowing performance.

* Correspondence: sives@skidmore.edu
Health and Exercise Sciences Department, Skidmore College, Saratoga Springs, NY, USA

Background

Rowing is a high-intensity sport, requiring high strength, power, anaerobic, and aerobic capacity [1–4]. Race times over the typical 2-km rowing race can range from 5.5 to 7 min in elite rowers, indicating a need for a variety of training intensities [1]. It has been estimated that aerobic metabolism contributes 67–84% of the energy requirement during racing [1], and this relative contribution of aerobic and anaerobic energy systems is the same for both on-the-water and ergometer rowing [5]. Because of the relatively high reliance on aerobic metabolism in racing performance [4, 5], endurance training dominates the training programs of most rowers [1]. However, there are multiple determinants of rowing performance [4], indicating that a rower's training program must encompass aerobic and anaerobic training, as well as training methods to develop peak power such as strength or power training. In fact, Ingham et al. [4] indicated that peak force and power over a maximal five-stroke test were two of the highest correlates to 2-km ergometer performance. As peak power correlates very highly with rowing performance, training for power is a part of many rowers' training programs [2] which may consist of strength training [6] or heavy rowing [7], performed concurrently with aerobic training. While strength training has been shown to enhance rowing performance [8–10], much less is known about the effect of power training, such as plyometrics, on rowing performance. Additionally, given the minimal equipment required to perform plyometrics versus weight training, plyometrics might have a greater potential for implementation.

There is a variety of ways to improve strength and power, and in many sports, plyometric training is used to increase movement speed and power [11]. Plyometric training is a type of physical conditioning that emphasizes the stretch-shortening cycle and typically involves both open and closed kinetic chain exercises, such as jumping or medicine ball throws [11]. A recent meta-analysis by Sáez-Sáez de Villarreal et al. [12] suggests that plyometric training is an effective method to improve strength and power, even over short periods (<10 weeks). Plyometric training improves power through increased neural drive, changes in muscle coordination, changes in the muscle tendon complex, and changes in muscle size and architecture [11]. It is known that neural adaptations account for strength increases in the early phases of strength training [13, 14]; however, major neural adaptations also occur with plyometric training and lead to the increases in explosive force production [15–17]. Plyometrics have also been shown to increase the cross-sectional areas of both type I and type II muscle fibers [18], without change to the myosin heavy chain ratios [16, 19]. Increased muscle preparatory activity and muscle activation have also been found, leading to plyometrics possibly even preventing injury [20]. However, the application of this training method has traditionally been applied to relatively narrow populations (e.g., football or track and field).

Previously, running economy, or the energy cost of running at a given work rate, has been shown to improve in response to plyometric training [21]. Running economy has even been suggested to be a better correlate of running performance than maximal oxygen consumption (VO_{2max}) [22]. Paavolainen et al. [23] were able to show that when endurance runners incorporated plyometric/explosive strength training into their training, 5-km running times and running economy were improved, and all without a change in VO_{2max}. This increase in running economy has been suggested to be due to an increase in stiffness of the musculotendinous system, which allows the body to momentarily store and utilize energy absorbed eccentrically by the force of landing [24], but neural mechanisms cannot be excluded as potential contributors [15, 16]. Thus, as plyometrics can improve endurance performance and power, with no chronic detriment when performed concurrently [23], plyometrics has the potential to be an effective means to improve performance in rowers, where the legs contribute significantly to generating stroke power.

To this end, Kramer et al. [3] investigated whether adding 20 min of plyometric training to rowing training would improve rowing performance. After 9 weeks of training, improvement in rowing performance, assessed via a 2.5-km time trial, did not differ between the control and experimental groups [3]. However, there were several limitations to this study: first, the training stimulus or volume of 20 min 3×/week may have been insufficient; second, the 2.5-km time trial (TT) is atypical of rowing; third, training volume was not matched between groups; fourth, the exercise selection was not optimal for rowers; and finally, rowing economy or power were not measured. Interestingly, while the previous study was unable to demonstrate a benefit of plyometrics on rowing performance [3], an estimated 50% of rowing coaches continue to include plyometric training into their training programs to improve rowing power [2]. Coaches that do use plyometrics often perform other strength training methods in addition, as concurrent training has been shown to increase rowing performance [10]. However, it remains to be seen whether plyometrics alone can improve rowing performance and thus validate their use by rowing coaches [7].

Therefore, the purpose of this study was to determine if 4 weeks of plyometric training, versus submaximal aerobic training matched for volume, would increase rowing economy, peak power, or performance in experienced youth rowers when combined with on-the-water training. We hypothesized that rowers who performed plyometric training would improve rowing economy, peak power, and performance over those conducting submaximal steady-state exercise.

Methods

Participants

Eighteen male rowers with a minimum of 1 year's competitive rowing experience were recruited from a local competitive (i.e., multiple state and national championship medals) high school rowing program. The participants had no previous experience with plyometric training. The experimental plyometric (PLYO) and the endurance (E) group each consisted of nine high-school-aged male rowers. The groups were matched with regard to pretraining 500-m times (endurance, E = 98.8 ± 5.8 s; PLYO = 99.8 ± 9.6 s, $p > 0.05$). As a result, there was also no difference in biological age or training age between groups. The physical characteristics of both groups are presented in Table 1. Unfortunately, recent 2000-m rowing performance times for the group were not available, but the team had achieved several state and national medals. All participants, and their legal guardians, provided written informed consent prior to inclusion in this study. This study was approved by the Institutional Review Board of Skidmore College and therefore was performed in accordance with the ethical standards set forth in the Declaration of Helsinki.

Intervention

The intervention lasted for 4 weeks, which is defined as a short-term plyometric period [11, 12] and is long enough to elicit significant physiological and/or performance changes [17, 25]. All testing and training was conducted during the fall competition season (September to November). These 4 weeks of training was also selected so that training could be completed before the major competitions for the rowers. Both groups performed 30 min of cross-training before on-the-water practice, 3 days/week, with 48 h in between sessions (e.g., Monday, Wednesday, and Friday). The PLYO group performed 30 min of plyometric exercise, while E performed steady-state cycling. All plyometric sessions contained exercises focusing on vertical explosiveness, such as box jumps, depth jumps, multiple box-to-box jumps, and double leg hops. Furthermore, as the rowing stroke involves opening of the trunk, backwards and overhead throws of medicine balls (10 lbs) were included to train explosive triple extensions. Sessions ranged from 100- to 150-ft contacts in week 1 to 125- to 170-ft contacts in week 4. Medicine ball exercise repetitions were periodized to progressive overload. The volume (number of foot contacts) conforms to recommended guidelines [26]. The full training program can be found in Table 2. A trained member of the research team oversaw every plyometric session and provided feedback on the quality of the movements.

The endurance group performed 30 min of steady-state cycling at ventilatory threshold at the same time as the experimental group. The "Talk Test" (cycling at an intensity at which a conversation was possible) was used to prescribe cycling intensity and has been shown to be a valid approximation of ventilatory threshold [27]. The athletes were also familiar with this method, as it was used at their club to prescribe low-intensity aerobic workouts. Cycling was used so that one group was not provided with a higher volume of rowing-specific training than the other and is also a common cross-training method for rowers. The endurance group was also supervised. After each group completed the 30 min of training, they proceeded to their on-the-water rowing practice. All subjects completed the same on-the-water workouts, and members from the PLYO and E groups rowed together in mixed boats. As all rowers were on the same team, outside of the training intervention (endurance or plyometric), rowing volume and intensity were identical for each member of the study.

Measurements

All measurements were taken during a single testing session on the Saturdays before and after the 4 weeks of training. Testing occurred over a 90-min period for each participant. All post-testing was performed at least 48 h since the last plyometric or biking session, allowing adequate recovery and avoiding undue influence of the last training session.

Upon arrival, participants had their stature (seca 217, UK), mass (Belfour Inc., WI, USA), and thigh and calf circumferences measured (Gulick tape measure). These measurements were taken by the same member of the research team for pre- and post-testing and were taken half way up the thigh and calf, as has been done in previous plyometric studies [28]. Rowing economy (RE) was assessed with a submaximal 8-min step test on a rowing ergometer (Model D, Concept2, VT, USA), which consisted of four 2-min stages at 90, 120, 150, and 180 W. The Concept2 rowing ergometer is considered to be an accurate rowing ergometer [29] and is the gold standard. Expired gases were collected using a one-way non-rebreathe mouthpiece to determine oxygen consumption (VO_2), a known measure

Table 1 The participant characteristics at baseline and following the 4-week intervention

	Control Group ($n = 8$)		Experimental Group ($n = 8$)	
	Pre	Post	Pre	Post
Age (year)	16 ± 0.6	16 ± 0.6	16 ± 0.8	16 ± 0.8
Stature (cm)	177 ± 4	177 ± 4	179 ± 6	179 ± 6
Mass (kg)	66.5 ± 9.4	66.2 ± 8.6	71.4 ± 6.5	71.8 ± 6.9
Thigh Circumference (cm)	49 ± 4.8	49 ± 3.0	52 ± 4.0	53 ± 3.5
Calf Circumference (cm)	35.4 ± 2.6	34.5 ± 2.5	35.1 ± 2.0	35.2 ± 1.9

Data are presented as mean ± SD

Table 2 The plyometric program performed for 30 min, 3 days a week, for 4 weeks

	Week 1	Week 2	Week 3	Week 4
Day 1				
Single leg push-off	3 × 8	3 × 10	3 × 10	3 × 10
Box jump	3 × 5	3 × 6	3 × 6	3 × 6
Depth jump	3 × 5	3 × 5	3 × 5	3 × 5
Squat jump	3 × 15	3 × 20	3 × 20	3 × 20
Backward throw	3 × 6	3 × 6	3 × 6	3 × 6
Overhead throw	3 × 5	3 × 6	3 × 6	3 × 6
Trunk rotation	3 × 5	3 × 6	3 × 6	3 × 6
Foot contacts	100	125	125	125
Day 2				
Double leg hops	3 × 5	4 × 5	4 × 5	4 × 5
5-5-5 squat	3 times	4 times	4 times	4 times
Front cone hops	4 cones, 5 times	4 cones, 5 times	4 cones, 5 times	4 cones, 5 times
Multiple box-to-box jumps	5 times	5 times	5 times	5 times
Wave squat	2 × 5	10 reps	10 reps	10 reps
Box jump	3 × 5	4 × 5	4 × 5	4 × 5
Foot contacts	150	170	170	170
Day 3				
Standing jump over barrier	3 × 5	4 × 5	4 × 5	4 × 5
Lateral jump over barrier	3 × 5	4 × 5	4 × 5	4 × 5
Single leg push-off	3 × 8	3 × 8	3 × 8	3 × 8
Depth jump	3 × 5	4 × 5	4 × 5	4 × 5
Pyramiding box hops	5 rounds	5 rounds	5 rounds	5 rounds
Backward throw	3 × 6	3 × 6	3 × 6	3 × 6
Overhead throw	3 × 5	3 × 5	3 × 5	3 × 5
Foot contacts	120	150	150	150

of energy expenditure (TrueOne 2400, Parvo Medics, Sandy, UT, USA). The accuracy of the O_2 analyzer is 0.1%, the flowmeter and analyzers were calibrated to less than 1% variance, and typical repeatability (coefficient of variation) in our lab for VO_2 is ~5%. VO_2 was obtained during the last 15 s of the 2-min stage, and based upon previous testing and pilot work, we determined participants were able to achieve steady state within the 2-min stages. Rating of perceived exertion (RPE) was measured using the Borgs Scale (RPE 0–10) [30]. Participants completed a 2-min warm-up and cooldown before and after the test, respectively.

After the RE measurements, participants rested for 30 min and then performed a maximal 500-m TT on the rowing ergometer. All participants were familiar with performing maximal 500-m trials as these were performed frequently as part of their normal training and/or performance assessments, prior to enrollment in the study, but none were performed during the intervention period. Stroke rate was not capped for the participants. Time, stroke rate, and average watts were measured during the TT. A 2-min warm-up and cooldown was completed before and after the TT, with participants asked to rest for another 30 min following the TT. Peak rowing power (RP) was then measured over three maximal trials of 15 s on the rowing ergometer. The recorded value for peak power was the highest wattage observed during the 15-s period. For both the RE and TT, the participants were instructed that they could self-select the ergometer resistances, which had to be the same for both the pre- and post-testing. However, as each rower was on the same team, they selected the same ergometer resistances (control 4.4 ± 0.2 vs. plyometrics 4.5 ± 0.0, arbitrary units, $p > 0.05$) which are also in accordance with US National Team testing guidelines. For the RP test, the resistance was set to the highest value (10) on the rowing ergometer.

Statistical Analysis

All statistics were performed using commercially available software (SPSS v. 23, Armonk, NY). Pre-planned t test comparisons were used to determine significance at baseline, in changes within the PLYO and E groups, and at post-test for stature, mass, circumferences, TT performance, and RP. In the case of violating normality, a non-parametric alternative method was employed. In addition, the magnitude of the change from pre-training to post-training was also determined using standardized differences in means (i.e., effect size, ES, Cohen's *d*) [31, 32]. Threshold values were established as *small* (0.2), *moderate* (0.6), *large* (1.2), and *very large* (2.0). A mixed-model analysis of variance (ANOVA) was used to determine differences in RE. Linear regression analysis was used to determine the slope of the line for VO_2 across work rate and the intercept for each individual. The level of significance was established at $p \leq 0.05$. To understand the potential relationships between rowing power, rowing economy, and performance, Pearson correlation coefficients were calculated. Data are reported as means ± standard deviation.

Results

Participant Characteristics

During the training period, one subject from the PLYO and one subject from the E group dropped out due to injuries, which were incurred during their on-the-water rowing training and were unrelated to the intervention. Acceptable adherence to the training program was set at 85%, and all remaining participants achieved this or higher. There were no differences in age, stature, mass, or thigh and calf circumferences between or within the groups at baseline prior to training ($p > 0.05$) (Table 1). There no were significant changes in any of the anthropometric measures within either group ($p > 0.05$); as such, at post-testing, there were no differences between the groups for the stature, mass, and thigh and calf circumferences ($p > 0.05$).

Rowing Economy

Rowing economy (Fig. 1) did not differ significantly between PLYO and E at all of the work rates before training. In response to training, the analysis of variance indicated no significant interaction effects for VO_2 values between the two groups at all of the work rates (90, 120, 150, 180 W, Fig. 1, $p > 0.05$) but a main effect for time was found to be significant ($p < 0.05$) indicating a generally lower VO_2 or energy cost from pre- to post-intervention. Additionally, linear regression analysis indicated no group differences in the slope (VO_2/watt relationship) at baseline, in response to training, or at post-intervention in either group (PLYO: $p = 0.17$, $p = 0.18$; E: $p = 0.2$, $p = 0.18$). RPE was also taken in the last minute of each stage, and there was a significant reduction in RPE following training in the PLYO group after training ($p = 0.05$), but not for the CON group (Fig. 2).

500-m Time Trial Performance

There was no difference in the 500-m times between the groups before training ($p = 0.32$). TT performance did not change for E after training ($p = 0.83$, ES = −0.08); however, the TT performance was significantly improved in PLYO (Fig. 3, $p \leq 0.05$, ES = −0.91). Furthermore, difference in TT performance was statistically different between the groups at post-testing. The average power output during the 500-m TT was not different between

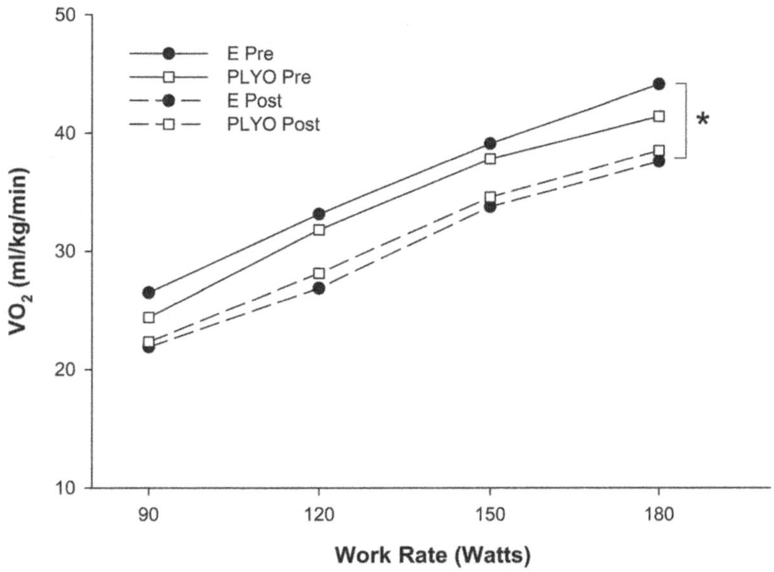

Fig. 1 Rowing economy of the endurance (*E*) and experimental (*PLYO*) groups recorded during an 8-min steady-state rowing step test (2-min stages at 90, 120, 150, and 190 W), before ($n = 9$/group) and after 4 weeks of plyometric training ($n = 8$/group). * indicates significant main effect of time (*pre* vs. *post*). Data are presented as means and error bars were omitted for visual clarity

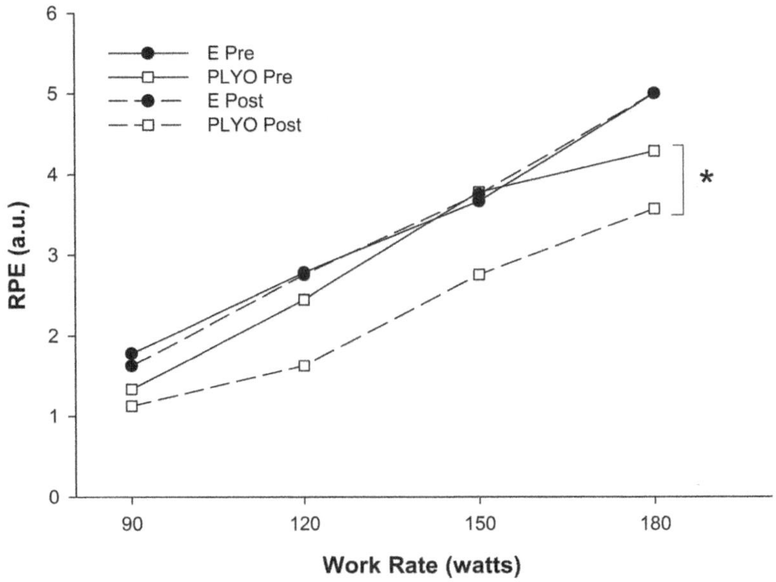

Fig. 2 Rating of perceived exertion (*RPE*) during the rowing economy test in the endurance (*E*) and experimental (*PLYO*) groups before ($n = 9$/group) and after 4 weeks of plyometric training ($n = 8$/group). * indicates significant main effect of time (*pre* vs. *post*). Data are presented as means and error bars were omitted for visual clarity

groups at baseline (363 ± 54 W vs. 372 ± 75 W, E vs. PLYO, respectively, $p = 0.77$), but PLYO significantly increased power output, and thus, the groups were significantly different post-training (368 ± 46 W vs. 414 ± 24 W, E vs. PLYO, respectively, $p = 0.02$, ES = −1.89). Finally, there were no group differences in the average stroke rate during the 500-m TT, at baseline (E 37 ± 4 strokes/min vs. PLYO 38 ± 3 strokes/min, $p = 0.52$), in response to training, or post-training (E 38 ± 4 strokes/min vs. PLYO 39 ± 5 strokes/min, $p = 0.52$).

Peak Rowing Power

There was no difference in RP between the groups before training ($p = 0.69$, ES = −0.07). After training, there was no change in RP within PLYO or E (Fig. 4; $p = 0.18$, ES = 0.14, $p = 0.12$, ES = 0.11). Although, there was a trend for a

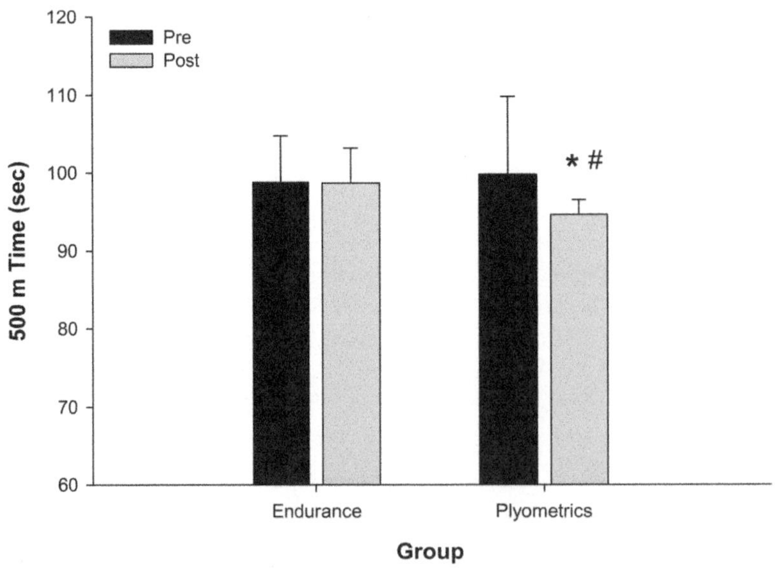

Fig. 3 The 500-m rowing ergometer time trial performance of the experimental (*PLYO*) and endurance (*E*) groups recorded before ($n = 9$/group) and after 4 weeks of plyometric training ($n = 8$/group). Data are expressed as means ± SD, * indicates significance within group compared to *pre* ($p \leq 0.05$)

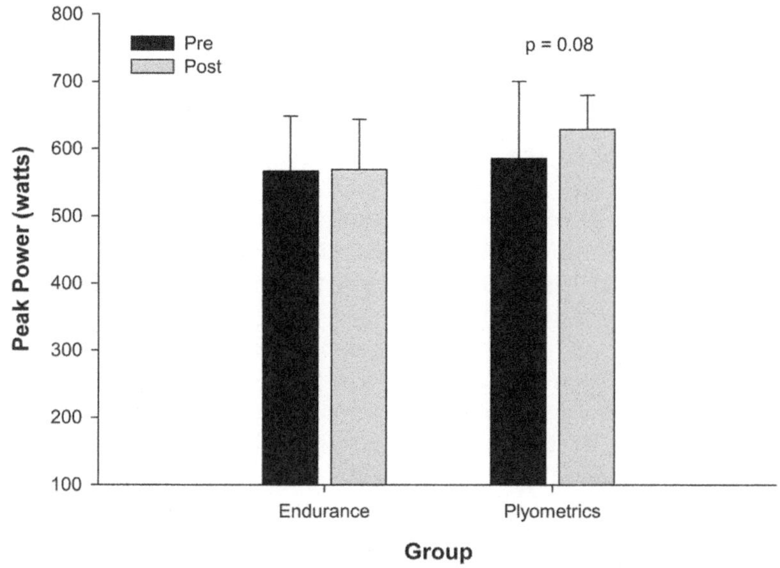

Fig. 4 Peak rowing power observed during three trials of 15-s maximal rowing ergometer tests in the experimental (*PLYO*) and endurance (*E*) groups, performed before ($n = 9$/group) and after 4 weeks of plyometric training ($n = 8$/group). Data are expressed as means ± SD

difference in RP between the groups following training ($p = 0.08$, ES = 0.66), with a tendency for greater power output in the PLYO group. RP was negatively correlated to VO_2 (energy expenditure) during work rates 90–180 W before training ($r = -0.549$, -0.879, -0.745, -0.736, $p = 0.34$, $p = 0.0$, $p = 0.001$, $p = 0.002$, for each work rate, respectively). In addition, post-training RP was negatively correlated to the VO_2/watt slope during the RE test ($r = -0.576$, $p = 0.039$). Finally, peak rowing power was negatively correlated with 500-m time performance before ($r = -0.92$, $p = 0.0$) and after training ($r = -0.78$, $p = 0.0$). Finally, the peak power responses were also highly reliable, and exploration of the three baseline trials indicated a significant reliability coefficient (Cronbach's $\alpha = 0.99$, $p = 0.00$).

Discussion

In the current study, we sought to determine if 4 weeks of plyometric training would increase rowing economy, peak power, or performance in experienced youth rowers when combined with on-the-water training. After the 4-week intervention, rowing economy for both groups was significantly improved, but no group differences were found. Peak rowing power was moderately changed as there was a tendency for difference between groups post-training with higher peak power in the plyometric group in response to this relatively short intervention. However, the main finding of this study is that the rowers who performed plyometric training significantly improved their 500-m TT, while this did not change for the endurance group. This study provides the first instance in which plyometric training significantly improved rowing sprint performance.

Plyometric Training and Rowing Economy

In the current study, rowing economy across work rate was significantly improved in both groups (Fig. 1), possibly indicating that plyometric and aerobic training had a similar effect on rowing economy. Previously, running economy has been shown to improve after plyometric training [21, 24, 28], and the reason for this improvement has been suggested to be increased musculotendinous stiffness (MTS) in the legs of runners [24]. A high MTS increases an individual's ability to absorb, harness, and recoil force during the stretch-shortening cycle, such as in running [33]. An increase in MTS is thus beneficial for a sport such as running, which involves an eccentric contraction when the runner's foot makes contact with the ground, where after plyometric training, the increased MTS results in more stored energy in the series elastic elements and reduces eccentric muscle demand. However, the beginning of the rowing stroke (known as the catch), is an anticipated motion in which the athlete is actually pulling themselves towards their feet, followed by a rapid press of the legs to apply power [34]. As there is not so much of a reactive movement, or ground reaction force in rowing when compared with running, increased MTS is likely less beneficial in rowing. Although, plyometric training has also been shown to increase muscle activation [20] and muscle force [35] and decrease ground reaction times [36] suggesting plyometrics might alter the work to rest ratio of rowing, through improved drive speed, allowing more time of the stroke cycle to be spent in recovery for a given stroke rate. Such a change, perhaps independent of economy, might correspond to improved boat speed, allowing for greater maintenance of the forward propulsion or "run" of the rowing shell in the water from each stroke. It is worth noting that these hypotheses warrant further investigation to confirm if this is, in fact, the case.

Plyometric Training and Rowing Power

Plyometric training has been suggested to improve power [37] in adults and in youth [38]. Results from the current study indicate that plyometric training in this athlete cohort (youth rowers), for this length of time (4 weeks), may elicit a moderate increase in rowing power (Fig. 4). This is in agreement with previous research as plyometrics are typically used to improve power [2, 11, 12]. It has been suggested by rowing biomechanics experts that elasticity stored in the tendons of rowers could be beneficial or initiating the drive sequence of the stroke [34]. The fact that the moderate improvement in rowing power did not reach statistical significance may be attributed to a number of potential factors. The training period was relatively short compared to other studies in the field of plyometrics, so with further training, there could have been a greater and/or significant change in rowing power. The sample size was also relatively small, possibly lacking the statistical power necessary to observe an increase in rowing power. Changes in RP also varied within the groups, suggesting that some individuals may have been better at performing the 15-s peak power ergometer test or possess the innate physiological traits or training acumen to achieve high rowing powers. Also, the motor coordination trained using plyometrics (jumping) is vastly different to the patterns used during the maximal peak power test, with a high rowing resistance. Furthermore, muscle coordination could have differed greatly between individuals due to the athletes being at varying stages of athletic maturity. However, it should be noted that with a greater sample size, and/or a longer training period, a significant difference in peak rowing power could be observed.

The peak rowing power test is a valuable test and predictor of rowing performance, as suggested by Ingham et al. [4]. However, the athletes whom Ingham et al. used were all elite rowers (current or former World Championship Finalists), who have a significantly higher athletic maturity and training history [4] when compared with the athletes in the current study. Therefore, the younger age and relatively lower training history (i.e., coordination and technical mastery) of the athletes utilized in the current study could explain the moderate improvement in rowing power. Specifically, these athletes may not have completed the physical and technical development to truly achieve maximum power, thus perhaps underestimating the possible changes with the training. However, we did find a significant inverse correlation between rowing power and rowing economy, that is, a greater rowing power was associated with lower energy expenditure for a given power output. This is suggestive that rowers with greater power may be more technically masterful and thus expend less energy during rowing.

Plyometric Training and Rowing Sprint Performance

Plyometric training has been shown to improve short running sprint performance [39], and results from the current study indicate that plyometric training is able to improve rowing sprint performance (Fig. 3). These findings are in contrast to a study performed by Kramer et al. in [3], in which 20 min of simple double leg plyometric exercises were added at the end of the strength training sessions completed by female collegiate rowers. Their rowing measures were a 2.5-km ergometer test, and the distance in meters achieved in 90 s. As a comparison with the current investigation, the 90-s rowing test is very similar to the 500-m TT. The average time for the plyometric group to perform the 500-m TT after training was ~95 s. Kramer et al. found no changes in the 90-s test after 9 weeks of training, whereas we observed a significant improvement in 500-m performance [3]. There are several potential reasons for this discrepancy.

The plyometric exercises used in the earlier study of Kramer et al. [3] were more simplistic than in the current investigation (e.g., no rotation or multiple jumps or upper body involvement). Indeed, the authors did indicate that the exercises they selected may not have been the best for improving rowing performance [3] and were performed following strength training, likely in a semi-fatigued state, suboptimal conditions for plyometric training. Additionally, in comparison to the study by Kramer et al., the current study contained more foot contacts (Table 2.) and focused on plyometric training versus steady-state training, matched for training volume (time) between groups. Kramer et al. did not match training volume [3]. To avoid this, training times were matched for volume of the dryland training in the present investigation. All on the water rowing training was also matched as all participants were members of the same team. Finally, Kramer et al. [3] recruited collegiate female rowers who were older than the high school male participants in the current study (mean age of 21 compared with a mean age of 16 years). As such, when prescribing plyometric training, it is important to consider factors such as performing these exercises in a non-fatigued state, foot contacts, and load in order to optimize any potential performance improvements.

Nonetheless, the current investigation was able to demonstrate that plyometric training improved 500-m rowing performance (Fig. 3). However, it remains to be seen if plyometric training is capable of improving rowing performance of a more gold standard distance, such as 2- or 6-km TT. As peak power was only moderately increased for the plyometric group, but rowing economy did not differ between pre- and post-training, the improvement in rowing performance could be due to increased rowing power but also to other mechanisms not measured in the current study (e.g., muscle coordination, activation, and rate of force development). Alternatively, the rating of perceived exertion, while not different prior to the intervention, was significantly reduced post-training in the PLYO group only (Fig. 2), which suggests a possible shift in maximal work rate, or the plyometric training may have increased the tolerance for work, thereby reducing perceived effort, and either phenomena might have contributed to the increased performance.

Experimental Considerations

The current study is not provided without limitation or further consideration. While the 500-m TT was shown to improve as a result of the plyometric training, the training program (three 30-min sessions/week) might be considered time consuming for coaches that are usually working under stringent time constraints. Although, the results from the current study indicate that plyometric training does not impair rowing economy; thus, if on-the-water or ergometer training is not available (e.g., weather or time constraints), plyometric training might serve as an effective substitute or adjunct.

As the purpose of the study was to highlight the effects of plyometric training, we cannot ascertain whether inclusion of strength training or strength training alone would provide additional or superior benefit. Plyometrics are often performed in conjunction with weight training (also known as complex training) and have been shown to cause greater improvements in power than either modality alone [40]. Whether or not complex training is beneficial for rowing performance has yet to be evaluated.

The 500-m TT measure used here is not the gold standard rowing performance test used by rowing coaches. The 2-km ergometer time trial is the most common rowing performance measure [1]. This test not only measures rowing ability, fitness, and technique but also mental fortitude. For this last reason, the 2-km test was not used to evaluate rowing performance of the young athletes in the current study. In young rowers, 2-km performances can vary greatly due to it being mentally challenging so the much shorter 500-m test was used to provide a more objective measure of whether the plyometric program improved rowing performance. Although it is worth mentioning that the reliability of the 500-m TT was not tested, the athletes were very accustomed to the test distance as it is included in training and assessment. Additionally, the athletes were not periodized for the 2-km test, which typically occurs in the spring season. As the 2-km test was not performed in the current study, further research is needed to definitively demonstrate whether improvements in 500-m performance due to plyometrics can be translated into the full 2-km test. The results of the current study can only be applied to youth males, and it remains to be seen if such training responses would be seen in older and/or more developed athletes. Although the 500-m test is not a gold standard measure for rowing, the fact that the athletes were able to significantly improve performance with plyometric training is important. First, because the athletes were able to improve their rowing sprint performance during a time in which no rowing sprint training was being undertaken, this might be a way to preserve anaerobic performance without detriment to aerobic performance (i.e., rowing economy). Second, coaches can also use the 500-m performance to estimate the 2000-m performance, as some coaches consider the wattage produced over 500 m to be 138% of 2000-m watts. Finally, more detailed exploration of the possible changes in muscle will provide greater insight into the training responses to plyometrics in rowers (e.g., hop test and vertical jump).

Conclusions

The purpose of this study was to determine whether plyometrics, a form of power training already used by rowing coaches, could improve rowing performance and the physiological measures of rowing economy and rowing power. Plyometrics significantly improved the 500-m TT rowing performance and moderately improved peak rowing power, but did not improve rowing economy, suggesting that improved rowing power and other factors could be responsible for the observed increased performance. These results suggest that plyometrics are able to improve rowing performance in young rowers and possibly in older/elite rowers and that rowing coaches should continue using this form of training. Plyometrics can be performed by coaches in conjunction with other methods of strength training or as a warm-up before beginning rowing-specific training. However, further research is needed to determine whether plyometrics can improve 2-km rowing performance and performance of other populations (i.e., elite rowers).

Acknowledgements

We are very grateful to the coaches and rowers of the Saratoga Rowing Association for allowing us to perform this investigation with them.

Authors' Contributions

JE-S, RE, SI, CE, and VO all made substantial contributions to the conception and design, acquisition of the data, or analysis and interpretation of the data. JE-S, RE, SI, CE, and VO were all involved in the drafting of the manuscript or in revising it critically for important intellectual content. JE-S, RE, SI, CE, and VO all agreed to be accountable for all aspects of the work in ensuring that questions related to the accuracy or integrity of any part of the work are appropriately investigated and resolved. JE-S, RE, SI, CE, and VO all approved the final version of the manuscript.

Competing Interest

Julian Egan-Shuttler, Rohan Edmonds, Cassandra Eddy, Veronica O'Neill, and Stephen J. Ives declare that they have no conflict of interest. No financial support was received for the conduct of this study or preparation of this manuscript. The findings and data presented in this study are presented honestly, without fabrication and data manipulation.

References

1. Mäestu J, Jürimäe J, Jürimäe T. Monitoring of performance and training in rowing. Sports Med. 2005;35(7):597–617.
2. Gee TI, Olsen PD, Berger NJ, Golby J, Thompson KG. Strength and conditioning practices in rowing. J Strength Cond Res. 2011;25(3):668–82.
3. Kramer JF, Morrow A, Leger A. Changes in rowing ergometer, weight lifting, vertical jump and isokinetic performance in response to standard and standard plus plyometric training programs. Int J Sports Med. 1993;14(8):449–54.
4. Ingham S, Whyte G, Jones K, Nevill A. Determinants of 2,000 m rowing ergometer performance in elite rowers. Eur J Appl Physiol. 2002;88(3):243–6.
5. de Campos MF, de Moraes Bertuzzi RC, Grangeiro PM, Franchini E. Energy systems contributions in 2,000 m race simulation: a comparison among rowing ergometers and water. Eur J Appl Physiol. 2009;107(5):615–9.
6. Kennedy MD, Bell GJ. Development of race profiles for the performance of a simulated 2000-m rowing race. Can J Appl Physiol. 2003;28(4):536–46.
7. Lawton TW, Cronin JB, McGuigan MR. Strength testing and training of rowers. Sports Med. 2011;41(5):413–32.
8. Haykowsky M, Syrotuik D, Taylor D, Bell G. The effect of high-intensity rowing and combined strength and endurance training on left ventricular systolic function and morphology. Int J Sports Med. 2007;28(06):488–94.
9. Izquierdo M, Exposito R, Garcia-Pallare J, Medina L, Villareal E. Concurrent endurance and strength training not to failure optimizes performance gains. Sci Sports Exerc. 2010;42:1191–9.
10. Young KC, Kendall KL, Patterson KM, Pandya PD, Fairman CM, Smith SW. Rowing performance, body composition, and bone mineral density outcomes in college-level rowers after a season of concurrent training. Int J Sports Physiol Perform. 2014;9(6):966–72. doi:10.1123/ijspp.2013-0428.
11. Markovic G, Mikulic P. Neuro-musculoskeletal and performance adaptations to lower-extremity plyometric training. Sports Med. 2010;40(10):859–95.
12. Sáez-Sáez de Villarreal E, Requena B, Newton RU. Does plyometric training improve strength performance? A meta-analysis J Sci Med Sport. 2010;13(5): 513–22.
13. Häkkinen K, Pakarinen A, Kallinen M. Neuromuscular adaptations and serum hormones in women during short-term intensive strength training. Eur J Appl Physiol Occup Physiol. 1992;64(2):106–11.
14. Moritani T, Herbert AD. Neural factors versus hypertrophy in the time course of muscle strength gain. Am J Phys Med. 1979;58(3):115–30.
15. Häkkinen K, Komi PV. Effect of explosive type strength training on electromyographic and force production characteristics of leg extensors muscles during concentric and various stretch-shortening cycle exercises. Scand J Sports Sci. 1985;7(2):65–76.
16. Kyröläinen H, Avela J, McBride JM, Koskinen S, Andersen JL, Sipilä S, et al. Effects of power training on muscle structure and neuromuscular performance. Scand J Med Sci Sports. 2005;15(1):58–64.
17. Rezaimanesh D, Amiri-Farsani P, Saidian S. The effect of a 4 week plyometric training period on lower body muscle EMG changes in futsal players. Procedia Soc Behav Sci. 2011;15:3138–42.
18. Potteiger JA, Lockwood RH, Haub MD, Dolezal BA, Almuzaini KS, Schroeder JM, et al. Muscle power and fiber characteristics following 8 weeks of plyometric training. J Strength Cond Res. 1999;13(3):275–9.
19. Pellegrino J, Ruby BC, Dumke CL. Effect of plyometrics on the energy cost of running and MHC and titin isoforms. Med Sci Sports Exerc. 2016;48(1):49–56.
20. Chimera NJ, Swanik KA, Swanik CB, Straub SJ. Effects of plyometric training on muscle-activation strategies and performance in female athletes. J Athl Train. 2004;39(1):24–31.
21. Turner AM, Owings M, Schwane JA. Improvement in running economy after 6 weeks of plyometric training. J Strength Cond Res. 2003;17(1):60–7.
22. Douglas L, Krahenbuhl GS. Running economy and distance running performance of highly trained athletes. Med Sci Sports Exerc. 1980;12(5):357–60.
23. Paavolainen L, Häkkinen K, Rusko H. Effects of explosive type strength training on physical performance characteristics in cross-country skiers. Eur J Appl Physiol Occup Physiol. 1991;62(4):251–5.
24. Spurrs RW, Murphy AJ, Watsford ML. The effect of plyometric training on distance running performance. Eur J Appl Physiol. 2003;89(1):1–7.
25. Lloyd RS, Oliver JL, Hughes MG, Williams CA. The effects of 4-weeks of plyometric training on reactive strength index and leg stiffness in male youths. J Strength Cond Res. 2012;26(10):2812–9.
26. Chu DA. Jumping into plyometrics. Champaign: Human Kinetics; 1992.
27. Persinger R, Foster C, Gibson M, Fater DC, Porcari JP. Consistency of the talk test for exercise prescription. Med Sci Sports Exerc. 2004;36(9):1632–6.
28. Paavolainen L, Häkkinen K, Hämäläinen I, Nummela A, Rusko H. Explosive-strength training improves 5-km running time by improving running economy and muscle power. American Physiological Society. 1999;86(5):1527–33.
29. Hopkins WG, Schabort EJ, Hawley JA. Reliability of power in physical performance tests. Sports Med. 2001;31(3):211–34.
30. Borg GA. Psychophysical bases of perceived exertion. Med Sci Sports Exerc. 1982;14(5):377–81.
31. Hopkins W, Marshall S, Batterham A, Hanin J. Progressive statistics for studies in sports medicine and exercise science. Med Sci Sports Exerc. 2009;41(1):3.
32. Cohen J. Statistical power analysis for the behavioral sciences. 2nd ed. Hillsdale: Lawrence Erlbaum; 1988.
33. Dalleau G, Belli A, Bourdin M, Lacour J. The spring-mass model and the energy cost of treadmill running. Eur J Appl Physiol Occup Physiol. 1998; 77(3):257–63.
34. Kleshnev V. Boat acceleration, temporal structure of the stroke cycle, and effectiveness in rowing. Proceedings of the Institution of Mechanical Engineers, Part P: Journal of Sports Engineering and Technology. 2010;224(1):63–74.
35. Carter AB, Kaminski TW, Douex Jr AT, Knight CA, Richards JG. Effects of high volume upper extremity plyometric training on throwing velocity and functional strength ratios of the shoulder rotators in collegiate baseball players. J Strength Cond Res. 2007;21(1):208–15.
36. Miller MG, Herniman JJ, Ricard MD, Cheatham CC, Michael TJ. The effects of a 6-week plyometric training program on agility. J Sports Sci Med. 2006;5(3):459.
37. Davies G, Riemann BL, Manske R. Current concepts of plyometric exercise. Int J Sports Phys Ther. 2015;10(6):760–86.
38. McCormick BT, Hannon JC, Newton M, Shultz B, Detling N, Young WB. The effects of frontal-and sagittal-plane plyometrics on change-of-direction speed and power in adolescent female basketball players. Int J Sports Physiol Perform. 2015;11(1):102–7.
39. Rimmer E, Sleivert G. Effects of a plyometrics intervention program on sprint performance. J Strength Cond Res. 2000;14(3):295–301.
40. Adams K, O'Shea JP, O'Shea KL, Climstein M. The effect of six weeks of squat, plyometric and squat-plyometric training on power production. J Appl Sport Sci Res. 1992;6(1):36–41.

A Placebo-Controlled Trial of Riboflavin for Enhancement of Ultramarathon Recovery

Martin D. Hoffman[1,2*], Taylor R. Valentino[3], Kristin J. Stuempfle[4] and Brandon V. Hassid[5]

Abstract

Background: Riboflavin is known to protect tissue from oxidative damage but, to our knowledge, has not been explored as a means to control exercise-related muscle soreness. This study investigated whether acute ingestion of riboflavin reduces muscle pain and soreness during and after completion of a 161-km ultramarathon and improves functional recovery after the event.

Methods: In this double-blind, placebo-controlled trial, participants of the 2016 161-km Western States Endurance Run were assigned to receive a riboflavin or placebo capsule shortly before the race start and when reaching 90 km. Capsules contained either 100 mg of riboflavin or 95 mg of maltodextrin and 5 mg of 10% ß-carotene. Subjects provided muscle pain and soreness ratings before, during, and immediately after the race and for the 10 subsequent days. Subjects also completed 400-m runs at maximum speed on days 3, 5, and 10 after the race.

Results: For the 32 (18 in the riboflavin group, 14 in the placebo group) race finishers completing the study, muscle pain and soreness ratings during and immediately after the race were found to be significantly lower ($p = .043$) for the riboflavin group. Analysis of the 400-m run times also showed significantly faster ($p < .05$) times for the riboflavin group than the placebo group at post-race days 3 and 5. Both groups showed that muscle pain and soreness had returned to pre-race levels by 5 days after the race and that 400-m run times had returned to pre-race performance levels by 10 days after the race.

Conclusions: This preliminary work suggests that riboflavin supplementation before and during prolonged running might reduce muscle pain and soreness during and at the completion of the exercise and may enhance early functional recovery after the exercise.

Keywords: Creatine kinase, Muscle fatigue, Muscle pain, Muscle soreness, Running

Key Points

- This study provides some evidence that riboflavin supplementation immediately before and during prolonged running may reduce muscle pain and soreness during and at the completion of the run.
- The study also offers some suggestion that riboflavin supplementation immediately before and during prolonged running might enhance functional recovery after the run.
- The findings should be considered preliminary and are based on a relatively small number of subjects but are particularly intriguing and warrant further investigation since the dose and dosing schedule might not have been optimal.

Background

Post-exercise muscle pain and soreness have been well documented in ultramarathon running [1–8]; however, the precise etiology and pathophysiology remain elusive. Presumably, the process begins with mechanical damage to the muscle and connective tissue; is followed by inflammation, swelling, and the production of free radicals; and culminates in the pain and soreness felt during and after exercise [9–11]. Markers of inflammation and

* Correspondence: mdhoffman@ucdavis.edu
[1]Department of Physical Medicine & Rehabilitation, Department of Veterans Affairs, Northern California Health Care System, Sacramento, CA, USA
[2]Ultra Sports Science Foundation, El Dorado Hills, CA, USA
Full list of author information is available at the end of the article

oxidative stress are known to be high following an ultramarathon [5, 7, 12–15].

Numerous pre- and post-exercise interventions using nutritional supplements and dietary strategies have been investigated for prevention or treatment of exercise-related muscle pain and soreness [10, 16]. Since the inflammatory response and free radical production with oxidative stress are likely involved in the mechanism leading to exercise-related muscle soreness, it seems plausible that supplementation with substances having anti-inflammatory or antioxidant properties may be an effective means of controlling such soreness. While research has provided some general support for the effectiveness of such substances in reducing exercise-related muscle soreness [10, 16], previous studies specific to ultramarathon running have demonstrated no effect. For instance, 6 weeks of vitamin E and C supplementation was found to have no effect on muscle damage, inflammatory markers, or muscle function recovery after a 50-km trail run [12, 13]. Furthermore, 3 weeks of supplementation with quercetin, another substance with known antioxidant properties, was not found to alter antioxidant capacity or oxidative damage, inflammation, muscle damage, or post-race muscle soreness from a 161-km ultramarathon [6, 15].

A common nutritional supplement that we believe has not been investigated for its effect on exercise-related muscle soreness is vitamin B2 (riboflavin). As for other flavonoids, riboflavin is known to exhibit antioxidant properties and protect tissue from oxidative damage [17–23]. Riboflavin is also important in cell repair and production and for protecting mitochondrial and other enzymes as a mitochondrial enzyme cofactor or cofactor precursor [24]. It is one of eight water-soluble B vitamins found in many foods and must be regularly supplied in the diet as it is not stored by the body [25]. Human trials have largely focused on the efficacy of riboflavin supplementation for migraine prophylaxis with favorable findings [26, 27]. Whether or not it might provide a protective role or enhanced recovery from exercise-induced skeletal muscle damage is unknown.

The purpose of this study was to investigate whether acute ingestion of riboflavin is effective at reducing muscle pain and soreness during and after completion of a 161-km ultramarathon, and in improving functional recovery after the event. The study was performed in association with the 161-km Western States Endurance Run (WSER) since this race is known to induce considerable muscle damage and pain [2, 3, 5–7, 28–32]. Based upon the evidence that riboflavin can protect tissue from oxidative damage and is important in cell repair, we hypothesized that riboflavin would be effective at reducing muscle pain and soreness and improving muscle recovery after this extreme level of exercise.

Methods

Study Design and Subjects

This double-blind, placebo-controlled trial was performed at the 2016 WSER, a 161.3-km ultramarathon through the Sierra Nevada Mountains of Northern California. The course is mostly single-track trail with 5500 m of cumulative climb and 7000 m of cumulative descent. Other race details have been provided elsewhere [33–36]. Nearby weather station ambient temperatures during the race ranged from a low of 1 °C at the start to a high of 34 °C. The San Francisco State University Institutional Review Board provided approval for the research with electronic consent obtained during online enrollment and formal consent obtained at race registration. Study participants completing the pre-race data collection were provided a t-shirt, and those completing the entire study were provided a $50 (USD) gift certificate.

Subject recruitment was by electronic notices sent to all race entrants 59 and 19 days before the race. Because of inadequate subject recruitment, additional subjects were recruited during race registration held the day before the race start.

All study participants were met during race registration for formal consenting, additional pre-race data collection, and review of expectations for participation. Subjects were then seen for further intervention before and during the race as outlined below. Immediately after race completion, subjects were escorted 30 m to a tent adjacent to the finish line where post-race data collection and a blood draw were performed. During the subsequent 10 days, the subjects recorded additional information that was then returned to the investigators electronically or by mail. They were sent an email the evening after the race reminding them of the post-race data collection and were provided an electronic copy of the data sheet at that time.

Subjects were asked to avoid any use of pain or non-steroidal anti-inflammatory drugs (NSAIDs) during the race. Additionally, subjects were asked to avoid use of pain medications or NSAIDs, compression garments, massage, electrical stimulation, and thermal modalities in the 10 days following the race. To check compliance, the post-race data form requested that they provide details about use of pain medications or NSAIDs during or after the race or any of the above interventions during the 10 days after the race. Subjects were also asked which group they thought they were in and why.

Intervention

Subjects were assigned to the riboflavin or placebo group in an alternating fashion based on the order of arrival to meet with the research team at race registration, with the on-site researchers and subjects being blinded to the group assignment. The subjects were told that they would receive either a placebo or an essential vitamin with flavonoid properties, but no other details of the supplement under study were provided until after data analysis had been completed.

All subjects received a capsule 0.5–1 h before the start of the race with a cup of water and were observed to swallow the capsule. They were also provided and observed to take another capsule at the 90-km aid station. Capsules were prepared by the investigators using riboflavin (Nature's Way Products, Inc., Green Bay, WI), maltodextrin (Now, Bloomingdale, IL), and 10% ß-carotene powder (BulkSupplements.com, Henderson, NV). The treatment group received capsules containing 100 mg of riboflavin, and the control group received capsules containing 95 mg of maltodextrin and 5 mg of 10% ß-carotene. Because riboflavin can cause urine to appear bright or fluorescent yellow [37] and might allow subjects to suspect they were in the treatment group, the small amount of ß-carotene was added to the placebo, as done in a prior placebo-controlled trial of riboflavin [27], since it can also cause a similar urine color change. The amount of ß-carotene in each capsule was approximately half of that in a single large raw baby carrot [38], so we recognize it was unlikely to cause marked urine discoloration, but it did allow us to legitimately tell the subjects that they might notice a discoloration of the urine regardless of their group assignment. We also recognized that ß-carotene is an antioxidant but felt that it would have no recognizable antioxidant effect at such a low dose.

Measurements

Body Weight

The body weight of each subject was obtained at race registration and immediately after finishing the race using the same scale (Sunbeam Products, Inc., Health o meter, model 349KLX, Boca Raton, FL) placed on a firm, level surface. For each measurement, the runner was clothed in running attire and shoes but had no other items on their body or in their hands.

Plasma Creatine Kinase Concentration

Plasma creatine kinase (CK) concentration was determined immediately post-race from a blood sample taken from the antecubital vein, with subjects seated in the upright position. The samples were centrifuged for 10 min at 3400 rpm within 10 min of collection and then stored in a cooler until transported to and analyzed by a clinical laboratory for plasma CK concentrations (Siemens Aktiengesellschaft, Dimension EXL, Munich, Germany).

Subjective Measurement of Muscle Pain and Soreness

Runners were asked to rate their perceived lower-body muscle pain and soreness according to a 10-point Likert scale with anchors of 1 (no soreness), 2.5 (dull, vague ache), 4 (slight soreness), 5.5 (more than slight soreness), 7 (sore), 8.5 (very sore), and 10 (unbearably sore). This approach has been previously used at the WSER [2–7] and elsewhere [39], and the values have been found to correlate with plasma CK concentrations [3–5]. Ratings were provided at race registration, during the race at the 48-, 90-, and 126-km checkpoints, at the finish prior to the blood draw, and each morning of the 10 days following the race after being up and moving around for approximately 30 min.

Functional Measurement

A 400-m run at maximal speed was used as a functional measurement, which we have previously used successfully [2, 3]. Those subjects enrolled in advance of race registration were asked to perform this test twice on separate days during the 21 days before the race, and all subjects were asked to perform the test on days 3, 5, and 10 after the race. Subjects were sent an electronic reminder the night before each post-race 400-m run. This test is functionally specific for running, but not overwhelmingly long and painful or so short and intense that it would be a high risk for inducing a strain injury. After an adequate warm-up, subjects were instructed to self-time the run, starting from a standing start. Subjects were asked to use the inside lane of a running track, assuring an accurate distance. In the event they did not have access to a track, they were allowed to utilize a level section of road that had been measured to the correct distance. They were asked to use the same site for all pre-race and post-race testing and under conditions without significant wind or other environmental variations.

Statistical Analyses

Comparison of treatment and control groups (age, sex, finish time, percent change in body mass from registration to immediately post-race, post-race plasma CK concentration, pre-race 400-m run time, average weekly running distance, highest weekly running distance, and longest training run) were made using unpaired *t* tests and the chi-square test. Main outcome variables (muscle pain and soreness rating and 400-m run time) were compared between groups with two-way (group × time) repeated measure analysis of variance (ANOVA) and Bonferroni post-tests. These data were tested for normality with the D'Agostino-Pearson normality test. The 400-m run time data were skewed and successfully normalized before analysis with the reciprocal function (i.e., transformed value = 1/original value). Statistical significance was set at $p < 0.05$.

A priori sample size determination was performed based on muscle pain and soreness ratings from previous research at the WSER [2–4]. Using a level of significance of $p < 0.05$, an expected common SD of 1.5 points, and 80% power, the predicted minimum sample size to determine a meaningful group difference of 1.5 points was 13 per group. Recent research at the WSER has shown attrition rate to be roughly 25–30% [2, 3, 40], so we aimed to recruit a minimum of 17 subjects per group.

Results

Of the 353 race entries, 44 runners enrolled in the study (22 in each group) and started the race. Of this group, 37 (84.1%, 20 in riboflavin group, 17 in placebo group) finished the race and 32 (18 in riboflavin group, 14 in placebo group) completed data collection. Of the 32 completing data collection, 8 had enrolled in advance of race registration and completed both pre-race 400-m run trials (5 in riboflavin group, 3 in placebo group). Overall race finish rate was 79.3% (280 of 353 starters), which was similar ($p = .55$) to that for the study participants.

Selected characteristics of the subjects completing the study are shown in Table 1. None of the examined characteristics differed between groups, including the post-race plasma CK concentrations. Furthermore, race finish rate (91 and 77% for the riboflavin and placebo groups, respectively) and study completion rate (82 and 64% for the riboflavin and placebo groups, respectively) did not differ statistically ($p = .4$ and $p = .3$, respectively) between groups. One subject in the placebo group failed to receive the capsule at 90 km, and two subjects in the riboflavin group reported emesis within an hour after taking the capsule at 90 km. All other subjects received both doses and were confirmed to not have had emesis during the hour after taking a capsule. Post-race exercise behavior appeared comparable between groups, and during the first 2 days post-race, none of our subjects reported exercise more taxing than running less than 2 km or some walking.

The findings relative to muscle pain and soreness ratings for those subjects completing the study are shown in Fig. 1. Analysis of the data across all time points revealed no significant group ($p = .14$) or group by time interaction ($p = .25$), but there was a significant ($p < .0001$) time effect. Post-race values were statistically similar to pre-race values by post-race day 5. The pre-race and race data for all subjects providing data through 90 km (21 and 20 in riboflavin and placebo groups, respectively) were also analyzed. There was a significant group by time interaction ($p = .023$) and time ($p < .0001$) effect, but no group effect ($p = .075$), and post-testing revealed a significantly lower value ($p < .01$) for the riboflavin group than the placebo group at 90 km. This finding prompted further exploratory analysis of the data for those subjects completing the study with exclusion of the pre-race and post-race data (i.e., considering only the ratings during the race and at the finish) that yielded a significant ($p = .043$) group effect, as well as a significant ($p < .0001$) time effect, but no significant ($p = .22$) interaction effect.

The post-race 400-m run times are shown in Fig. 2. Significant time ($p < .0001$) and group ($p = .016$) effects were found, but no significant ($p = .60$) interaction effect was evident. Post-testing revealed significant group differences ($p < .05$) at post-race days 3 and 5. For the 8 subjects who had completed 400-m runs prior to the race, the post-race day 10 times were not statistically different ($p = .10$) from the pre-race times (mean ± SD,

Table 1 Selected characteristics of the two study groups

Characteristic	Riboflavin ($n = 18$)	Placebo ($n = 14$)
Age (years)	44 ± 8	46 ± 7
Sex (% men)	83	79
Average weekly running distance (km)[a]	83 ± 20	94 ± 20
Highest week running distance (km)[a]	135 (126–156)	129 (120–142)
Longest training run or race (km)[a]	80 (66–92)	80 (56–97)
Body mass change from registration to post-race (%)	−3.6 ± 2.1	−2.6 ± 2.0
Finish time (hours)	27.26 ± 2.36	27.08 ± 2.88
Used any pain medication during the race (%)	50	36
Used any pain medication in 10 days post-race (%)	33	43
Post-race plasma CK (U/L)	6804 (3536–24,592)	12,819 (7560–46,965)

Data are reported as mean ± SD, a percentage, or median (interquartile range) if the data were skewed for either group

[a]Distances are during the 3 months prior to the race. No significant group differences were present

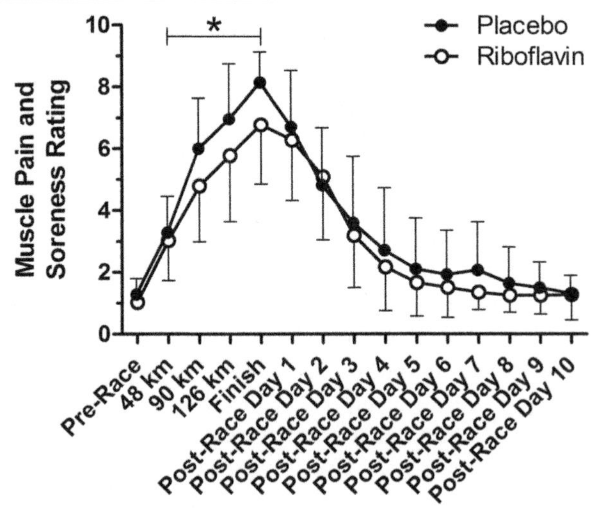

Fig. 1 Mean lower-body muscle pain and soreness ratings for the 2 groups. *$p = .043$ for group comparison considering only the during-race and finish data. *Error bars* represent 1 SD and are shown only in 1 direction for clarity

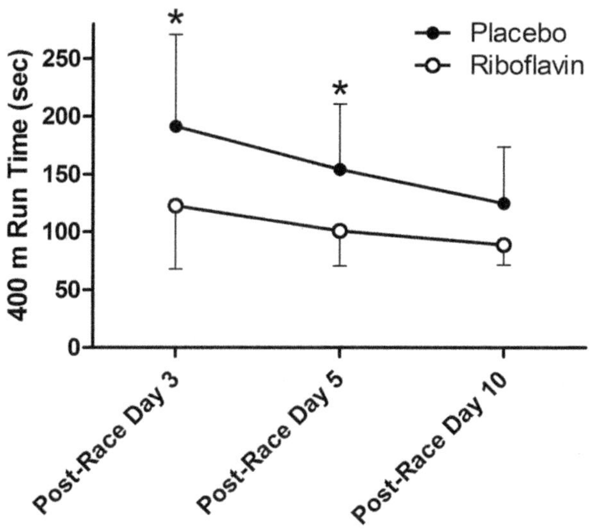

Fig. 2 Mean 400-m run times for the 2 groups. *$p < .05$ for post-testing group comparison. *Error bars* represent 1 SD and are shown only in 1 direction for clarity

82 ± 9, 80 ± 10, and 85 ± 7 s for pre-race trial 1, pre-race trial 2, and post-race day 10, respectively).

As shown in Table 1, pain medication use during the race was not different between groups but was at 50% among the riboflavin group and 36% among the placebo group. Considering the 9 subjects in the riboflavin group who reported using pain medication during the race, 7 used a NSAID and 2 used acetaminophen at a mean (range) of 29% (12–62%) of the maximum recommended 24-h dose. Of the 6 subjects in the placebo group who reported using pain medication during the race, 1 used a NSAID and 4 used either acetaminophen, paracetamol, or paracetamol with codeine at a mean (range) of 39% (10–75%) of the maximum recommended 24-h dose. Comparison of muscle pain and soreness ratings between subjects who used pain medication during the race with those not using pain medication during the race revealed no suggestion of a group or interaction effect, whether considering all time points ($p = .43$ and $p = .61$ for group and interaction effects, respectively) or just the ratings during the race and at the finish ($p = .98$ and $p = .82$ for group and interaction effects, respectively).

Subjects who received riboflavin correctly suspected they had received the treatment 50% of the time, whereas 23% of the placebo group incorrectly thought they were in the treatment group. These rates of suspicion about being in the treatment group were not statistically different ($p = .16$). There were 3 subjects in the riboflavin group and 1 subject in the placebo group who noted a yellow urine color.

Discussion

This work is a preliminary examination of riboflavin for potential benefits of reducing muscle pain and soreness during and after strenuous exercise and at enhancing recovery from strenuous exercise. The findings suggest that the vitamin may have some benefits. Indeed, riboflavin supplementation immediately before and midway during prolonged exercise appeared to be linked with reduced muscle pain and soreness during and at the completion of the exercise, and there was some evidence for enhanced functional performance during the initial several days after the exercise. While the findings require cautious interpretation, they are adequately interesting to warrant further investigation.

Given that post-race plasma CK concentrations were similar between groups, there is no evidence from this work that riboflavin acts by reducing muscle cell rupture. Rather, it would seem that it must act by altering the physiological response to exercise in other manners. While the underlying mechanism of action cannot be established from this study, it seems conceivable that the antioxidant properties of riboflavin [17–23] could explain reduced muscle pain and soreness during exercise, although the lack of reduced muscle pain and soreness during recovery does not seem consistent with this mechanism. On the other hand, the mitochondrial protective function of riboflavin [24] might be a plausible explanation for the riboflavin group demonstrating enhanced functional recovery without improvement in muscle pain and soreness during the recovery period.

Participants of the WSER are generally well-trained and experienced ultramarathon runners given that a recent qualifying ultramarathon is required to gain entry into the race. In this regard, they were conditioned for this type of activity and were adapted for controlling and responding to significant muscle injury from prolonged running. It is possible that an effect of riboflavin could be even greater in a group of subjects who are more naïve to strenuous exercise.

We chose to provide two 100-mg doses of riboflavin which were received immediately prior to exercise and around 11–16 h later during the approximately 20–30 h it took to complete the race. This dose and schedule were chosen because we felt it would be feasible to achieve subject cooperation and that any effectiveness should still be evident even if this was not the optimal dose or dosing schedule. The doses we provided were well above the recommended dietary allowance for riboflavin of 1.3 mg/day for adult men and 1.1 mg/day for adult women [41]. While the body absorbs little riboflavin from single doses beyond 27 mg [42], the vitamin appears safe at much higher doses [41] and riboflavin supplements are typically available in 100-mg capsules with recommendations to take 1–2 per day. Plasma concentrations of riboflavin and flavocoenzymes have been shown to peak around 2 and 3.5 h, respectively, after a single 60-mg dose of riboflavin, but the plasma concentrations remain elevated for hours [42]. Considering this information, it is possible that a lower dose at more frequent intervals might be more effective and would be recommended for future studies of this nature if feasible in the study environment.

The present findings indicate that muscle pain and soreness ratings of our subjects had returned to pre-race levels by 5 days after the race. For the subsample of 8 subjects who performed the pre-race 400-m runs, their times at 10 days after the race were statistically similar to pre-race times, although mean times were still ~5% slower at 10 days after the race. Our prior work at the WSER had also demonstrated that muscle pain and soreness ratings had statistically returned to baseline by post-race day 5, but 400-m run times were not examined in that study beyond post-race day 5 at which time pre-race performance had not been fully recovered [3]. In the present work, we extended the post-race time period of examination to 10 days and found that this appears to be close to the timeframe of 400-m run recovery. This is not intended to suggest that athletes are fully recovered from a 161-km ultramarathon within 10 days or shortly thereafter but rather that our subjective measure of resting muscle pain and soreness and our objective measure of 400-m speed had nearly recovered during this relatively short time period.

The WSER serves as an excellent environment to induce muscle pain and damage as evident from prior work at the race [2, 3, 5–7, 28–32]. This is confirmed with the present work in which muscle pain and soreness ratings at the end of the race averaged ~7–8 on the 10-point scale (sore to very sore) and median post-race plasma CK concentrations were ~7000–13,000 U/L. However, subject recruitment is a challenge in performing research of this nature in a competition setting such as the WSER. This is reflected in the number of subjects we were able to recruit. In particular, it is unfortunate that the number of subjects completing the pre-race 400-m runs was so low, which limits the robustness of our interpretation of the findings relative to functional recovery. While the treatment and placebo groups appeared to be well matched and blinding appeared to be adequate in this study, we cannot be certain that the groups were well matched for baseline performance at the 400-m run.

We acknowledge some other limitations with this study resulting largely from constraints related to the study being performed at a competition. Perhaps most importantly is that a sizable percentage of the subjects (50 and 36% in the riboflavin and placebo groups, respectively) used pain medication during the race and some used pain medication in the 10-day post-race period. The use of NSAIDs during this event has been common, ranging from 32 to 57% among those participating in our prior research [3, 34, 43]. Interestingly, earlier work has demonstrated that NSAID use during the race was not effective at controlling post-race muscle soreness [4] though the effect of NSAIDs on muscle pain and soreness during the race has not been systematically examined. Among the present subjects using pain medication during the race, the usual dosage was relatively low compared with the maximal recommended dose during 24 h. Not surprisingly, our separate comparison of muscle pain and soreness ratings between subjects who used pain medication during the race and those not using pain medication during the race revealed no suggestion of an effect of the pain medication on this variable. Thus, given these considerations, it seems unlikely that the use of pain medication during the race confounded the present finding of lower muscle pain and soreness during and at the completion of the race among the riboflavin group compared with the placebo group. Another potential study limitation is that, because we did not assess dietary practices of the subjects, it is conceivable that one group had a greater intake of anti-oxidants than the other. Additionally, the 400-m runs were unsupervised and self-timed, but this was the most feasible approach and we believe this study population was capable of maximally exerting themselves during unsupervised trials and correctly recording the times. Finally, we also recognize that some might consider it ideal to have measured pre-race plasma CK concentrations and to examine the pre-race to post-race change in plasma CK concentration rather than just the post-race value. But, since these runners would have reduced training prior to the race, we would expect pre-race plasma CK concentrations to have been very low relative to the post-race values, as previously demonstrated [4–7], so not using the pre-race to post-race change would not have altered our interpretation of the findings for this variable.

Conclusions

From this work, we conclude that there is some evidence that riboflavin supplementation immediately before and midway through prolonged running may reduce muscle pain and soreness during and at the completion of the exercise and that there is some suggestion that riboflavin might enhance functional recovery after the exercise. We acknowledge that this study is a preliminary examination of riboflavin for this purpose and involved a small number of subjects in which the dose and dosing schedule might not have been optimal. As such, the findings appear intriguing and warrant additional investigation of riboflavin as a means to reduce muscle pain during exercise and to enhance post-exercise recovery.

Abbreviations
ANOVA: Analysis of variance; CK: Creatine kinase; NSAID: Nonsteroidal anti-inflammatory drug; SD: Standard deviation; WSER: Western States Endurance Run

Acknowledgements
This research could not have been accomplished without the help of numerous volunteers. We thank Sutter Auburn Faith Hospital for laboratory services; John Fors, NP, Tracy Beth Høeg, MD, PhD, and Sonja A. Wilkey, MD, for phlebotomy services; and the following individuals for assistance with data collection: Dr. Jeffrey A. Chan, Kelly Cronin, George Daniel Cross, Casey Curl, Maria Gonzalez, Jasmine Magallanes, and Tiffany Anne Morales. The contents reported here do not represent the views of the Department of Veterans Affairs or the US Government.

Funding
The work was funded by the Western States Endurance Run Foundation and the Rossi Family Foundation and is also the result of work supported with resources and the use of facilities at the VA Northern California Health Care System.

Authors' Contributions
MDH and KJS conceived and designed the experiments. MDH, KJS, and TRV secured funding for the research. TRV, KJS, and BVH performed the experiments. MDH analyzed the data and prepared the manuscript. All authors discussed and revised the manuscript and approved the final manuscript.

Competing Interests
Martin D. Hoffman, Taylor R. Valentino, Kristin J. Stuempfle and Brandon V. Hassid have no conflicts of interest.

Author details
[1]Department of Physical Medicine & Rehabilitation, Department of Veterans Affairs, Northern California Health Care System, Sacramento, CA, USA. [2]Ultra Sports Science Foundation, El Dorado Hills, CA, USA. [3]Department of Kinesiology, San Francisco State University, San Francisco, CA, USA. [4]Health Sciences Department, Gettysburg College, Gettysburg, PA, USA. [5]School of Medicine, University of Maryland, Baltimore, MD, USA.

References

1. Frey W, Wassmer P, Frey-Rindova P, Braun D, Schwarz F, Arnold M, et al. Muscle aches and biochemical changes following a ultra-marathon in the cold—modification by diclofenac. Schweiz Z Med Traumatol. 1994;2:30–6.
2. Hoffman MD, Badowski N, Chin J, Stuempfle KJ. A randomized controlled trial of massage and pneumatic compression for ultramarathon recovery. J Orthop Sports Phys Ther. 2016;46(5):320–6.
3. Hoffman MD, Badowski N, Chin J, Stuempfle KJ, Parise CA. Determinants of recovery from a 161-km ultramarathon. J Sports Sci. 2017;35(7):669–77.
4. McAnulty S, McAnulty L, Nieman DC, Morrow J, Dumke C, Henson D. Effect of NSAID on muscle injury and oxidative stress. Int J Sports Med. 2007;28(11):909–15.
5. Nieman DC, Dumke CL, Henson DA, McAnulty SR, Gross SJ, Lind RH. Muscle damage is linked to cytokine changes following a 160-km race. Brain Behav Immun. 2005;19(5):398–403.
6. Nieman DC, Henson DA, Davis JM, Dumke CL, Gross SJ, Jenkins DP, et al. Quercetin ingestion does not alter cytokine changes in athletes competing in the Western States Endurance Run. J Interferon Cytokine Res. 2007;27(12):1003–11.
7. Nieman DC, Henson DA, Dumke CL, Oley K, McAnulty SR, Davis JM, et al. Ibuprofen use, endotoxemia, inflammation, and plasma cytokines during ultramarathon competition. Brain Behav Immun. 2006;20(6):578–84.
8. Visconti L, Capra G, Carta G, Forni C, Janin D. Effect of massage on DOMS in ultramarathon runners: a pilot study. J Bodyw Move Ther. 2015;19(3):458–63.
9. Bryne C, Twist C, Eston R. Neuromuscular function after exercise-induced muscle damage. Sports Med. 2004;34(1):49–69.
10. Connolly DA, Sayers S, McHugh MP. Treatment and prevention of delayed onset muscle soreness. J Strength Cond Res. 2003;17(1):197–208.
11. Eston RG, Mickleborough J, Baltzopoulos V. Eccentric activation and muscle damage: biomechanical and physiological considerations during downhill running. Br J Sports Med. 1995;29(2):89–94.
12. Mastaloudis A, Morrow JD, Hopkins DW, Devaraj S, Traber MG. Antioxidant supplementation prevents exercise-induced lipid peroxidation, but not inflammation, in ultramarathon runners. Free Radic Biol Med. 2004;36(10):1329–41.
13. Mastaloudis A, Traber MG, Carstensen K, Widrick JJ. Antioxidants did not prevent muscle damage in response to an ultramarathon. Med Sci Sports Exerc. 2006;38(1):72–80.
14. Nieman DC, Dumke CI, Henson DA, McAnulty SR, McAnulty LS, Lind RH, Morrow JD. Immune and oxidative changes during and following the Western States Endurance Run. Int J Sports Med. 2003;24(7):541–7.
15. Quindry JC, McAnulty SR, Hudson MB, Hosick P, Dumke C, McAnulty LS, et al. Oral quercetin supplementation and blood oxidative capacity in response to ultramarathon competition. Int J Sport Nutr Exerc Metab. 2008;18(6):601–16.
16. Sousa M, Teixeira VH, Soares J. Dietary strategies to recover from exercise-induced muscle damage. Int J Food Sci Nutr. 2014;65(2):151–63.
17. Christensen H. Riboflavin can protect tissue from oxidative injury. Nutr Rev. 1993;51(5):149–50.
18. Hultquist D, Xu F, Quandt KS, Shlafer M, Mack CP, Till GO, et al. Evidence that NADPH-dependent methemoglobin reductase and administered riboflavin protect tissues from oxidative injury. Am J Hematol. 1993;42(1):13–8.
19. Iwanaga K, Hasegawa T, Hultquist DE, Harada H, Yoshikawa Y, Yanamadala S, et al. Riboflavin-mediated reduction of oxidant injury, rejection, and vasculopathy after cardiac allotransplantation. Transplantation. 2007;83(6):747–53.
20. Lee ES, Corfe BM, Powers HJ. Riboflavin depletion of intestinal cells in vitro leads to impaired energy generation and enhanced oxidative stress. Eur J Nutr. 2013;52(5):1513–21.
21. Ogura R, Katsuki T, Daoud AH, Griffin AC. Anti-oxidative effects of vitamin B2-butyrate on the cardiac mitochondrial disorders induced by adriamycin. J Nutr Sci Vitaminol (Tokyo). 1982;28:329–34.
22. Sanches SC, Ramalho LN, Mendes-Braz M, Terra VA, Cecchini R, Augusto MJ, et al. Riboflavin (vitamin B-2) reduces hepatocellular injury following liver ischaemia and reperfusion in mice. Food Chem Toxicol. 2014;67:65–71.
23. Seekamp A, Hultquist DE, Till GO. Protection by vitamin B2 against oxidant-mediated acute lung injury. Inflammation. 1999;23:449–60.
24. Liu J, Ames BN. Reducing mitochondrial decay with mitochondrial nutrients to delay and treat cognitive dysfunction, Alzheimer's disease, and Parkinson's disease. Nutr Neurosci. 2005;8:67–89.
25. Kennedy DO. B vitamins and the brain: mechanisms, dose and efficacy-a review. Nutrients. 2016;8(2):68.
26. Boehnke C, Reuter U, Flach U, Schuh-Hofer S, Einhäupl KM, Arnold G. High-dose riboflavin treatment is efficacious in migraine prophylaxis: an open study in a tertiary care center. Eur J Neurol. 2004;11(7):475–7.
27. Schoenen J, Jacquy J, Lenaerts M. Effectiveness of high-dose riboflavin in migraine prophylaxis. A randomized controlled trial. Neurology. 1998;50(2):466–70.
28. Hoffman MD, Ingwerson JL, Rogers IR, Hew-Butler T, Stuempfle KJ. Increasing creatine kinase concentrations at the 161-km Western States Endurance Run. Wilderness Environ Med. 2012;23(1):56–60.
29. Hoffman MD, Stuempfle KJ. Sodium supplementation and exercise-associated hyponatremia during prolonged exercise. Med Sci Sports Exerc. 2015;47(9):1781–7.
30. Hoffman MD, Stuempfle KJ. Muscle cramping during a 161-km ultramarathon: comparison of characteristics of those with and without cramping. Sports Med Open. 2015;1(1):8. Epub 2015 May 21.
31. Hoffman MD, Stuempfle KJ, Fogard K, Hew-Butler T, Winger J, Weiss RH. Urine dipstick analysis for identification of runners susceptible to acute kidney injury following an ultramarathon. J Sports Sci. 2013;31(1):20–31.
32. Kasmer ME, Wren JJ, Hoffman MD. Foot strike pattern and gait changes during a 161-km ultramarathon. J Strength Cond Res. 2014;28(5):1343–50.
33. Hoffman MD, Fogard K. Factors related to successful completion of a 161-km ultramarathon. Int J Sports Physiol Perform. 2011;6(1):25–37.
34. Hoffman MD, Stuempfle KJ, Rogers IR, Weschler LB, Hew-Butler T. Hyponatremia in the 2009 161-km Western States Endurance Run. Int J Sports Physiol Perform. 2012;7(1):6–10.
35. Hoffman MD, Wegelin JA. The Western States 100-Mile Endurance Run:

participation and performance trends. Med Sci Sports Exerc. 2009;41(12):2191–8.
36. Parise C, Hoffman MD. Influence of temperature and performance level on pacing a 161-km trail ultramarathon. Int J Sports Physiol Perform. 2011;6(2):243–51.
37. Kenefick RW, Heavens KR, Dennis WE, Caruso EM, Guerriere KI, Charkoudian N, et al. Quantification of chromatographic effects of vitamin B supplementation in urine and implications for hydration assessment. J Appl Physiol (1985). 2015;119(2):110–5.
38. US Department of Agriculture, Agricultural Research Service, Nutrient Data Laboratory. USDA National Nutrient Database for Standard Reference, Release 28. Version Current: September 2015. https://ndb.nal.usda.gov/ndb. Accessed 5 Jan 2017.
39. Smith L, Brunetz MH, Chenier TC, McCammon MR, Houmard JA, Franklin ME, et al. The effects of static and ballistic stretching on delayed onset muscle soreness and creatine kinase. Res Q Exerc Sport. 1993;64(1):103–7.
40. Stuempfle KJ, Valentino T, Hew-Butler T, Hecht FM, Hoffman MD. Nausea is associated with endotoxemia during a 161-km ultramarathon. J Sports Sci. 2016;34(17):1662–8.
41. Institute of Medicine. Dietary reference intakes for thiamin, riboflavin, niacin, vitamin B6, folate, vitamin B12, pantothenic acid, biotin, and choline. Washington, DC: The National Academies Press; 1998. doi:10.17226/6015.
42. Zempleni J, Galloway JR, McCormick DB. Pharmacokinetics of orally and intravenously administered riboflavin in healthy humans. Am J Clin Nutr. 1996;63:54–66.
43. Hoffman MD, Fogard K, Winger J, Hew-Butler T, Stuempfle KJ. Characteristics of 161-km ultramarathon finishers developing exercise-associated hyponatremia. Res Sports Med. 2013;21:164–75.

The analysis of knee joint loading during drop landing from different heights and under different instruction sets in healthy males

Dmitry Verniba[1,2,3*], Jason D. Vescovi[2], David A. Hood[2,3] and William H. Gage[1,2,3]

Abstract

Background: Mechanical loading during exercise has been shown to promote tissue remodeling. Safe and accessible exercise may be beneficial to populations at risk of diminished bone and joint health. We examined the effect of drop height and instruction on knee loading during a drop-landing task and proposed a task that makes use of drop heights that may be appropriate for rehabilitation purposes and functional in daily life to examine transient knee joint loads.

Methods: Twenty males (22.0 ± 2.8 years) performed drop landings from 22 cm (low) and 44 cm (high) heights, each under three instructions: "land naturally" (natural), "softly" (soft), and "stiffly" (stiff). Knee compression force and external flexion moment were estimated using three-dimensional inverse dynamics and normalized to body mass.

Results: Peak knee compression force was larger ($p < 0.001$) for high (17.8 ± 0.63 N/kg) than low (14.8 ± 0.61 N/kg) heights. There was an increase ($p < 0.001$) in the knee compression force across soft (11.8 ± 0.40 N/kg), natural (17.0 ± 0.62 N/kg), and stiff (20.2 ± 0.67 N/kg) instructions. Peak knee flexion moment in high-natural (2.12 ± 0.08 Nm/kg) was larger ($p < 0.001$) than in high-soft (1.88 ± 0.08 Nm/kg), but lower than in high-stiff (2.23 ± 0.08 Nm/kg). No differences in peak knee flexion moment were observed across instructions for the low height.

Conclusions: We propose a drop-landing task that creates a scalable increase in knee compression loading. The absence of increased knee flexion moment with drop from the low height, compared to high, suggests that individuals could perform the task without incremental risk of knee injury. This task could be used in future studies to examine the effect of acute bouts of mechanical loading on bone and cartilage metabolism.

Keywords: Biomechanics, Drop landing, Physical activity, Force, Moment

Key Points

- The current drop-landing task creates an increase in knee compression loading with instruction to land stiffly.
- The absence of increased knee flexion moment during landing from a 22 cm height (household stair) suggests that individuals could perform the task without an increased risk of knee joint injury.
- The current task could be used in future studies to examine the effect of acute bouts of mechanical loading on bone and cartilage metabolism, and bone and joint health.

Background

The effects of physical activity and resulting mechanical loads on bone health and articular cartilage integrity have implications for many groups including military [1], athletes [2], postmenopausal women [3], children [4], older adults [5], and clinical populations such as

* Correspondence: verniba@yorku.ca
[1]Orthopaedic Neuromechanics Laboratory, Sherman Health Science Research Centre, York University, Toronto, Ontario, Canada
[2]Muscle Health Research Centre, York University, Toronto, Ontario, Canada
Full list of author information is available at the end of the article

individuals with osteoarthritis [6] and individuals with stroke [7]. Researchers have reported positive, site-specific adaptations to bone mineral density in response to chronic exposure to activities associated with high mechanical loads (volleyball, basketball) compared to other types of activities (running, swimming) [8, 9]. In contrast, prolonged absence of mechanical loading (bed rest) leads to disuse osteoporosis [10]. Similarly, the health of articular cartilage is maintained through natural formation and degradation processes [11]. Short-term and acute responses of skeletal and articular cartilage metabolism to physical activity have been reported [12–14]; however, findings across studies are difficult to compare because the types of activities and research methodology are not standardized [14]. Traditionally, animal models have been used to examine the effects of mechanical loading on bone and articular cartilage [15, 16]; however, a comparable and standardized model to assess the acute response of bone and cartilage turnover to various levels of mechanical loading has not yet been clearly defined in humans [17]. To improve clinical utility of exercise that may result in a net formation of bone and cartilage in humans, it is important to have a standardized approach that allows researchers to examine responses, to quantify doses of mechanical loads, and to determine if a dose-response exists [14].

In developing an exercise, it is critical that risk of injury is not unduly elevated. It has been suggested that most acute knee joint soft tissue injuries are non-contact in nature, that is, the injury results from a person's own movement and not a contact with an object or a person [18]. Further, it has been shown that excessive sagittal knee joint moment during landing may result in ligament injury [19, 20]. Instructions related to how to execute the landing have been shown to affect joint loading during drop landing [21–23], but no research has examined the influence of instruction set on loading during drop landings from a relatively low height. Researchers have previously described lower limb joint loading during drop landings from relatively large heights (e.g., >59 cm) in younger people [24], but these heights are prohibitive for individuals recovering from a joint injury or those with existing degenerative joint conditions.

The purpose of the current study was (1) to explore a drop-landing task that makes use of drop heights that may be more appropriate for rehabilitation purposes and are functional in daily life and (2) to examine transient knee joint loads during the drop-landing response to examine the effect of drop height and instruction cues on knee joint loads, with a focus to evaluating the potential for incremental injury risk during the task. The drop-landing task may then be useful for rehabilitation and strengthening purposes, and in providing a task in which loading can be controlled in examining metabolic responses to joint loading in human participants.

Methods

Participants

Participants were excluded if they reported a history of neurological or musculoskeletal disorders; or an injury, pain or surgery on their lower body or back in the six months prior to participation. Twenty healthy males (age 22.0 ± 2.8 years, height 1.72 ± 0.1 m, body mass 83.2 ± 14.9 kg; mean ± SD) were included. The local institutional research ethics board provided approval of the methods used in this study. The study was performed in accordance with the ethical standards of the Declaration of Helsinki. All participants provided informed consent prior to participation. A sample size calculation was based on preliminary data obtained with the first 10 participants; results indicated that a total of 20 participants would provide adequate statistical power (>80%).

Setup and Protocol

Participants wore their own athletic shoes in order to improve ecological validity of the study. Infrared reflective markers were placed on the bony landmarks [25], to produce a 6-segment kinematic model: pelvis, left and right thigh, left and right shank, and left and right foot [26]. The three-dimensional kinematic model created using Visual3D software (v4.84.0, C-Motion Inc., Ontario) has been shown to produce results of good to excellent reliability during a similar drop-landing protocol [27]. All offline processing was conducted using Visual3D, which was successfully utilized in previously published works [28–31]. Marker movement was recorded using a 7-camera motion capture system (MX40, Vicon, Colorado). Marker position was sampled at a frequency of 100 Hz and filtered offline using a digital Butterworth 4th order low-pass filter with a 6 Hz cutoff. The filter cutoff frequency was determined using residual analysis of the difference between filtered and unfiltered signals [32] over 0.5–25 Hz range in 0.5 Hz steps with right ankle marker position data from a randomly selected trial recorded for the first four participants; the average cut-off frequency was used.

All trials were initiated with participants standing on an elevated platform at either of two heights: 22 cm (low) and 44 cm (high). The low height was consistent with the height of one riser for typical household stairs, while the high was consistent with the height of two risers. Participants were asked to step outwards off the platform with the rear leg straight and drop such that both feet simultaneously contacted two force plates (OR6-7, AMTI, Massachusetts), with one foot on each force plate. To standardize upper body movement between participants and conditions, participants were asked to lace fingers and maintain their hands over the abdomen during all trials. To avoid participants using different strategies when leaving the elevated platform, the investigator demonstrated the step-off technique and instructed participants explicitly to not jump off or lower themselves. Force plate signals were sampled at 1000 Hz and filtered offline using a Butterworth 4th order low-pass filter with an 8 Hz cutoff. The filter cutoff frequency was determined using a residual analysis approach [32] over 0.5–25 Hz range in 0.5 Hz steps with vertical ground reaction force (GRF) signal from a randomly selected trial recorded for the first four participants; the average cutoff frequency was used. A similar drop-landing methodology has been previously validated and utilized by Niehoff et al. [33] to examine joint loading in response to drop landing in a similar cohort.

Participants performed 10 drop-landing trials in each of six conditions, which were defined by combinations of two heights ("low", "high") and three instruction sets ("soft", "natural" and "stiff"), for a total of 60 drop-landing trials. On average, participants performed one drop per minute per block of conditions. In addition, rest/recovery breaks were provided between each of the conditions to ameliorate the effects of fatigue. All participants completed the natural trials first, for both platform heights. For the natural instruction, participants were instructed to land on the force plates in whatever manner felt comfortable and natural–"land as naturally as possible". The order of platform heights (low, high) was counterbalanced across the participants. Following the completion of the low and high trials under the natural instruction, all participants performed drop-landing trials under the soft and stiff instructions from the low and high heights (low-soft, low-stiff, high-soft, and high-stiff), which were arranged in random order. In the soft landing, participants were instructed to "land softly, absorbing the force at landing"; in the stiff landing, participants were instructed to "land stiffly, without absorbing the force at landing". The investigator demonstrated the soft landing technique with exaggerated flexion at the knee and the stiff landing technique with reduced flexion at the knee. Participants reported that they replicated soft and stiff landings with exaggerated and reduced knee flexion as demonstrated.

Measures of Interest

To confirm the change in the kinematics and kinetics of landing between drop-landing heights and instruction conditions, knee flexion angle and vertical GRF during landing were calculated. All measures of interest, except the knee angle, were normalized to participant's body mass. Peak knee flexion angle and peak GRF were then reported.

To investigate the effect of different drop heights and landing instructions on knee joint loading the following measures were calculated bilaterally: knee joint compression force, knee joint flexion moment, knee joint abduction moment, and knee joint external rotation moment. Joint compression force was operationally defined as joint reaction force that acted along the longitudinal axis at the proximal end of the leg segment. The values for knee abduction and external rotation moment were reported at the peak knee flexion moment, in order to aid the estimation of the knee joint soft tissue injury risk. In this study, net external moments, which represent the external load on the joint, were described. Ankle, knee, and hip joint power as well as ankle and hip sagittal moment were calculated bilaterally, and the values of each were reported at the time of peak knee flexion moment to describe neuromuscular control during landing.

The measures of interest were averaged across the lower limbs for each trial following the analysis which confirmed no bilateral differences. All measures were calculated in Visual3D using the validated marker set reported earlier, and three-dimensional inverse dynamics algorithms [27, 34]; and resolved into the proximal segment coordinate system. All inertial segment properties were estimated from anthropometric data as per Dempster et al. [35].

Statistical Analysis

All statistical analyses were conducted using JMP (v8.0, SAS Institute, North Carolina). A two-factor (*height* [low/high] X *instruction* [soft/natural/stiff]) mixed effects (*participant*–random effect, *height* and *instruction*–fixed effect) repeated measures analysis of variance (rmANOVA) was used to test for differences in the dependent measures between drop-landing conditions. Contrast analyses with Tukey HSD correction were performed to compare means and test interactions.

Fatigue can affect measures obtained using the inverse dynamics approach resulting in the order effect. To examine the potential order effect on knee joint compression and flexion moment, the first three consecutive trials of the third condition were compared with the last three consecutive trials for the sixth condition, across the low-soft, low-stiff, high-soft, and high-stiff condition blocks. A one-way (*order* [first/last]) mixed effects rmANOVA (*order*–fixed effect, *participant*–random effect) was conducted separately for each main measure of interest. The effect size was reported using generalized eta squared (η_G^2) and considered trivial (<0.02), small (0.2–0.12), moderate (0.13–0.25), and large (≥0.26) [36].

Results

The Analysis of the Trial/Condition Order Effect

There was no significant effect of order for the peak knee compression force or the peak knee flexion moment.

Peak Kinematic and Kinetic Measures

Knee Flexion Angle

There was no significant interaction effect, but the main effects of height and instruction were significant (Table 1). Peak knee flexion angle was larger for the high drop height than for the low. Peak knee flexion angle was greater under the soft instruction than under both natural and stiff instruction; peak knee flexion angle under the natural instruction was greater than under the stiff (Table 2).

Vertical nGRF

There was no significant interaction effect, but the main effects of height and instruction were significant (Table 1). Peak ground reaction force (nGRF) was larger for the high drop height than for the low. Peak nGRF increased with instruction to land stiffly, from soft to natural to stiff (Table 2).

Knee Compression Force

There was no interaction effect, but the main effects for height and instruction were significant (Table 1). Peak knee compression force was larger for the high drop height than for the low. Peak compression knee force increased with instruction to land stiffly, from soft to natural to stiff (Figs. 1a and 2a).

Knee Flexion Moment

There was a significant interaction effect observed (Table 1). Peak knee flexion moment was not different between the low-soft, low-natural, and low-stiff conditions. Peak knee flexion moment in the high-soft condition was larger than in the low-soft, low-natural, and low-stiff condition, but lower than in the high-natural and high-stiff condition, which were not different from each other (Figs. 1b and 2b).

Measures Reported at the Peak Knee Flexion Moment

Knee Abduction Moment

There was no significant interaction effect or main effect of instruction; however, the main effect of height was significant (Table 1). Knee abduction moment was larger for the high drop height than for the low (Table 2).

Knee External Rotation Moment

There was no significant interaction effect, but the main effects for height and instruction were significant (Table 1). Knee external rotation moment was larger for the low drop height than for the high. Knee external rotation moment was lower under the soft instruction than under both natural and stiff, which were not different from each other (Table 2).

Table 1 Summary of the statistical analyses

Peak measures	Interaction df(2,38)				Height *df*(1,19)				Instruction *df*(2,38)			
	F	*p* value	Effect size		*F*	*p* value	Effect size		*F*	*p* value	Effect size	
Knee flexion angle (°)	1.6	0.21	0.01	T	206.2	<0.01	0.30	L	103.0	<0.01	0.57	L
Vertical nGRF (N/kg)	0.5	0.64	<0.01	T	104.8	<0.01	0.27	L	86.8	<0.01	0.53	L
Knee compression force (N/kg)	0.1	0.89	<0.01	T	68.0	<0.01	0.17	M	90.8	<0.01	0.53	L
Knee flexion moment (Nm/kg)	16.5	<0.01	0.05	S	230.2	<0.01	0.45	L	15.8	<0.01	0.05	S
Measures at the peak knee flexion moment												
Knee abduction moment (Nm/kg)	2.4	0.10	0.01	T	44.3	<0.01	0.14	M	0.2	0.82	<0.01	T
Knee external rotation moment (Nm/kg)	2.2	0.13	0.01	T	14.7	<0.01	0.06	S	5.8	<0.01	0.02	T
Ankle flexion moment (Nm/kg)	2.6	0.08	0.01	T	105.1	<0.01	0.37	L	0.5	0.60	0.01	T
Hip extension moment (Nm/kg)	1.1	0.36	<0.01	T	1.7	0.21	0.01	T	6.5	<0.01	0.05	S
Ankle power (W/kg)	5.3	0.01	0.03	S	85.7	<0.01	0.48	L	3.3	<0.05	0.05	S
Knee power (W/kg)	9.4	<0.01	0.03	S	139.3	<0.01	0.63	L	7.0	<0.01	0.06	S
Hip power (W/kg)	10.3	<0.01	0.06	S	2.8	0.11	0.04	S	12.2	<0.01	0.07	S
Measures of trial order effect	Order df(1,19)											
	F	*p* value	Effect size									
Peak knee compression force (N/kg)	0.2	0.701	<0.01	T								
Peak knee flexion moment (Nm/kg)	0.56	0.465	0.01	T								

The effect sizes are reported using generalized eta squared. *T* trivial, *S* small, *M* moderate, *L* large

Table 2 Summary of the results which were not included in the figures

Peak measures	Low						High					
	Soft		Natural		Stiff		Soft		Natural		Stiff	
Knee flexion angle (°)	75.49	(2.39)	51.31	(2.75)	45.17	(1.95)	87.71	(2.70)	67.26	(2.88)	59.17	(1.71)
Vertical nGRF (N/kg)	12.71	(0.32)	18.18	(0.78)	22.36	(1.03)	17.24	(0.66)	23.05	(0.99)	26.60	(1.06)
Measures at the peak knee flexion moment												
Knee abduction moment (Nm/kg)	0.52	(0.29)	0.47	(0.26)	0.44	(0.34)	0.7	(0.36)	0.76	(0.39)	0.75	(0.42)
Knee external rotation moment (Nm/kg)	0.04	(0.07)	0.07	(0.12)	0.05	(0.12)	−0.05	(0.14)	−0.02	(0.14)	0.02	(0.17)
Ankle flexion moment (Nm/kg)	0.88	(0.04)	0.83	(0.05)	0.74	(0.11)	1.19	(0.06)	1.21	(0.06)	1.16	(0.07)
Hip extension moment (Nm/kg)	0.18	(0.11)	0.41	(0.14)	0.56	(0.20)	0.09	(0.12)	0.35	(0.20)	0.56	(0.22)

Mean (SE)

Ankle Flexion Moment

There was no significant interaction effect or main effect of instruction; however, the main effect of height was significant (Table 1). Ankle flexion moment was larger for the high drop height than for the low (Table 2).

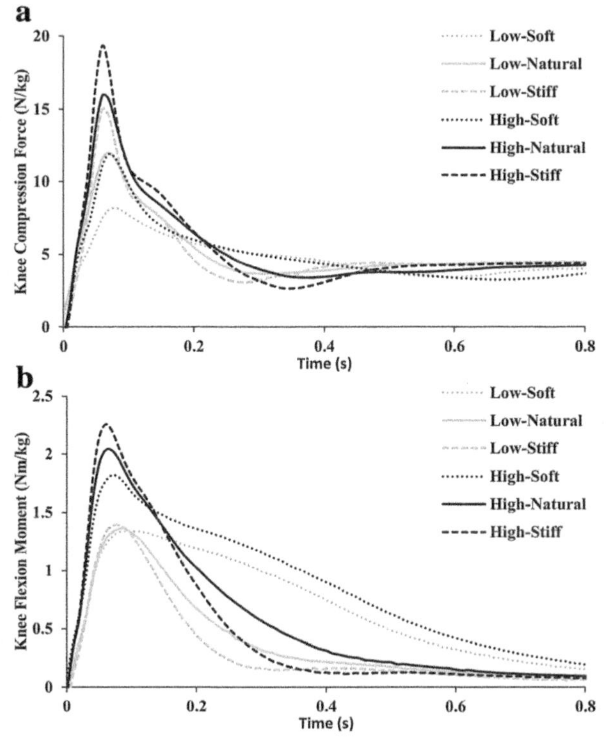

Fig. 1 Averaged ($n = 20$) time series for the body mass-normalized knee joint compression force (**a**) and flexion moment (**b**) as a result of a drop from both low and high heights. The compression force peaks for both drop heights and all three instructions are temporally aligned at approximately 0.07 s. The flexion moment peaks are temporally aligned at approximately 0.07 s for the low-stiff, high-soft, high-natural, and high-stiff conditions; while the peaks for the low-soft and low-natural conditions are temporally aligned at approximately 0.09 s

Hip Extension Moment

There was no significant interaction effect or main effect of height; however, the main effect of instruction was significant (Table 1). Hip extension moment was smaller for the soft condition than for the natural and stiff, which were not different from each other (Table 2).

Ankle Power

There was a significant interaction effect observed (Table 1). Ankle negative power (energy absorption) was

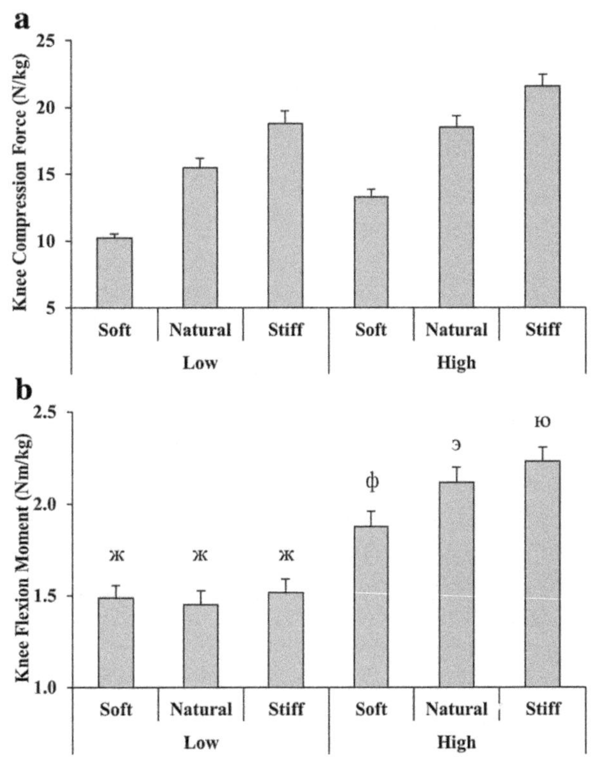

Fig. 2 **a** Peak normalized knee joint compression force and **b** peak normalized external knee joint flexion moment. The *error bars* are SE. **a** Both main effects of height and instruction were significant. **b** Significant interaction effect between height and instruction was observed. Levels not connected by the same symbol are significantly different

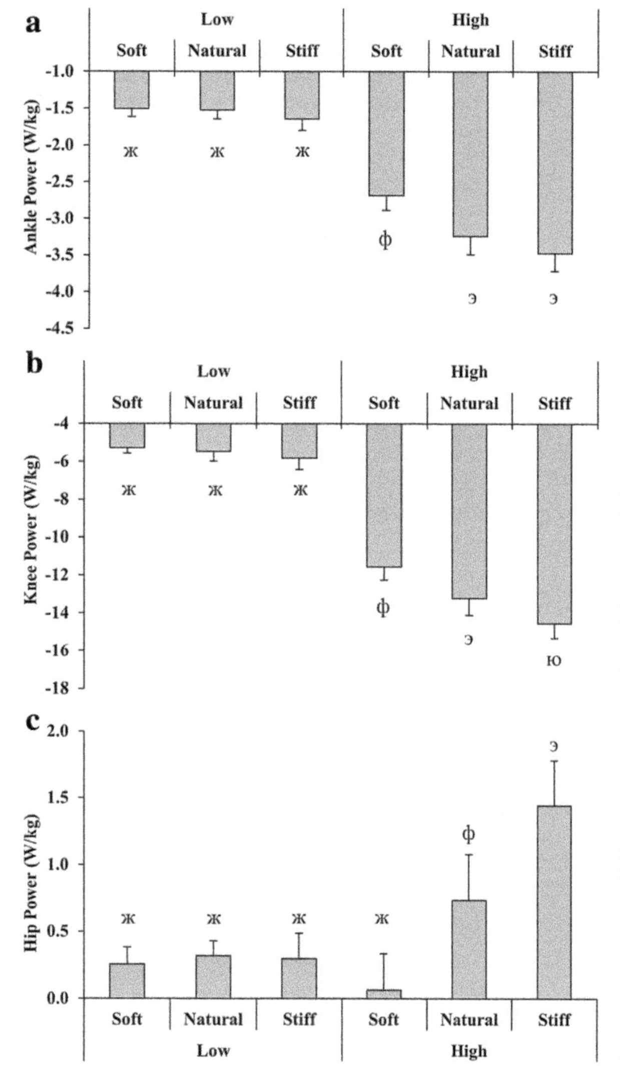

Fig. 3 Normalized joint power measured at the peak knee joint flexion moment for **a** ankle, **b** knee, and **c** hip. The *error bars* are SE. Significant interaction effects between height and instruction were observed in **a**–**c**. Levels not connected by the same symbol are significantly different. The negative power represents energy absorption and eccentric activation. The positive power represents energy generation and concentric activation

not different between instructions for the low height. Ankle negative power was greater for the high height for all instructions and increased from soft to natural and stiff, which were not different (Fig. 3a).

Knee Power

There was a significant interaction effect observed (Table 1). Knee negative power was not different between instructions for the low height. Knee negative power was greater for the high height for all instructions and increased from soft to natural to stiff instruction (Fig. 3b).

Hip Power

There was a significant interaction effect observed (Table 1). Hip positive power (energy generation) was not different between instructions for the low height. Hip positive power was smaller in high-natural condition than in high-stiff, but larger than in high-soft and all of the low instruction conditions, which were not different from each other (Fig. 3c).

Discussion

The current study suggested a drop-landing task that makes use of drop heights that may be appropriate for rehabilitation purposes and are functional in daily life. This study examined transient knee joint loads during the drop-landing response and the effect of drop height and instruction cues on knee joint loads. Further, this study took steps toward a development of standardized exercise task to examine the effect of acute bouts of mechanical loading on bone and cartilage metabolism in humans, since previous research has been focused on animal models [15, 16]. Consistent with previous literature [24, 30], we found that the knee joint compression force increased with drop height and the instruction to land stiffly. Though sagittal knee joint moment scaled with instruction at the high height, it did not change with instruction set at the low height, suggesting that while instruction can increase knee joint compression at the low height, knee joint moment and perhaps; therefore, joint injury risk are not increased with the instruction set at the low height. Precautions were taken to standardize drop-landing task; demonstrations of step-off and landing techniques were provided. The results suggest relatively low, approximately 7%, variability within subjects in the measure of peak sagittal knee angle across conditions (Table 2).

Knee compression force was modulated by instruction; Fig. 2a suggests that compression force can be reduced by approximately 50% if the soft instruction is used, or increased by approximately 30% if the stiff instruction is used, relative to the natural landing instruction. As compression force has been associated with promoting tissue remodeling [12], the exercise task we proposed could improve bone and joint health. Since increased joint moment is associated with ligament injury [8], the absence of increased knee moment suggests that individuals could perform drop-landing task from the low height as opposed to high height without incremental risk of joint injury.

The Effect of Drop Height on Lower Limb Joint Kinetics and Kinematics

The increase in the intensity of the drop-landing task at the greater drop-height resulted in elevated knee flexion angle during landing, vertical GRF, and knee joint compression force. The current findings are in agreement with previous research, which has demonstrated greater peak knee flexion angle and peak vertical GRF when landing from 60 cm compared with 20 cm [37, 38]. The aforementioned biomechanical measures all increase to attenuate impact forces during landing phase. While average frontal and transverse plane moment, which were consistent with previously reported values [39, 40], were found to be statistically different between heights with moderate and small effect size, respectively, the values were smaller than those experienced by young adults in sport setting (abduction moment 1.3 Nm/kg and external rotation moment 0.2 Nm/kg) [41, 42]; and likely not clinically relevant.

The Effect of Instruction on Lower Limb Joint Kinetics and Kinematics

The results revealed the scaling of vertical nGRF, knee joint flexion angle, and compression force with increased landing stiffness. Consistent with the current results, previous research has indicated that instruction to land softly, as opposed to stiffly, from 40 cm resulted in lower vertical nGRF and larger knee joint flexion angle [22]. Additionally, the magnitude and timing of the peak knee compression force (Fig. 1a) were comparable to previously published data [43]. Finally, the force profiles for instruction condition signals were qualitatively comparable between the low and high drop height (Fig. 1a), which was consistent with our expectations.

The Effect of Drop Height and Instruction on Lower Limb Joint Kinetics and Kinematics

The increase in drop height and landing stiffness resulted in increased knee joint compression force. The compression force increased from soft to natural to stiff instruction for both low and high drop heights and was greater for the high drop height (Fig. 2a). Since the increase in landing stiffness produced a linear scaling of the ground reaction force and the knee compression force, it is reasonable to suspect that a similar pattern between drop height and landing stiffness would be observed in the knee flexion moment, i.e., the increase in the flexion moment from soft to natural to stiff for the low and high heights. However, this was not the case. While the instruction to increase landing stiffness from the high height did result in the increase of the knee flexion moment, there was no difference in the moment observed with this instruction during landing from the low height.

The lower limb power analysis revealed that at the peak knee flexion moment, both the ankle and the knee showed negative power (Fig. 3a and b) and flexion joint moments (Fig. 2b; Table 2), indicating energy absorption and eccentric activation of the associated musculature, which is consistent with previous research [23]. In contrast to previous reports [23], however, the current study revealed positive hip joint power (Fig. 3c) and extension moment (Table 2), indicating concentric activation rather than eccentric. The concentric activation about the hip likely served to rotate the trunk forward and bring the body's center of mass closer to the knee joint center in order to reduce the flexion moment at the knee by decreasing the effective length of the moment arm. A shorter moment arm, given that the ground reaction force magnitude was unchanged, would produce a lesser flexion moment about the knee joint. Importantly, in the low height condition, all three joints showed no difference in power magnitude across all levels of instruction, which suggests an equal rate of energy transfer between levels of instruction observed for each of the three joints (Fig. 3). In contrast, at the high height, the rate of energy absorption (the ankle and knee; Fig. 3a and b) and energy generation (the hip; Fig. 3c) increased across instruction levels in all three joints. The difference in patterns between heights as seen across instruction levels in the knee flexion moment and power measures may be driven by the kinetic energy absorption demand. Kinetic energy absorption demand was larger during landing from the high height than from the low; hence, the instruction condition produced a more pronounced energy absorption response at the high drop height than at the low. Considering that the hip showed positive power and that there was a significant interaction effect between the drop height and instruction condition with positive hip power increasing across instruction levels at the high height, but not at the low, it appears as though neuromuscular control of the hip at the low height reduced the loading effect at the knee. However, despite the increase in the positive hip power at the high height, it appears, the capacity of the hip joint to attenuate or obviate the development of additional moment at the knee became relatively less pronounced, as the hip joint became unable to efficiently reduce knee joint flexion moment. The dissimilarity between the previously reported data and the current findings with respect to hip power is likely because previous studies often reported peak joint power, while the current paper reported joint power values measured at the peak knee flexion moment. The peak values of measures of interest may often be temporally misaligned with one another and the event of interest, which in this paper was defined as the peak knee flexion moment. Hence, in order to explain why the peak knee flexion moment did not change with instruction at the low height, when it has increased significantly at the high height, we investigated joint power measured specifically at the peak knee flexion moment.

Clinical Implications

Studies agree that the majority of soft tissue knee injuries are non-contact and occur during sudden deceleration and/or landing maneuvers [19]. The literature suggests that loading through the quadriceps may be one of the mechanisms leading to knee joint ligament injury, as the quadriceps muscle activity producing sagittal moment has been shown to generate large shear force pulling tibia anteriorly on femur [20, 44]. In this study, knee compression forces as well as sagittal moments were larger in the high drop height. In the low height, however, while the knee compression force increased with instruction, the instruction did not influence the knee flexion moment. Since an increase in the knee flexion moment may increase the risk of joint injury, it appears that the knee joint compression force, and thus, perhaps tissue stimulation toward cartilage formation, during landing from a lower 22 cm height (consistent with a household stair) can be increased using an instruction to land more stiffly without suggestion of increase in the risk of knee joint injury as the knee flexion moment did not increase with landing stiffness.

Limitations

The current study is limited by inclusion of male participants only. Future research should include female participants, as due to the anatomical differences, the kinetics and kinematics of the lower limb may differ between sexes. Further, the current study is limited by the use of an inverse dynamics approach. The authors recognize that the bone-on-bone force does not correspond directly to joint compression force calculated using inverse dynamics approach [32]. The inverse dynamics approach does not consider muscle activation force, which adds to the compression force in the knee. Previous research has shown comparable knee loads during stair climb to the current findings during the low-soft condition, while the tibiofemoral bone-on-bone force was 3.5-fold larger when compared to joint reaction force [45]. Nevertheless, the inverse dynamics approach is a feasible and simpler alternative to techniques used to quantify joint bone-on-bone loading [46]. The future work should include muscle force modeling to improve joint compression force estimation. Lastly, a relatively large number of trials collected in this study may have resulted in participant fatigue despite that participants received rest/recovery breaks. Fatigue can affect measures obtained using the inverse dynamics approach resulting in the order effect. We mitigated the effect of fatigue by counterbalancing the first two blocks of trials across participants and randomly assigning the last four trial blocks. With the follow-up analysis, we showed no difference between the earlier and later trial means which suggests that fatigue, if present, did not affect the measures of interest.

Conclusions

The drop-landing task creates an increase in knee joint compression loading that can be scaled using specific instructions. Use of 22 cm height may be safer and beneficial for joint and bone injury rehabilitation, as it represents a height that is much lower than previously discussed in the literature, and is representative of a standard stair height and therefore functionally accessible. Our aim is to utilize the outcomes of the current study in future work aimed at establishing a standardized task to examine the effect of acute bouts of mechanical loading on bone and cartilage metabolism.

Acknowledgements

The authors would like to thank Frank Rizqo for his assistance with data collections. The authors would also like to thank Janessa Drake for proofreading the manuscript.

Funding

This work was supported by Canadian Institutes of Health Research catalyst grant 2010-06-01. The funds were used to purchase necessary laboratory supplies.

Authors' contributions

DV participated in the design of the study; carried out the data acquisition, analysis and interpretation of the results; and drafted the manuscript. JV, DH, and WG participated in the conception and design; analysis and interpretation of the results; drafting and revisions of the manuscript for important intellectual content. All authors read and approved the final manuscript.

Competing interests

Dmitry Verniba, Jason Vescovi, David Hood, and William Gage declare that they have no conflict of interest.

Author details

[1]Orthopaedic Neuromechanics Laboratory, Sherman Health Science Research Centre, York University, Toronto, Ontario, Canada. [2]Muscle Health Research Centre, York University, Toronto, Ontario, Canada. [3]School of Kinesiology and Health Science, York University, Toronto, Ontario, Canada.

References

1. Finestone A, Milgrom C. How stress fracture incidence was lowered in the Israeli army: a 25-yr struggle. Med Sci Sports Exerc. 2008;40(11 Suppl):S623–9. doi:10.1249/MSS.0b013e3181892dc2.
2. Louboutin H, Debarge R, Richou J, et al. Osteoarthritis in patients with anterior cruciate ligament rupture: a review of risk factors. Knee. 2009;16(4): 239–44. doi:10.1016/j.knee.2008.11.004.
3. NAMS. Management of osteoporosis in postmenopausal women: 2010 position statement of The North American Menopause Society. Menopause. 2010;17(1):25–54. doi:10.1097/gme.0b013e3181c617e6. quiz 55-6.
4. Fuchs RK, Bauer JJ, Snow CM. Jumping improves hip and lumbar spine bone mass in prepubescent children: a randomized controlled trial. J Bone Miner Res. 2001;16(1):148–56. doi:10.1359/jbmr.2001.16.1.148.
5. Ozcivici E, Luu YK, Adler B, et al. Mechanical signals as anabolic agents in bone. Nat Rev Rheumatol. 2010;6(1):50–9. doi:10.1038/nrrheum.2009.239.

6. Rannou F, Poiraudeau S. Non-pharmacological approaches for the treatment of osteoarthritis. Best Pract Res Clin Rheumatol. 2010;24(1):93–106. doi:10.1016/j.berh.2009.08.013.
7. Lau RW, Pang MY. An assessment of the osteogenic index of therapeutic exercises for stroke patients: relationship to severity of leg motor impairment. Osteoporos Int. 2009;20(6):979–87. doi:10.1007/s00198-008-0773-1.
8. Bass SL, Saxon L, Daly RM, et al. The effect of mechanical loading on the size and shape of bone in pre-, peri-, and postpubertal girls: a study in tennis players. J Bone Miner Res. 2002;17(12):2274–80. doi:10.1359/jbmr.2002.17.12.2274.
9. Creighton DL, Morgan AL, Boardley D, Brolinson PG. Weight-bearing exercise and markers of bone turnover in female athletes. J Appl Physiol (1985). 2001;90(2):565–70.
10. Takata S, Yasui N. Disuse osteoporosis. J Med Invest. 2001;48(3-4):147–56.
11. Goldring MB, Marcu KB. Cartilage homeostasis in health and rheumatic diseases. Arthritis Res Ther. 2009;11(3):224. doi:10.1186/ar2592.
12. Liang MT, Braun W, Bassin SL, et al. Effect of high-impact aerobics and strength training on BMD in young women aged 20–35 years. Int J Sports Med. 2011;32(2):100–8. doi:10.1055/s-0030-1268503.
13. Mundermann A, Dyrby CO, Andriacchi TP, King KB. Serum concentration of cartilage oligomeric matrix protein (COMP) is sensitive to physiological cyclic loading in healthy adults. Osteoarthritis Cartilage. 2005;13(1):34–8. doi:10.1016/j.joca.2004.09.007.
14. Maimoun L, Sultan C. Effects of physical activity on bone remodeling. Metabolism. 2011;60(3):373–88. doi:10.1016/j.metabol.2010.03.001.
15. Congdon KA, Hammond AS, Ravosa MJ. Differential limb loading in miniature pigs (Sus scrofa domesticus): a test of chondral modeling theory. J Exp Biol. 2012;215(Pt 9):1472–83. doi:10.1242/jeb.061531.
16. Hsieh YF, Wang T, Turner CH. Viscoelastic response of the rat loading model: implications for studies of strain-adaptive bone formation. Bone. 1999;25(3):379–82.
17. Lester ME, Urso ML, Evans RK, et al. Influence of exercise mode and osteogenic index on bone biomarker responses during short-term physical training. Bone. 2009;45(4):768–76. doi:10.1016/j.bone.2009.06.001.
18. Marshall SW. Recommendations for defining and classifying anterior cruciate ligament injuries in epidemiologic studies. J Athl Train. 2010;45(5):516–8. doi:10.4085/1062-6050-45.5.516.
19. Dai B, Herman D, Liu H, Garrett WE, Yu B. Prevention of ACL injury, part I: injury characteristics, risk factors, and loading mechanism. Res Sports Med. 2012;20(3-4):180–97. doi:10.1080/15438627.2012.680990.
20. DeMorat G, Weinhold P, Blackburn T, Chudik S, Garrett W. Aggressive quadriceps loading can induce noncontact anterior cruciate ligament injury. Am J Sports Med. 2004;32(2):477–83.
21. McNair PJ, Prapavessis H, Callender K. Decreasing landing forces: effect of instruction. Br J Sports Med. 2000;34(4):293–6.
22. Myers CA, Torry MR, Peterson DS, et al. Measurements of tibiofemoral kinematics during soft and stiff drop landings using biplane fluoroscopy. Am J Sports Med. 2011;39(8):1714–22. doi:10.1177/0363546511404922.
23. Zhang SN, Bates BT, Dufek JS. Contributions of lower extremity joints to energy dissipation during landings. Med Sci Sports Exerc. 2000;32(4):812–9.
24. Devita P, Skelly WA. Effect of landing stiffness on joint kinetics and energetics in the lower extremity. Med Sci Sports Exerc. 1992;24(1):108–15.
25. C-Motion. Marker Set Guidelines. C-Motion Wiki Documentation [Website]. 2015; www.c-motion.com/v3dwiki/index.php?title=Marker_Set_Guidelines#cite_note-Serge-1. Accessed 29 Dec 2016.
26. Leardini A, Sawacha Z, Paolini G, Ingrosso S, Nativo R, Benedetti MG. A new anatomically based protocol for gait analysis in children. Gait Posture. 2007;26(4):560–71. doi:10.1016/j.gaitpost.2006.12.018.
27. Ford KR, Myer GD, Hewett TE. Reliability of landing 3D motion analysis: implications for longitudinal analyses. Med Sci Sports Exerc. 2007;39(11):2021–8. doi:10.1249/mss.0b013e318149332d.
28. Alenezi F, Herrington L, Jones P, Jones R. The reliability of biomechanical variables collected during single leg squat and landing tasks. J Electromyogr Kinesiol. 2014;24(5):718–21. doi:10.1016/j.jelekin.2014.07.007.
29. Wang H, Frame J, Ozimek E, Leib D, Dugan EL. The effects of load carriage and muscle fatigue on lower-extremity joint mechanics. Res Q Exerc Sport. 2013;84(3):305–12. doi:10.1080/02701367.2013.814097.
30. Nagano H, Tatsumi I, Sarashina E, Sparrow WA, Begg RK. Modelling knee flexion effects on joint power absorption and adduction moment. Knee. 2015. doi:10.1016/j.knee.2015.06.016
31. Verniba D, Vergara ME, Gage WH. Force plate targeting has no effect on spatiotemporal gait measures and their variability in young and healthy population. Gait Posture. 2015;41(2):551–6. doi:10.1016/j.gaitpost.2014.12.015.
32. Winter DA. Biomechanics and motor control of human movement. 3rd ed. Hoboken, New Jersey: John Wiley & Sons; 2005.
33. Niehoff A, Muller M, Bruggemann L, et al. Deformational behaviour of knee cartilage and changes in serum cartilage oligomeric matrix protein (COMP) after running and drop landing. Osteoarthritis Cartilage. 2011;19(8):1003–10. doi:10.1016/j.joca.2011.04.012.
34. C-Motion. Inverse Dynamics. C-Motion Wiki Documentation [Website]. 2013; www.c-motion.com/v3dwiki/index.php?title=Inverse_Dynamics. Accessed 29 Dec 2016.
35. Dempster WT, Gabel WC, Felts WJ. The anthropometry of the manual work space for the seated subject. Am J Phys Anthropol. 1959;17:289–317.
36. Bakeman R. Recommended effect size statistics for repeated measures designs. Behav Res Methods. 2005;37(3):379–84.
37. Bobbert MF, Huijing PA, van Ingen Schenau GJ. Drop jumping. II. The influence of dropping height on the biomechanics of drop jumping. Med Sci Sports Exerc. 1987;19(4):339–46.
38. Peng HT. Changes in biomechanical properties during drop jumps of incremental height. J Strength Cond Res. 2011;25(9):2510–8. doi:10.1519/JSC.0b013e318201bcb3.
39. Herman DC, Barth JT. Drop-jump landing varies with baseline neurocognition: implications for anterior cruciate ligament injury risk and prevention. Am J Sports Med. 2016;44(9):2347–53. doi:10.1177/0363546516657338.
40. Tran AA, Gatewood C, Harris AH, Thompson JA, Dragoo JL. The effect of foot landing position on biomechanical risk factors associated with anterior cruciate ligament injury. J Exp Orthop. 2016;3(1):13. doi:10.1186/s40634-016-0049-1.
41. Jones PA, Herrington LC, Graham-Smith P. Technique determinants of knee joint loads during cutting in female soccer players. Hum Mov Sci. 2015;42:203–11. doi:10.1016/j.humov.2015.05.004.
42. Frank B, Bell DR, Norcross MF, Blackburn JT, Goerger BM, Padua DA. Trunk and hip biomechanics influence anterior cruciate loading mechanisms in physically active participants. Am J Sports Med. 2013;41(11):2676–83. doi:10.1177/0363546513496625.
43. Torry MR, Shelburne KB, Peterson DS, et al. Knee kinematic profiles during drop landings: a biplane fluoroscopy study. Med Sci Sports Exerc. 2011;43(3):533–41. doi:10.1249/MSS.0b013e3181f1e491.
44. Markolf KL, O'Neill G, Jackson SR, McAllister DR. Effects of applied quadriceps and hamstrings muscle loads on forces in the anterior and posterior cruciate ligaments. Am J Sports Med. 2004;32(5):1144–9. doi:10.1177/0363546503262198.
45. Costigan PA, Deluzio KJ, Wyss UP. Knee and hip kinetics during normal stair climbing. Gait Posture. 2002;16(1):31–7.
46. D'Lima DD, Fregly BJ, Patil S, Steklov N, Colwell Jr CW. Knee joint forces: prediction, measurement, and significance. Proc Inst Mech Eng H. 2012;226(2):95–102.

Permissions

All chapters in this book were first published in SM, by Springer International Publishing AG.; hereby published with permission under the Creative Commons Attribution License or equivalent. Every chapter published in this book has been scrutinized by our experts. Their significance has been extensively debated. The topics covered herein carry significant findings which will fuel the growth of the discipline. They may even be implemented as practical applications or may be referred to as a beginning point for another development.

The contributors of this book come from diverse backgrounds, making this book a truly international effort. This book will bring forth new frontiers with its revolutionizing research information and detailed analysis of the nascent developments around the world.

We would like to thank all the contributing authors for lending their expertise to make the book truly unique. They have played a crucial role in the development of this book. Without their invaluable contributions this book wouldn't have been possible. They have made vital efforts to compile up to date information on the varied aspects of this subject to make this book a valuable addition to the collection of many professionals and students.

This book was conceptualized with the vision of imparting up-to-date information and advanced data in this field. To ensure the same, a matchless editorial board was set up. Every individual on the board went through rigorous rounds of assessment to prove their worth. After which they invested a large part of their time researching and compiling the most relevant data for our readers.

The editorial board has been involved in producing this book since its inception. They have spent rigorous hours researching and exploring the diverse topics which have resulted in the successful publishing of this book. They have passed on their knowledge of decades through this book. To expedite this challenging task, the publisher supported the team at every step. A small team of assistant editors was also appointed to further simplify the editing procedure and attain best results for the readers.

Apart from the editorial board, the designing team has also invested a significant amount of their time in understanding the subject and creating the most relevant covers. They scrutinized every image to scout for the most suitable representation of the subject and create an appropriate cover for the book.

The publishing team has been an ardent support to the editorial, designing and production team. Their endless efforts to recruit the best for this project, has resulted in the accomplishment of this book. They are a veteran in the field of academics and their pool of knowledge is as vast as their experience in printing. Their expertise and guidance has proved useful at every step. Their uncompromising quality standards have made this book an exceptional effort. Their encouragement from time to time has been an inspiration for everyone.

The publisher and the editorial board hope that this book will prove to be a valuable piece of knowledge for researchers, students, practitioners and scholars across the globe.

List of Contributors

Sam Robertson
Centre for Exercise and Sport Science, Deakin University, Geelong, Victoria, Australia
Institute of Sport Exercise and Active Living (ISEAL), Victoria
University, Footscray Park campus, PO Box 14428, Melbourne, Victoria 8001, Australia

Peter Kremer and Jacqueline Tran
Centre for Exercise and Sport Science, Deakin University, Geelong, Victoria, Australia

Brad Aisbett
Centre for Physical Activity and Nutrition Research, Deakin University, Burwood, Victoria, Australia

Ester Cerin
Centre for Physical Activity and Nutrition Research, Deakin University, Burwood, Victoria, Australia
School of Public Health, The University of Hong Kong, Hong Kong, China

Leandro Kansuke Oharomari and Anderson Marliere Navarro
Department of Food and Nutrition, Pharmaceutical Sciences College, Araraquara, São Paulo, Brazil

Camila de Moraes
School of Physical Education and Sport of Ribeirão Preto, University of São Paulo, Ribeirão Preto, São Paulo, Brazil

Riccardo Lo Martire
Division of Physiotherapy, Department of Neurobiology, Care Sciences, and Society, Karolinska Institutet, Alfred Nobels allé 23 100, Huddinge 141 83,Sweden
Department of Physiology and Pharmacology, Karolinska Institutet,Stockholm, Sweden
Department of Aeronautical and Vehicle Engineering,KTH Royal Institute of Technology, Stockholm, Sweden

Kristofer Gladh
Division of Physiotherapy, Department of Neurobiology, Care Sciences, and Society, Karolinska Institutet, Alfred Nobels allé 23 100, Huddinge 141 83, Sweden
Department of Physiology and Pharmacology, Karolinska Institutet, Stockholm, Sweden

Anton Westman
Division of Physiotherapy, Department of Neurobiology, Care Sciences, and Society, Karolinska Institutet, Alfred Nobels allé 23 100, Huddinge 141 83, Sweden
Department of Physiology and Pharmacology, Karolinska Institutet, Stockholm, Sweden
Department of Anesthesia and Intensive Care, Karolinska University Hospital, Huddinge, Sweden

Björn O. Äng
Division of Physiotherapy, Department of Neurobiology, Care Sciences, and Society, Karolinska Institutet, Alfred Nobels allé 23 100, Huddinge 141 83, Sweden
School of Education, Health and Social Studies, Dalarna University,Falun, Sweden

Seema Malhotra, Kiran Preet, Shweta Rawat, Sayar Singh, Inderjeet Singh, L. Robert Varte,Tirthankar Chatterjee, M. S. Pal and Soma Sarkar
Defence Institute of Physiology and Allied Sciences (DIPAS), Ministry of Defence. Government of India, Lucknow Road, Delhi 110054, India

Arvind Tomar
Defence Research and Development Establishment (DRDE). Ministry of Defence, Government of India, Jhansi Road, Gwalior 474002, Madhya Pradesh, India

Kazushige Goto
Faculty of Sport and Health Sciences, Ritsumeikan University, 1-1-1, Nojihigashi, Kusatsu, Shiga 525-8577, Japan
Graduate School of Sport and Health Science, Ritsumeikan University, Kusatsu, Shiga 525-8574, Japan

Sahiro Mizuno and Ayaka Mori
Graduate School of Sport and Health Science, Ritsumeikan University, Kusatsu, Shiga 525-8574, Japan

Andrew J. Gardner and Christopher R. Levi
Centre for Stroke and Brain Injury, School of Medicine and Public Health, University of Newcastle, Callaghan, New South Wales, Australia
Hunter New England Local Health District Sports Concussion Program, John Hunter Hospital, Newcastle, New South Wales, Australia

Grant L. Iverson
Department of Physical Medicine and Rehabilitation, Harvard Medical School, Spaulding Rehabilitation Hospital, Boston, MA, USA
Mass General Hospital for Children Sport Concussion Program, Boston, MA, USA Home Base, A Red Sox Foundation and Massachusetts General Hospital Program, Boston, MA, USA

E. Couvé-Deacon, D. Postil, O. Barraud, C. Duchiron, D. Chainier and M.C. Ploy
University Limoges, UMR, 1092 Limoges, France
INSERM, UMR, 1092 Limoges, France
CHU Limoges, Laboratory of Bacteriology-Virology-Hygiene, 2 avenue Martin Luther King, 87042 Limoges, cedex, France

A. Labrunie and P.M. Preux
CHU Limoges, Centre d'Epidémiologie de Biostatistique et de Méthodologie de la Recherche, Limoges, France

N. Pestourie
CHU Limoges, Laboratory of Bacteriology-Virology-Hygiene, 2 avenue Martin Luther King, 87042 Limoges,cedex, France

B. François
University Limoges, UMR, 1092 Limoges, France
INSERM, UMR, 1092Limoges, France
INSERM, CIC-1435, F-87000 Limoges, France. 5CHU Limoges,Centre d'Epidémiologie de Biostatistique et de Méthodologie de la Recherche, Limoges, France

Andrew J. Gardner
Centre for Stroke and Brain Injury, School of Medicine and Public Health, University of Newcastle, Callaghan, Australia
Priority Research Centre for Stroke and Brain Injury, Level5, McAuley Building, Calvary Mater Hospital, Waratah, NSW 2298, Australia

David R. Howell
The Micheli Center for Sports Injury Prevention, Waltham, MA, USA
Division of Sports Medicine, Department of Orthopaedics, Boston Children's Hospital, Boston, USA
Brain Injury Center,Boston Children's Hospital, Boston, MA, USA

Christopher R. Levi
Centre for Stroke and Brain Injury, School of Medicine and Public Health, University of Newcastle, Callaghan, Australia
Hunter New England Local Health District Sports Concussion Program, John Hunter Hospital, Newcastle, New South Wales, Australia

Grant L. Iverson
Center for Health and Rehabilitation, Department of Physical Medicine and Rehabilitation, Harvard Medical School, 79/96 Thirteenth Street, Charlestown Navy Yard, Charlestown, MA, USA
Spaulding Rehabilitation Hospital, Charlestown, USA
MassGeneral Hospital for Children™ Sport Concussion Program, and HomeBase, A Red Sox Foundation and Massachusetts General Hospital Program, Boston, MA, USA

Ann-Sofie Bakshi and Johanna Gripenberg
STAD, Centre for Psychiatry Research, Department of Clinical Neuroscience,Karolinska Institutet, & Stockholm Health Care Services, Stockholm County Council, Norra Stationsgatan 69, SE-1113-64 Stockholm, Sweden

Yasmina Molero
STAD, Centre for Psychiatry Research, Department of Clinical Neuroscience,Karolinska Institutet, & Stockholm Health Care Services, Stockholm County Council, Norra Stationsgatan 69, SE-1113-64 Stockholm, Sweden
Department of Medical Epidemiology and Biostatistics, Karolinska Institutet, Stockholm, Sweden

Andrew Brinkley, Hilary McDermott, Rachel Grenfell-Essam and Fehmidah Munir
School of Sport, Exercise and Health Sciences, National Centre for Sport and Exercise Medicine, Loughborough University, Loughborough, Leicestershire LE11 3TU, UK

Lewis Anthony Gough, Sanjoy Kumar Deb, Andy Sparks and Lars Robert McNaughton
Sports Nutrition and Performance Group, Department of Sport and Physical Activity, Edge Hill University, Ormskirk, Lancashire L39 4QP, UK

A. Boussuges and K. Ayme
UMR MD2, Dysoxie-Suractivité, Aix-Marseille Université et Institut de Recherche
Biomédicale des Armées (IRBA), Faculté de Médecine Nord,Marseille, France

G. Chaumet
Altrabio, Lyon, SA, France

E. Albier and M. Borgnetta
Institut National de Plongée Professionnelle, Port de la Pointe Rouge, Marseille, France

O. Gavarry
Laboratoire HandiBio EA 4322, Université de Toulon, La Garde, France

Brendan T. Barrett, Alice G. Cruickshank and Alex Mankowska
1School of Optometry and Vision Science, University of Bradford, Bradford, UK.

Jonathan C. Flavell
School of Optometry and Vision Science, University of Bradford, Bradford, UK.
Department of Psychology, University of York, York, UK

Simon J. Bennett
School of Sport and Exercise Science, Liverpool John Moores University, Liverpool, UK

Julie M. Harris
School of Psychology and Neuroscience, University of St Andrews, St Andrews, UK

John G. Buckley
School of Engineering, University of Bradford, Bradford, UK

Christopher J. Gaffney
Institute of Biomedical Problems (IBMP), Moscow, Russia.
Centre of Human & Aerospace Physiological Sciences (CHAPS), King's College London, Faculty of Life Sciences & Medicine, Guy's Campus, London SE1 1UL, UK

Elena Fomina, Dennis Babich, Vladimir Kitov and Konstantin Uskov
Institute of Biomedical Problems (IBMP), Moscow, Russia

David A. Green
Centre of Human & Aerospace Physiological Sciences (CHAPS), King's College London, Faculty of Life Sciences & Medicine, Guy's Campus, London SE1 1UL, UK
KBRwyle, European Astronaut Centre, Linder Höhe, D-51147 Cologne, Germany

Kyle R. Barnes
Department of Movement Science, Grand Valley State University, 1 Campus Drive, Allendale, MI 49401, USA

Jessica N. Janecke
Office of Undergraduate Research andScholarship, Grand Valley State University, 1 Campus Drive, Allendale, MI49401, USA

Flavio A. Cadegiani and Claudio E. Kater
Adrenal and Hypertension Unit, Division of Endocrinology and Metabolism,Department of Medicine, Escola Paulista de Medicina, Universidade Federalde São Paulo (EPM/UNIFESP), R. Pedro de Toledo 781 - 13th floor, São Paulo,SP 04039-032, Brazil

Toby Mündel, Marine Machal, Darryl J. Cochrane and Matthew J. Barnes
School of Sport and Exercise, Massey University, Private bag 11 222,Palmerston North 4442, New Zealand

Julian D. Egan-Shuttler, Rohan Edmonds, Cassandra Eddy, Veronica O'Neill and Stephen J. Ives
Health and Exercise Sciences Department, Skidmore College, SaratogaSprings, NY, USA

Martin D. Hoffman
Department of Physical Medicine & Rehabilitation, Department of Veterans
Affairs, Northern California Health Care System, Sacramento, CA, USA
UltraSports Science Foundation, El Dorado Hills, CA, USA

Taylor R. Valentino
Department of Kinesiology, San Francisco State University, San Francisco, CA, USA

Kristin J. Stuempfle
Health Sciences Department, Gettysburg College, Gettysburg, PA, USA

Brandon V. Hassid
School of Medicine, University of Maryland, Baltimore, MD, USA

Dmitry Verniba and William H. Gage
Orthopaedic Neuromechanics Laboratory, Sherman Health Science Research Centre, York University, Toronto, Ontario, Canada

Muscle Health Research Centre, York University, Toronto, Ontario, Canada
School of Kinesiology and Health Science, York University, Toronto, Ontario, Canada.

Jason D. Vescovi
Muscle Health Research Centre, York University, Toronto, Ontario, Canada

David A. Hood
Muscle Health Research Centre, York University, Toronto, Ontario, Canada
School of Kinesiology and Health Science, York University, Toronto, Ontario, Canada

Index